THE TREE
DISPENSARY

THE TREE
DISPENSARY

Christina Stapley

AEON

First published in 2021 by
Aeon Books Ltd
PO Box 76401
London
W5 9RG

Copyright © 2021 by Christina Stapley

The right of Christina Stapley to be identified as the author of this work has been asserted in accordance with §§ 77 and 78 of the Copyright Design and Patents Act 1988.

All rights reserved. No part of this publication may be reproduced, stored in a retrieval system, or transmitted, in any form or by any means, electronic, mechanical, photocopying, recording, or otherwise, without the prior written permission of the publisher.

British Library Cataloguing in Publication Data

A C.I.P. for this book is available from the British Library

ISBN: 978-1-91350-472-4

Typeset by Medlar Publishing Solutions, Pvt Ltd., India
Printed in Great Britain

www.aeonbooks.co.uk

The intent of this book is solely informational and educational. The information and suggestions in this book are not intended to replace the advice or treatments given by health care professionals. The authors and publisher have made every effort to present accurate information. However, they shall be neither responsible nor liable for any problem that may arise from information in this book.

Contents

Dedication and Acknowledgements   vii
Foreword   viii
INTRODUCTION   1

SPRING

    Ash   7
    Beech   19
    Birch   29
    Blackthorn   41
    Elderflower   53
    Hawthorn   65
    Horse chestnut   77
    Quince   87
    Rosemary   99
    Willow   111

SUMMER

    Barberry   125
    Black Mulberry   137
    Elderberry   147
    Fig   157
    Limeflower   169
    Oak   179
    Walnut   189

AUTUMN

    Crab Apple   203
    Cramp Bark   213
    Medlar   223
    Pear   233
    Rowan   243
    Sea Buckthorn   251
    Sweet Chestnut   261

WINTER

    Bay   273
    Hazel   283
    Holly   295
    Ivy   305
    Juniper   317
    Scots Pine   331

Bibliography   343
Biography for Christina Stapley   349
Index   351

Dedication and Acknowledgements

This book is dedicated to my grandchildren, Elliott, Tighe, Carys, Samuel, and Natasha, hoping the trees of today may thrive throughout their lifetimes and beyond.

I would like to offer particular thanks to three colleagues. My dear friend Ruth Mannion-Daniels who has given tremendous support in many ways, ever since I first told her of my concept for this book. My friend and colleague in herbal history as well as herbalism, Anne Stobart, for her support and assistance on my visit to Holt Wood Medicinal Forest and since; and my friend Barbara Lewis who read the manuscript, advised, supported my work and much more. They have all accompanied me on this journey of discovery. I would like to thank my friends Linda and David Papworth for their continued encouragement and David for his excellent photographs of the birds in this book. My thanks also goes to the staff at the Weald and Downland Living Museum, for without my workshops and tree walks there, this book might never have been written.

Foreword

During my training as a herbalist, I searched unsuccessfully for an in-depth book on trees in herbal medicine. Already a historical researcher and growing thirteen trees offering herb harvests, I found the more encyclopaedic books available did not encourage my interest. At the time, however, I had much to learn in other areas of medicine.

My real fascination with trees grew from researching in preparation for tutoring a historical herb workshop. *The A–Z of Medicinal Trees.* The workshop was held at the Weald and Downland Living Museum where there were fine examples of many of my own trees and several more. The interest attracted by that first and subsequent day courses and guided tree walks, when I was asked so many questions, encouraged me to delve further into their histories.

More than that, it brought a change in me. For years as a herbalist I had been walking about looking down for what was growing around my feet. The emphasis changed to looking up and I was delighted by the exquisite detail of tiny female flowers on trees, which I simply could not believe I had completely missed before.

I took photographs, pressed herbarium samples, harvested for a wider range of recipes and studied trees in my collection of old herbals. I increased my collection of items turned or carved from their wood. I listened to sap rushing up inside the trunks in spring, paid attention to the variation in sound that the rustling leaves make at different seasons, and felt the slippery sap covered inner surface between the wood and bark as I peeled it away for harvests. I watched associated birds, insects and animals and experimented with barks, catkins and leaves to produce dyes. The varying shades produced at different seasons and from trees in different environments is a valuable source of information in itself, revealing chemical changes as the trees react to their annual cycle and habitat.

Never again will a tincture or dried herb of tree origin be simply a name on the label and list of constituents, actions and indications. I hope as you read this book, written from personal experience and interaction with the trees growing around us, you also will feel a stronger connection and wish to explore, plant and care for them yourselves.

THE TREE
DISPENSARY

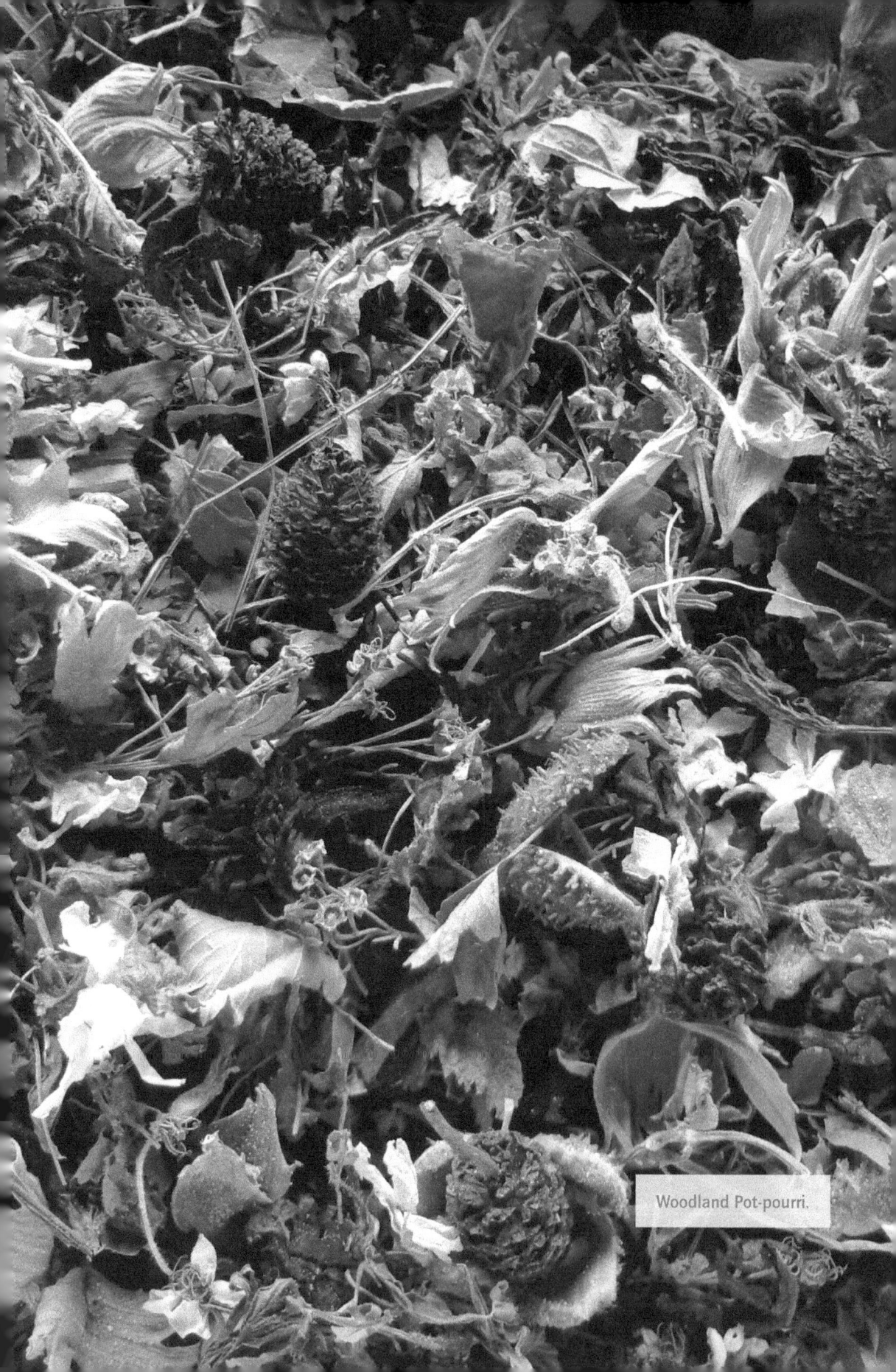

Woodland Pot-pourri.

INTRODUCTION

The Tree Dispensary presents a personal appreciation of the trees as the author has experienced them through everyday life, as a herb historian and herbalist.

"Getting to Know the Tree" sections cover a wide area of general knowledge from cultivation experience to cookery, wines, crafts, and folklore.

In the histories, having been trained by my archivist father to go to primary sources, I have allowed these to dominate the text. Voices from the past speak for themselves from my library of original herbals, rather than presenting a modern view of the past.

The herbalist's reference section is material selected from information that I compiled as a handy reference when prescribing and has additions from my own observations. In this, dosages and constituents are taken from a wide variety of sources including:-

Barker J. *The Medicinal Flora of Britain and Northwestern Europe.* (Winter Press. 2001).
Barnes J. et al. *Herbal Medicines* (Pharmaceutical Press. 2nd edition. 2002).
Bartram T. *Bartram's Encyclopedia of Herbal Medicine.* (Robinson. 1998).
Blumenthal et al. *Herbal Medicine. Expanded Commission E monographs.* (Integrative Medicine Commission. 2000).
Bone K. A *Clinical Guide to Blending Liquid Herbs.* (Churchill Livingstone. 2003).
British *Herbal Pharmacopoeia.* (British Herbal Medicine Association. 1983).
Burlando B. et al. *Herbal principles in Cosmetics.* (CRC Press. 2010).

Chiej R. *The Macdonald Encyclopedia of Medicinal Plants.* (Macdonald Publishing. London. 1984).

Duke J.A. *Handbook of Phytochemical Constituents of GRAS herbs and other Economic Plants.* (CRC Press LLC. 2001).

Duke J.A. *Handbook of Medicinal Herbs* (CRC Press LLC. 2nd edition. 2002).

Hoffmann D. *The New Holistic Herbal.* (Element. 1990).

Mills S. & Bone K. *Principles & Practice of Phytotherapy.* (Churchill Livingstone. 2000).

Schultz et al. *Rational Phytotherapy.* (Springer. 2004).

Wren R.C. *Potter's Encyclopaedia of Botanical Drug and Preparations.* (Daniel, U.K. 1998).

Weiss R.F. M.D. *Herbal Medicine.* (Thieme. 2nd edition revised and expanded. 2000).

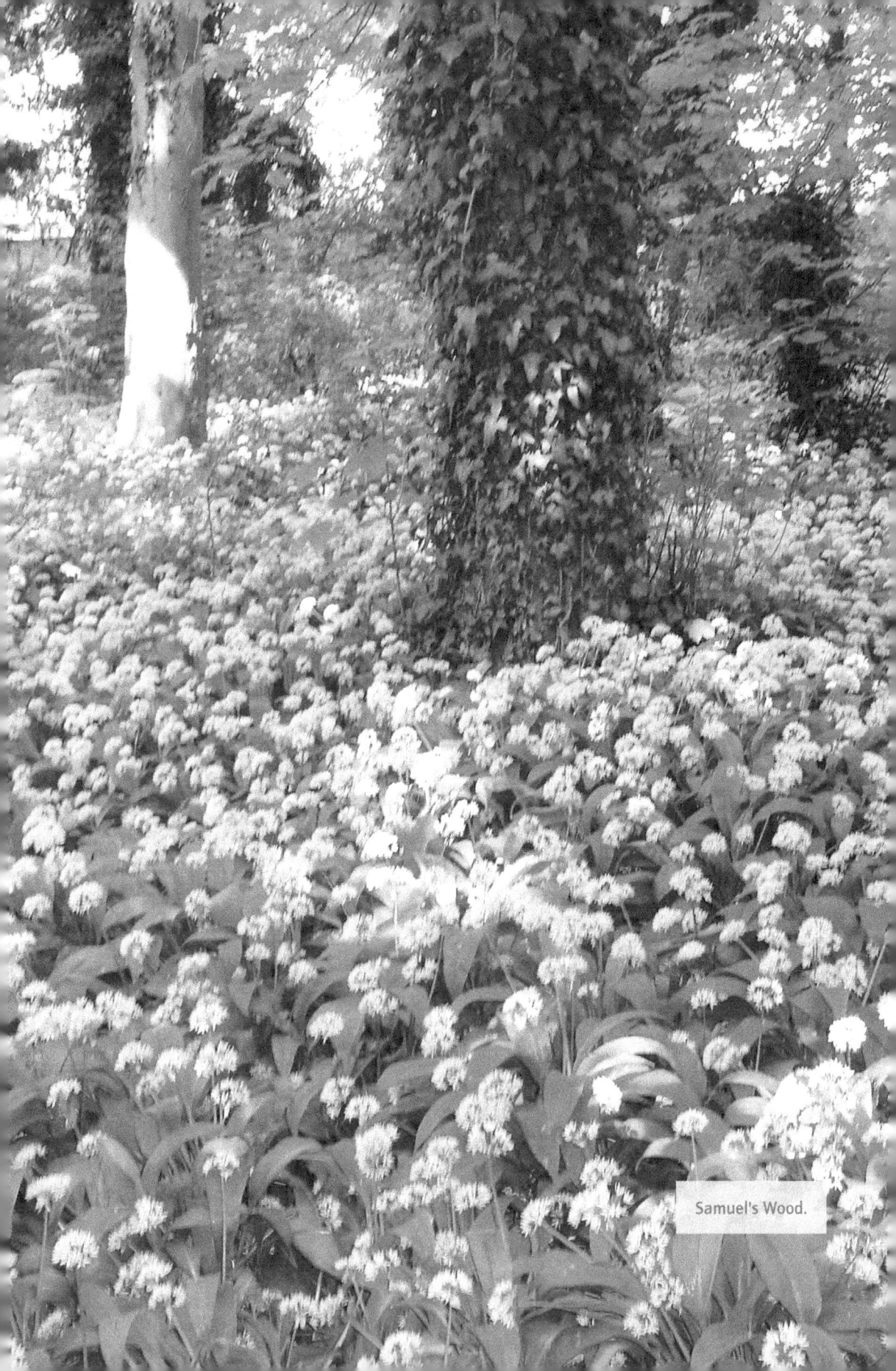
Samuel's Wood.

SPRING

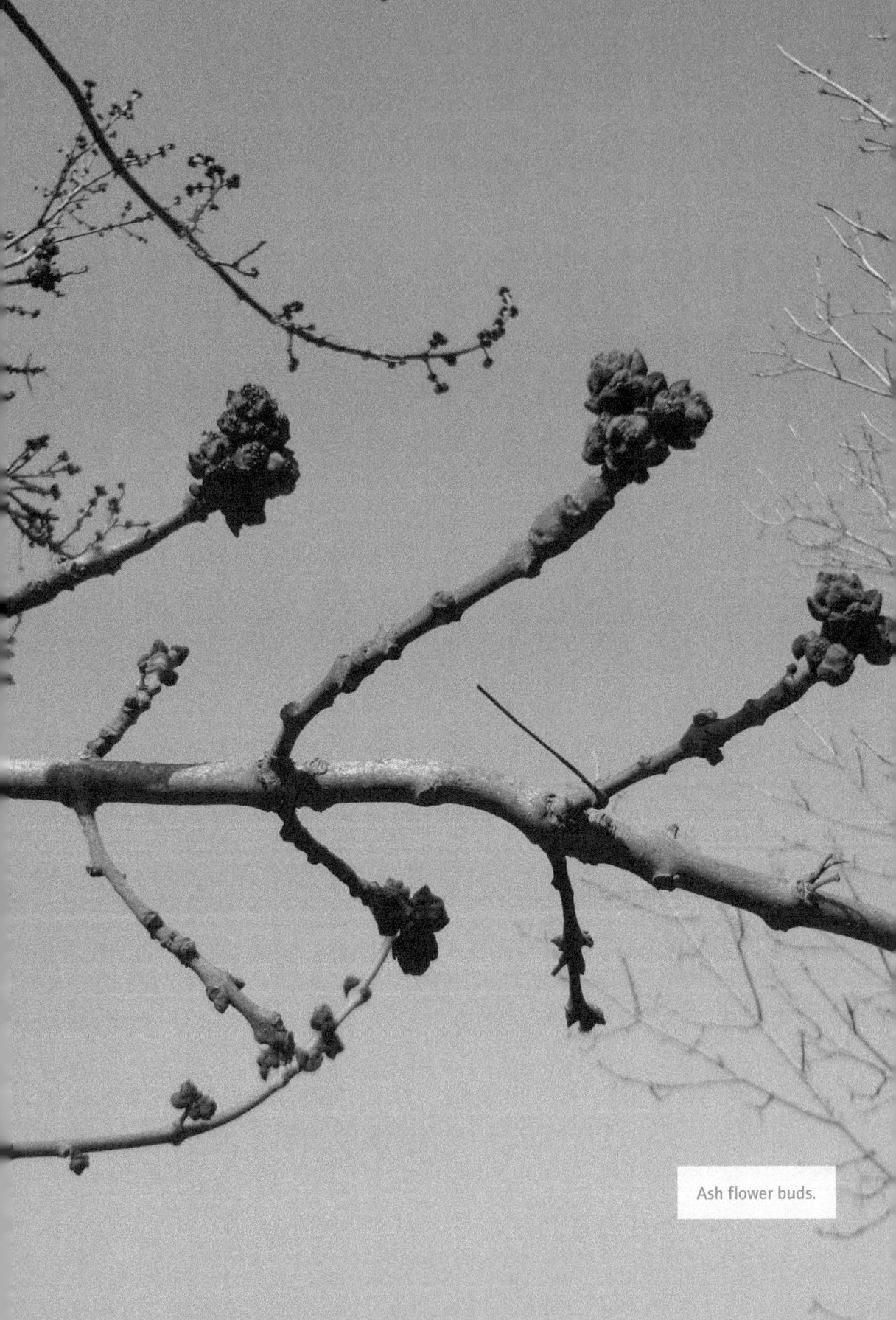

Ash flower buds.

Ash

Fraxinus excelsior – Ash – Oleaceae

ASH – Usefulness – The fruits can be pickled when young. They contain edible oil, similar to sunflower oil.[1] The leaves, fruits, bark and sap have medicinal properties. The wood can be turned and has been greatly used since prehistoric times. From the handle of the "Iceman's" dagger in the Bronze Age to wheelbarrows and frames for the Mosquito bomber.[2] Ash trees and the environment they provide support a wide range of wildlife, from the brown fritillary butterfly to bullfinches and the dormouse. Ash wood burns well, with little smoke. The ashes give potash and the bark has been used for tanning calf-skins. The leaves contain a green colouring and can be used as an over-dye on blues to give green.

Dangers – Ash trees are currently threatened by Chalara dieback, a disease caused by a fungus called *Hymenoscyphus fraxineus*. As the crown of the tree dies back it is usually deadly to the tree. Ash keys should not be fed in large quantities to domestic animals.

Getting to Know the Ash Tree – The black knobbly balls produced on year-old twigs and branches during winter make native ash trees easy to identify. I paid them little attention however, until one spring walking in the hills I found myself staring in wonder at a branch in full flower.

At the time I did not even associate it with the ash, only being familiar with the leaves and the possible height of over a hundred feet of these fast-growing, yet fairly long-lived trees. The identification really

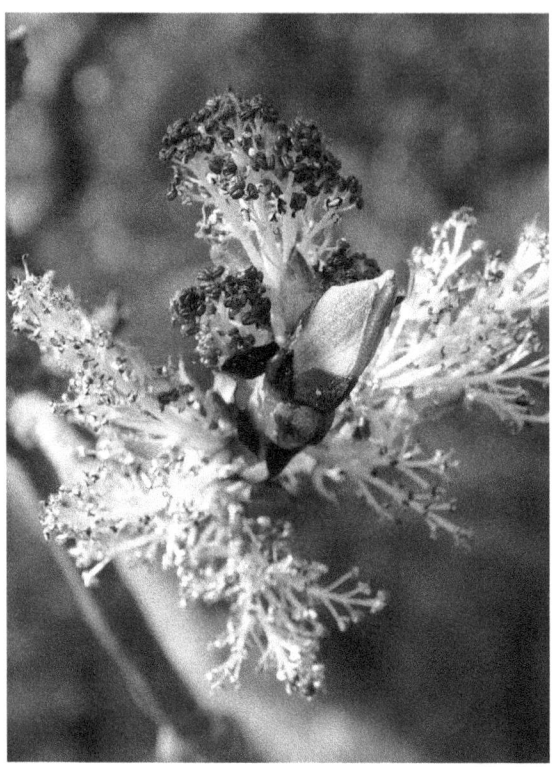
Ash flowering.

surprised me. I had never realised the ash could be so fascinating. Perhaps I should have known that a tree with the importance in folklore and magic of the ash must have something very special about it.

The following year I was careful to watch for the opening of the flowers. Coming before the leaves in April, when partly opened, the panicles first reminded me of a stem of purple sprouting broccoli with maroon beads on the tips. Returning to view their progress, several days later, I saw the flowers were now opening out like mini seaweed with yellow branches having purple tipped pistils. The ovary, which will become the fruit, develops between the two pollen carrying stamens. Each flower is bi-sexual, but the male part dies before the female ovary of that flower develops, ensuring that each is cross-pollinated from other trees. Since they are wind-pollinated they do not need petals.

The leaves commonly have eight to twelve leaflets in pairs, growing straight from the central stem with an added odd one at the end, although an occasional even numbered leaf occurs. They may seem slightly dull after the flowers, but have attracted a good deal of folklore, with even numbered leaves gathered for love divination. Additionally they have medicinal use and were also picked as a tea substitute in the nineteenth century. Diuretic and mildly purgative properties of the leaves should be kept in mind if you try this at home.

On days when I have taught hedgerow basketry and we used young, flexible ash branches, I recall how delighted the goat was to eat all the leaves left over. Young shoots and leaves have also been fed to deer. Should cows eat them, as apparently happened in the Godalming area in the early nineteenth century, butter from their milk was described as rank. However, cattle have been fed on the bark in Lancashire in past times when grass was scarce. A note of caution on ruminating animals, eating ash is listed in notes on poisons found in veterinary practice, with "acute impaction of the rumen" recorded. The amount eaten was not specified.[3]

Along with the leaves, the young, still tender and abundant clusters of seeds, known as ash keys have always been harvested to be powdered and prepared for medicine or pickled to accompany salads. In past years on historical woodland workshop days, I have introduced others to picking ash keys and making the pickle in white wine vinegar, sweetened with sugar. Ash fruits were also called in the seventeenth century peterkeyes or kitkeyes, each containing the seed near the stalk. In autumn the keys fly in the wind from the tree, twisting like tiny propellers and taking the seeds sometimes over long distances. With the aid of these, ash trees have a marked tendency to spread their young into gardens, and especially into gravelled paths, where they are not welcome, and so the ash has tended to be looked upon almost as a weed by many gardeners.

Neither past uses in medicine and cookery, nor the popularity of the wood for everything from tool handles to snooker cues seems to recommend it to modern ears. Transport has much to thank the ash for. The wood has provided frames for horse-drawn coaches, the Mosquito bomber plane, and the Morris traveller car. Ash has also provided veneer in interior fittings on trains[4] and had a role in boat-building. Cabinet makers named the interestingly patterned veined wood "green ebony".

In the north, many place names contain the Nordic term "ask" commemorating ash coppices or nurseries from the Middle Ages.[5] Askham Bryan is one. Ash trees were coppiced in the past and cut on a twelve to fifteen year rotation to give hop-poles, and building materials. Outer and inner layers of the light-coloured bark have both been used in medicine. Also the lye or wash from the ashes of the burnt wood can be used as a shampoo for dandruff, or an application to treat ringworm.[6]

Unpopular as it may be with some gardeners, over the past twenty or so years the occurrence of the fungal disease, ash dieback, that threatens ash in Britain, has made many turn to consider the role of ash in the environment. The leaves are important as a food for many species of moth, including the coronet and privet hawk-moth. After a long life, the deadwood of the ash supports the lesser stag-beetle, and the lovely, rare brown fritillary butterfly is attracted to the ash. Where it grows in the under-storey of woods, alongside the hazel, ash is host to dormice. Ash trees also provide nesting sites for birds from the larger owls and woodpeckers down to smaller redstarts and nuthatches.

Legends and Folklore. The saying, "if the ash before the oak we are going to have a soak, if the oak before the ash we will only have a splash" remains familiar to many even today. It refers to which tree will open leaves first. This is almost always the oak, as the ash is late with the flowering period coming earlier. Folklore of the ash is so much greater than simple weather lore. The ash is the eternal World Tree or tree of life in Norse legend. This Yggdrasil reaches across all nine worlds in Norse mythology with three great roots supporting it. Under one is the well of wisdom, under another is the Scandinavian Hades, and by the third root is a spring where the gods meet in council. The fate of men is determined by the Norns, maidens who dwell close to this root.[7]

Beliefs in the strength of the ash lingered on in Scotland over the centuries. The tree as protector against shrews, which were believed to cause lameness by running over the foot of a person or animal, is an extraordinary tale. The cure was supposed to be brought about by capturing a shrew that was then entombed inside an ash tree. The tree was asked for help and as it healed over the place where the shrew had been placed, so the lameness was expected to be healed.[8] Gilbert White mentions this practice in the late eighteenth century.

While some believed the broomsticks of witches were made of ash, as with other useful trees, there is another set of folklore declaring the ash to be protective against witches and magic. In Ireland, ash wood was burned to keep the devil away and in Scotland in the eighteenth century John Lightfoot recorded new-born babies being given sap from the ash to protect them from witches and goblins.[9] The ritual of passing a sick child through a hoop made by bending an ash sapling is recorded in the early 1800s[10] and again over a hundred years later.[8] There is far more in legend and folklore than I can recount here.

Notes

1. Chiej R. *The Macdonald Encyclopedia of Medicinal Plants.* (Macdonald Publishing. London. 1984). 135.
2. Warren P. *British Native Trees, past and present uses.* (Wildeye. 2006). 47.
3. Fröhne D. Pfander H. *A Colour Atlas of Poisonous Plants.* (Wolf Science. 1983). 232.
4. Lewington A. *Plants for People.* (Eden Project Books. 2003). 247.
5. McLean T. *Medieval English Gardens.* (Barrie & Jenkins. 1989). 244.
6. Scott. M. (ed), *An Irish Herbal.* K'Eogh. (1735). (Aquarian. 1986). 24.
7. Baker St. Barbe. *Trees A Book of the Seasons.* (Lindsay Drummond Ltd. 1948). 1.
8. Freethy R. *From Agar to Zenry.* (Crowood Press. 1985). 65.
9. Grigson G. *The Englishman's Flora.* (The Folio Society. 1987). 272.
10. Green T. *Universal Herbal or Botanical Dictionary.* 2 vols, (Caxton, London. 2nd edition. 1824). Vol. 1. 578.

ASH – History of Medicinal Use

Ash is a native tree of the British Isles, which spread during the dominance of mixed oak woodland in very early times. Both the wood and the charcoal from ash trees are easily recognised and have been recorded from settlements during the Mesolithic period onwards. The highest numbers quoted by Godwin are from the north-west and Somerset on limestone areas. As well as charcoal finds, ash was also discovered to have been used in building track-ways, foundations for buildings and providing shafts and handles of tools and weapons.

The Anglo-Saxon period was a time when medicinal baths were used and these were made using tree barks and herbs. Ash and willow barks have anti-inflammatory properties and these could be applied in salves to ease wounded or inflamed parts of the body. Ash continued to be used into the second millennium for poulticing multiple injuries with fractures and bruising. We find the bark and flowers of the ash in the *Chirurgia* or book on surgery, written by the most important surgeon of Bologna, Theodoric (1205–1298) in 1277. Surgeons of this period knew ash as a mild styptic, repercussive to remove offensive matter and a regenerative agent, supporting growth of new tissue.[1]

In a manuscript of recipes from the fourteenth century, one has the fascinating title of "driving away wind in the ears". This title may of course be referring to inflammation in the ear from being in cold wind, or that may just be my modern mind working overtime. The branch from an ash tree is taken still green and placed in the full heat of the fire so that the sap will

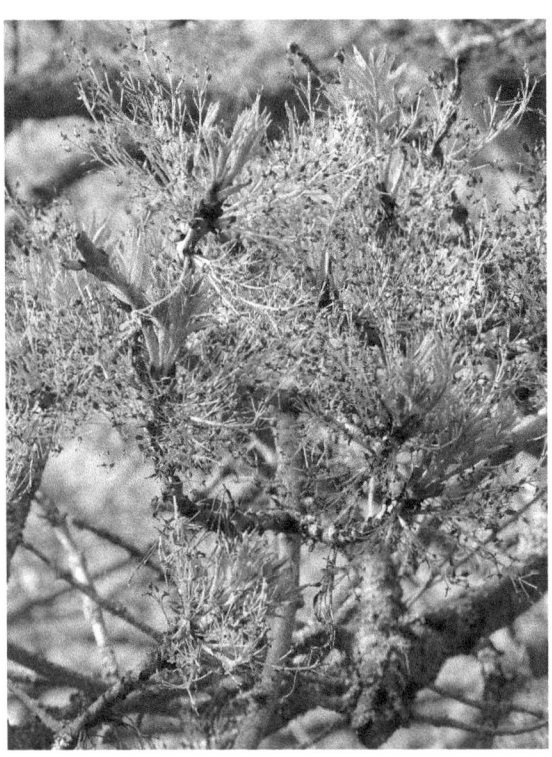
Ash with last flowers and leaf buds now opening.

ooze out from the ends. This warm sap is put into the ear each night until the patient is cured.[2] The same method of gathering ash sap, which then has the addition of fat and other herbs, appears a century later in another ear treatment.[3] This time it is for an evil ear. We can only surmise as to whether this term refers to a build up of wax or an abscess. The second seems likely as ash was also used to treat festering areas producing pus, particularly in the mouth.

References to ash being used against serpents and their bites occur in the sixteenth century. Gerard recommends the ash as a diuretic to aid weight loss and with added nutmeg to provoke urine. Culpeper tells us the ash tree is governed by the sun and writes scathingly about the belief that adders are afraid of ash leaves and the tree. He supposes this has come from Pliny and Gerard. Culpeper points out that he has seen proof that adders have no such fear. He then approves the diuretic uses and repeats the great antidote of Matthiolus of Siena (sixteenth century doctor and naturalist) against poison and pestilence. This includes ash tree seeds and Culpeper writes, "I am very loath to leave out this medicine, which if it were stretched out, and cut in thongs, would reach round the world." (p.338).[4]

Just four years after the publication of Culpeper's herbal, Coles gives us the classification of ash leaves and bark in his *Paradise of Plants*; dry and moderately hot, with the seed, which he also refers to as keys, as hot and dry in the second degree. Again this is a moderate degree, not particularly heating. He recommends all parts of the tree including the roots for their diuretic properties in treating dropsy. Coles repeats all that we have read before but instead of only preparing the bark in vinegar as a poultice, he adds an alternative recipe to boil the leaves and bark in oil before applying to the stomach. Then he writes that the seeds, husks removed, not only help stitch in the side from wind, but are commended for rickets. They were also powdered with nutmegs to increase "natural seed and stir up bodily lust" (p.306).[5] He does not question the use against serpent bites.

In the 1694 *Bates Dispensatory*, edited by the doctor and self-styled professor of physic, William Salmon, we find ash keys included with water cress, pine tops and more, in a distilled water against scurvy. This aspect of use of the ash keys made them a popular country pickle. Many culinary recipes follow over the next two centuries. In the same year,

Pechey prescribes the juice of the leaves and tender twigs as a morning diuretic and the powdered seeds in wine for dropsy. He adds that the salt of the ash provokes sweat and urine.

In the following century, Miller in his *Botanicum Officinale* places more emphasis on treating the spleen and liver, as well as the stone. He records the bark being given successfully in other countries to treat intermittent fevers. In Ireland in 1735, Ke'ogh writes of the inner bark for treating fevers and the wood ash being applied to ringworm.[6] In 1790, Meyrick gives the strong leaf tea as a purge and repeats William Withering, affirming that the bark sometimes cures the ague. He backs up this claim for ash with fevers by including the statement by the physician Vander Mye from the previous century that the distilled water had been given in pestilential diseases with success.[7]

Summary. Use of ash bark dominates the early recipes, leaves also providing a diuretic drink. Belief in ash as a protector and treatment for serpent bites was criticised by Culpeper, but lived on in folklore. Other diuretic treatments for dropsy and urinary stones, and use as a mild purge for the liver and spleen continue throughout the history of ash use. All parts of the tree found their way into recipes, with outward applications as well as teas, distilled water and alcoholic extractions. Ash keys gain in popularity for their content of vitamin C in treating scurvy from the end of the seventeenth century. Ash is absent from several nineteenth-century herbals. However, in 1916 the leaves are still being gathered for treatments and this time gout is mentioned.[8] See Herbalists' Reference for the modern view.

Recipes

Extracted from A Collection of Receipts. 1746. "For a Dropsy. Take the Leaves of Ash-trees, as soon as they begin to come out, and double distil them; give nine Spoonfuls of this Water, with one Spoonful of Mustard-seed, in the Morning; and at four or five in the Afternoon, give a Spoonful of Mustard-seed, in the like Quantity of White-wine: This is recommended as never failing. When the Distemper is taken at first, rest from taking it for ten Days, and then begin again." (p.241).[9]

Notes

1. Rosenman L.D. MD. *A Medieval Surgical Pharmacopoeia and Formulary. 1170–1325.* (San Francisco. 1999). 43.
2. Henslow G. Rev. Prof. M.A. *Medical Works of the Fourteenth Century.* (Burt Franklin. New York. 1972). Ms.D. 133.
3. Dawson W. (ed), *A Leechbook of the XVth Century.* (Macmillan & Co. 1934). 99. (266).
4. Culpeper N. *Culpeper's Complete Herbal and English Physician Enlarged.* (London. 1815 edition). 14. 337.
5. Coles W. *The Paradise of Plants.* (1657). 306.
6. Scott M. (ed), *An Irish Herbal.* [original Ke'ogh 1735]. (Aquarian 1986). 24.
7. Meyrick W. *The New Family Herbal.* (Birmingham. 1790). 21.
8. Teetgen A.B. *Profitable Herb-Growing and Collecting.* (London.1916). 176.
9. Anon. *A Collection of Receipts.* (Printed for the Executrix of Mary Kettilby. 1746). 241.

FRAXINUS EXCELSIOR – Herbalists' Reference

The Parts of Ash Used for Medicine – The sap is harvested in early spring, the bark can be harvested a little later from two to three year old twigs. The fruits or keys are the next harvest and should still be green and quite soft. The leaflets are harvested without the stalk, in May or June.

Dosage and Forms – One heaped teaspoon of leaf to each cup of boiling water. Infuse for fifteen minutes. Dose: half a cup three times daily. Syrup of the fruits may also be made.

Constituents – The bark of ash contains salicylates. Other parts contain flavone glycosides, resins, tannin, mannitol, and fruit acids.

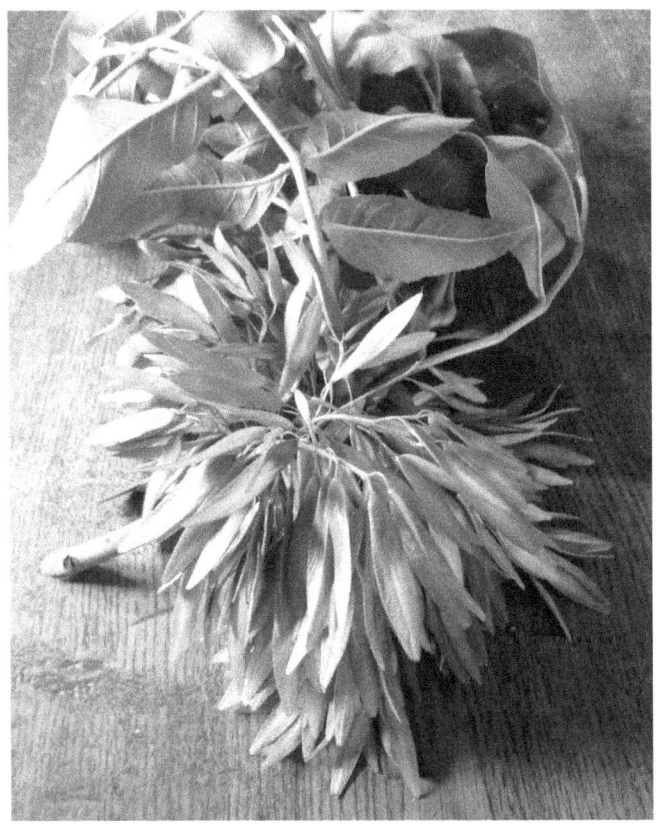

Ash keys and leaves.

Actions and Uses – The action of ash is largely to stimulate kidney function with resulting diuresis, which is helpful in oedema. Promoting excretion of uric acid indicates ash to treat gout and rheumatic conditions. As ash also has a diaphoretic effect, stimulating blood circulation to the periphery of the body, this makes it useful if the patient is feverish. The anti-inflammatory effect can be classed as moderate and is due to the coumarins inhibiting T-cells and prostaglandin biosynthesis.[1]

Precautions and Contraindications. Do not use the bark if the patient has a salicylate allergy.

Note

1. Mills S. & Bone K. *Principles & Practice of Phytotherapy.* (Churchill Livingstone. 2000). 149.

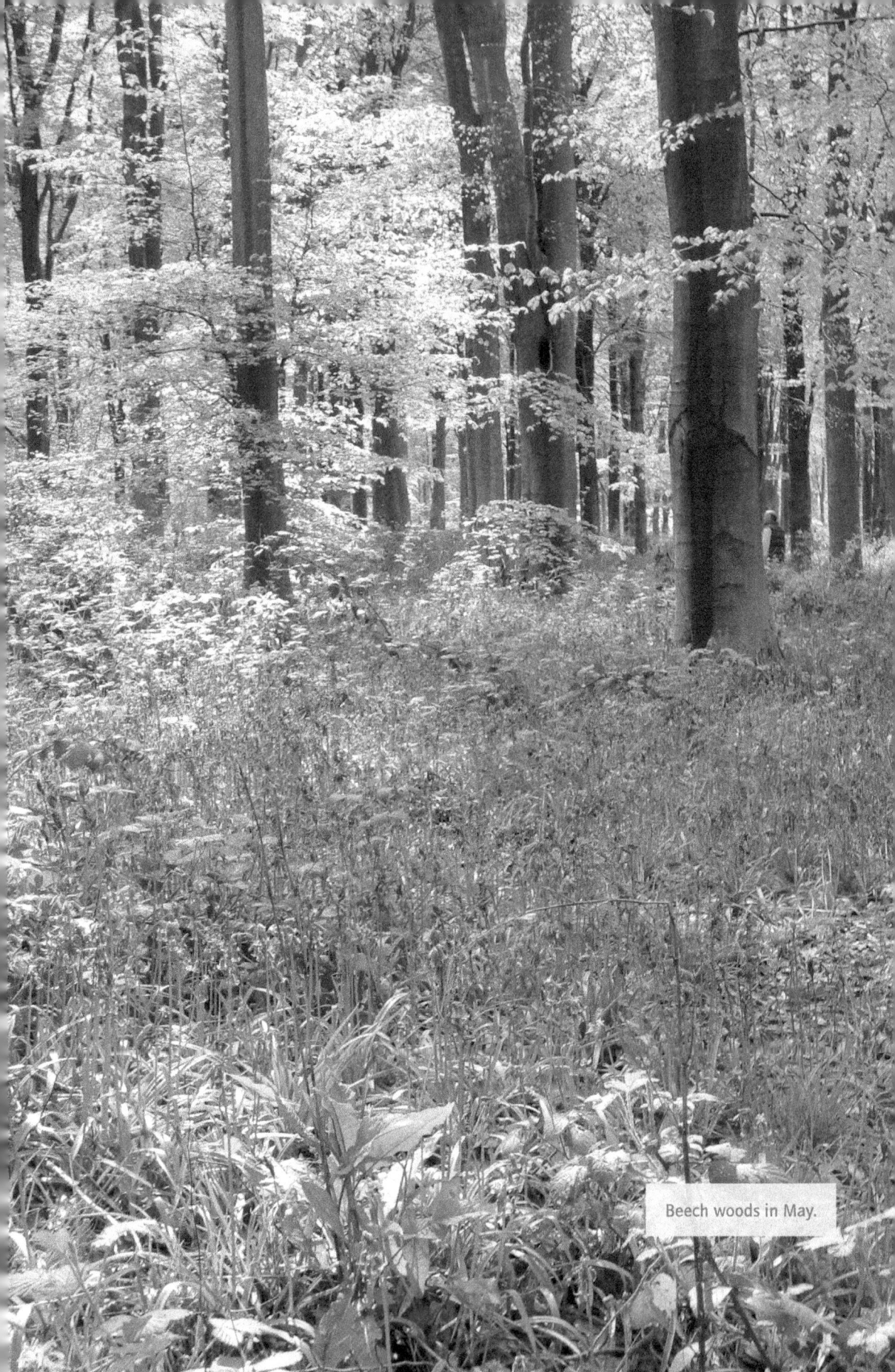
Beech woods in May.

Beech

Fagus sylvatica – Beech – Fagaceae

BEECH – Usefulness – The oil and nuts are nutritious. The nuts have been famine food and the oil from them burned in oil lamps. The new leaves make a once popular liqueur. Beech nuts have been an important food for pigs. Parts of the beech tree were formerly used medicinally. Ash from burning the branches has been a hair dye and used in making glass. Wood from the tree has been valued for making furniture and turns well. Baskets can be made from the bark. Hedges of beech are valued in gardens because of their habit of keeping their brown leaves through winter, which makes a good screen.

Dangers – The nuts contain saponins and oxalic acid, which are mostly insoluble. When eaten they may cause indigestion and are considered toxic in large amounts.[1] Use of beech tar for skin conditions has been discontinued due to toxicity to the kidneys.[2]

Getting to Know the Beech Tree – It has been my great delight for a number of years to visit nearby beech woods late in April or early in May, when the bluebells are out. The tall majesty of soaring beech trees reaching heavenwards, towards the sunlight, never fails to inspire me. With the encouragement of other trees forcing them upwards, beech can grow to forty five metres (148 feet).[3] Spotting the tiny saplings directly beneath them is another pleasure, for unlike acorns falling from oaks, which have help from squirrels and jays to give their progeny a wider spread, beech nuts are always found beneath the parent tree.

This gives us closely placed trees, tall and elegant in their growth with smooth bark, as if their youthful skin remains for longer than that of other trees. It also means that the canopy of leaves shuts out light that would otherwise support varied plant growth beneath. The bluebells and fungi are generally the most likely companions to beech trees. This may be death cap fungi or the more welcome truffles. Shallow-rooted, beech has a particularly reliant relationship with mycorrhizal fungi to supply nutrients and is susceptible when growing alone to be uprooted by high winds. If the tree survives long enough, without being crowded by others, it may achieve a wide girth, and at that point seems to attract the attention of lovers who see its bark as the perfect material for carving their initials and hearts. These it will display for the rest of their lives and more, as it may live for 200-300 years. Several kinds of fungus may also attack older trees, including honey fungus and bracket fungi.

The male flowers are the most familiar, hanging in bunches of fluffy tassels from the ends of the branches. The smaller female flowers are higher up the branch, appearing almost as fluffy balls and are very attractive. In past centuries the hairy nature of the flowers, leaves and husks was interpreted as a sign that the tree offered hair treatments. The thin nuts were burned and their ashes mixed with honey to apply to the scalp for thinning hair and scaly dandruff. This sticky application might be washed off with the boiled decoction of the nuts. A decoction of the bark was applied as a hair dye and charcoal from the wood used by dyers. The wood ash contains a high proportion of potash and charcoal from the wood has been used for making gunpowder![4]

Beyond trees and plants, books are my next love and the fact that early books might be leather-bound over thin sheets of beech-wood and printers' fonts were carved of beech, makes me appreciate the tree even more. In early spring I watch for the distinctive pointed leaf buds with their bronze coloured scales protecting the opening leaf. The new leaf is silky with long hairs.

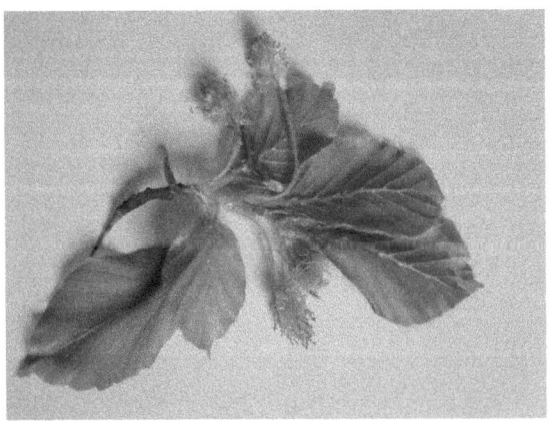

Male and female beech flowers.

Soon afterwards I can collect freshly opened beech leaves from my garden for beech-leaf gin. The fresh green colouring they impart seems to capture the essence of spring. The very young leaves have also been eaten and, over a longer period into the year, used to make cooling compresses. The Greek *Phago* gives the name *Fagus* meaning "I eat" but whether this referred to the leaves or nuts is unclear. Regardless, consumption of a large quantity at once is not good for health.

The copper beech leaves have not been eaten or used in the same way. The sight of a row of copper beeches can be magnificent in the early summer sunshine, and one particular line of them never fails to delight me as we pass them in Hampshire on the A272 between Winchester and Petersfield.

The height of mature beech is impressive at twenty-five to forty metres (eighty to 130 feet). Record-breaking beeches planted in 1745 over a length of 500 yards next to the A93 in Perth and Kinross are recorded by Adams.[5] Such straight growth and length of timber with few knots in the wood has ensured considerable use for building ships, floorboards for houses, cogs for mill machinery, furniture, particularly Windsor chairs, and even musical instruments, such as the harpsichord. The bark meanwhile has not been wasted, being used to make baskets.

It is the beech nuts that have most household use. In some years in Britain they are very thin and poor, being much thicker and more useful when grown in a warmer climate on the Continent. There the cake left from pressing the oil can provide a cattle food. Pulp remaining from pressing is not for human consumption, but the oil is good. With warmer weather giving fattened nuts, they have even been harvested to produce beech butter in this country.[6] The oil pressed from the nuts is tasty, odourless and a good substitute for olive oil in salad dressings and cooking. Pressing the oil at home is practical only if you can harvest over a kilo of the nuts. In centuries past when there was sufficient harvest, oil lamps burned beechnut oil and the oil also gave water-resistant polish to furniture. Beech nuts can be roasted and ground to make a coffee substitute, which perhaps is better taken in the small amounts you are likely to be able to process.

Like oaks, beeches do not produce a great harvest of their fruits every year, saving their energy for real bumper crops every two or three years. This strategy is to ensure that at that time the many animals that find beech nuts irresistible cannot possibly eat all of them. Some will be left to grow as young trees. As the nuts have such high nutritional value, pigs, deer, mice, squirrels, and pheasants are all attracted by them. Although they like the nuts, it has been observed that deer do not eat the young trees, which do manage to grow in parkland where deer live.

Gathering beech husks in quantity for use in Christmas decorations is an easy matter in autumn. They are very attractive secured in bunches, and decorated with gold balls in the centres for addition to wreaths. Sprays of the autumn leaves can also be preserved in glycerine, to great effect for flower arranging.

Legends and Folklore. It was once believed that the wind of Thor, god of thunder, could be heard in the rustling leaves making it the best tree to stand beneath during a thunderstorm, as it was less likely to be struck by lightning than an oak. In France and Bavaria where this idea was investigated over 17 years, observation supported it as fact.[7] The distinctive mark left on the bark where old growth has ceased seemed to the superstitious to be a sign of the evil eye.[8]

Notes

1. Fröhne D. Pfander H. *A Colour Atlas of Poisonous Plants.* (Wolf Science. 1983). 136.
2. Barker J. *The Medicinal Flora of Britain and Northwestern Europe.* (Winter Press. 2001). 18.
3. Lewington A. *Plants for People.* (Eden Project Books. 2003). 179.
4. Grieve. M. *A Modern Herbal.* (1st published 1934 Jonathan Cape. Saavas. 1984). 92.
5. Adams M. *The Wisdom of Trees.* (Head of Zeus Ltd. 2014). 146.
6. Phillips R. *Wild Food.* (Pan Books. 1983). 149.
7. DeCleene M. & Lejeune M.C. *Compendium of Symbolic and Ritual Plants in Europe.* (Man and Culture Publishers, Ghent. Belgium. 2003). 143.
8. Vickery R. *Oxford Dictionary of Plant-Lore.* (Oxford University Press. 1997). 28.

BEECH – History of Medicinal Use

Although it has been claimed that the beech was introduced by the Romans, evidence of beech pollen from Hampshire has shown its presence in Britain from 6,000BC.[1] Beech tends to be under-represented as it has a low pollen production, but records also include charcoal from Neolithic sites onwards and use in a Neolithic trackway in Somerset. Frequency of records is much higher in the area of a line from the Wash to the Bristol Channel.[2]

Gerard's enlarged herbal (Johnson, 1633) notes that Dioscorides classes the beech with the oak. Pliny prescribed beech leaves for infections, beech ash in ointment for bladder stones, and mixed with honey for scabies. The first mention of medicinal use in Britain comes in the Anglo-Saxon Leechbooks. However, this is not directly for beech but use of a fern that grows on the roots of the tree to be applied to heal a rupture.[3] Hildegard of Bingen in *Physica* also includes something growing on the tree. This time it is a mushroom, which must be eaten cooked, to warm the stomach and remove mucus. The fungus is described as hot. Of the tree itself Hildegard writes of magical incantation, ritual, and prayers to be undertaken while cutting branches with new leaves for treating jaundice. Other recipes involve the roots and acorns.[4]

In a fifteenth century Leechbook we find a recipe for treating sick, and presumably painful ears with the juice of beech leaves mixed with vinegar.[5] This would be very astringent alone, but then powdered quicklime is added, before the liquid is strained, and introduced

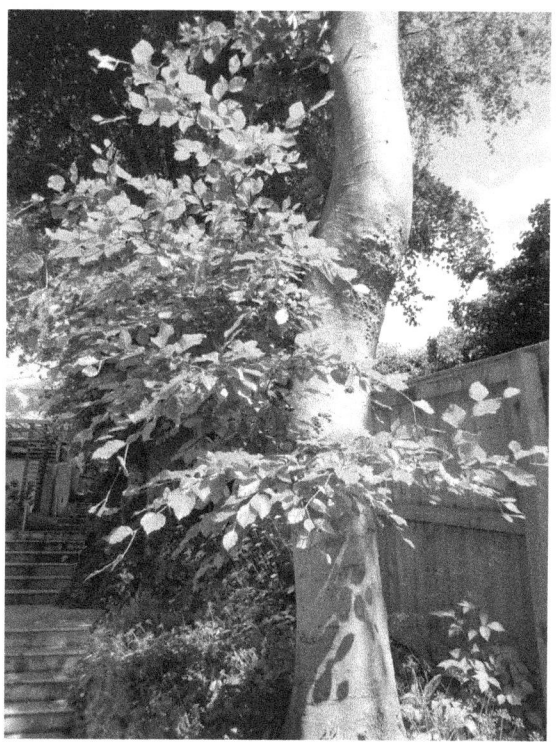

A slender beech with young leaves.

while hot into the ear. This is definitely not a recipe to repeat today. A hundred years later Gerard gives us rather more sensible recommendations for using the cooling properties of the leaves and astringency of the tannins in the mast or kernels.

Culpeper classes the beech as a plant of Saturn, repeating the cooling and binding nature of the leaves for hot swellings and use of the water gathered in beech hollows for scurf or running sores in man and beast. He adds instructions to boil the leaves for a poultice, or to include them in an ointment. Coles, thorough as ever, gives us all that has been written before, with the added detail that the nuts are burned to give ashes and these are mixed with honey and applied for scurvy head. There is one new recipe for the leaves, buds and bark to be sodden in red wine, or running water, to make what appears to be a Sitz bath for menorrhagia or a prolapsed womb. A drink of the decoction in red wine with cinnamon and sugar is given internally following this.

Much later, in the nineteenth century we note beech tar has found its way into some Pharmacopoeias as the best source of a type of creosote distilled from the wood.[6] This substance is unlike the creosote used for painting on fences, although the smell was similar. It was obtained by destructive distillation of the wood and was used externally in a similar manner to other tars to treat skin diseases.[7] Use has since been discontinued, due to toxicity to the kidneys.[8]

Summary. From the earliest mentions, there is a theme of using the astringency of the tree parts to treat skin diseases and infestations. This included scabies, weeping eczema, blistered skin, and dandruff. Potency was added by the guaiacol in beech tar, which was prepared in more recent times. The other main use has been of the leaves, applied either in a compress, wash, or ointment, for their cooling and binding properties. Beech tar is no longer prescribed due to concerns on safety. See also Herbalists' Reference.

Recipe

Extracted from Leechcraft. The Olde English Herbarium 78. "**Fern** *ffelix*. 2. For that a young man be ruptured take this same plant where it grows on the root of a beech tree, pound with lard and smear a cloth therewith and bind it to the pain so that meanwhile he be turned upwards, on the fifth day he shall be healed." (p.323).[3]

Notes

1. Mabey R. *Flora Britannica* (concise edition). (Chatto & Windus. 1998). 93.
2. Godwin Sir H. *History of the British Flora*. (Cambridge University Press. 2nd edition. 1975). 273, 275.
3. Pollington S. *Leechcraft*. (Anglo Saxon Books. 2000). 323. *Olde English Herbarium*. 78.
4. Throop P. (trans), *Hildegard von Bingen's Physica*. (Healing Arts Press. 2000). 52, 80, 122–4, 171.
5. Dawson W. (ed), *A Leechbook of the XVth Century*. (Macmillan & Co. 1934). 101, (269).
6. Flückiger F.A. & Hanbury D. F.R.S. *A History of Drugs*. (Macmillan & Co. 1879.). 623.
7. Todd R.G. (ed), *Extra Pharmacopoeia Martindale*. 25th edition. (Pharmaceutical Press. 2nd edition. 1967). 1421.
8. Barker J. *The Medicinal Flora of Britain and Northwestern Europe*. (Winter Press. 2001). (18).

FAGUS SYLVATICA – Herbalists' Reference

The Parts of Beech Used for Medicine – Bark from the young branches is gathered for use or drying in early spring. Oil from the seeds.[1]

Dosage and Forms – Decoction, capsules.

Constituents – Guaiacol, creosol, cresolin, tannin, phlorol.

Actions and Uses – As with many barks, that of the beech can supply an astringent, antiseptic decoction for use as a mouthwash. This may help with pain from receding gums, which could present as toothache (the tar was formerly packed into an aching tooth). It also has expectorant properties, may help to reduce fever, and has been given to treat bronchitis. Chiej lists the bark as additionally antacid. However, there are herbs that are better researched and possibly more efficient in these roles.

Topical Application – Beech tar was used in general medicine until the late twentieth century.[2] Weiss still lists it as available at the turn of

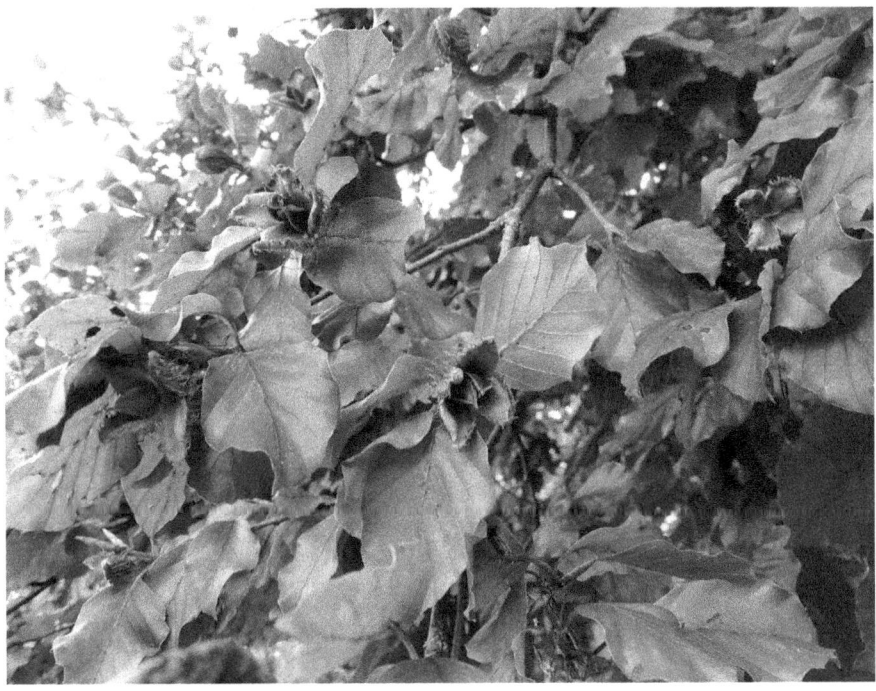

Beech seeds in their husks.

the century, but adds a warning about the effects on the kidneys of long term use of several wood tars.

Contraindications and Precautions – Beech tar distilled from the branches was once used topically to treat skin conditions and dandruff, as well as internally. This is no longer prescribed due to the discovery of a toxic action in the liver.

Comment. Considering the actions and uses of beech, there are more readily available, safer herbal alternatives. However, it has perhaps been typical that the strongest acting preparation was adopted by later medicine. The beech tar was then identified as toxic and discarded.

Notes

1. Bown D. *The RHS Encyclopedia of Herbs.* (Dorling Kindersley. 1996). 282.
2. Todd R.G. (ed), *Extra Pharmacopoeia Martindale.* (Pharmaceutical Press. 25th edition. 1967). 1421.

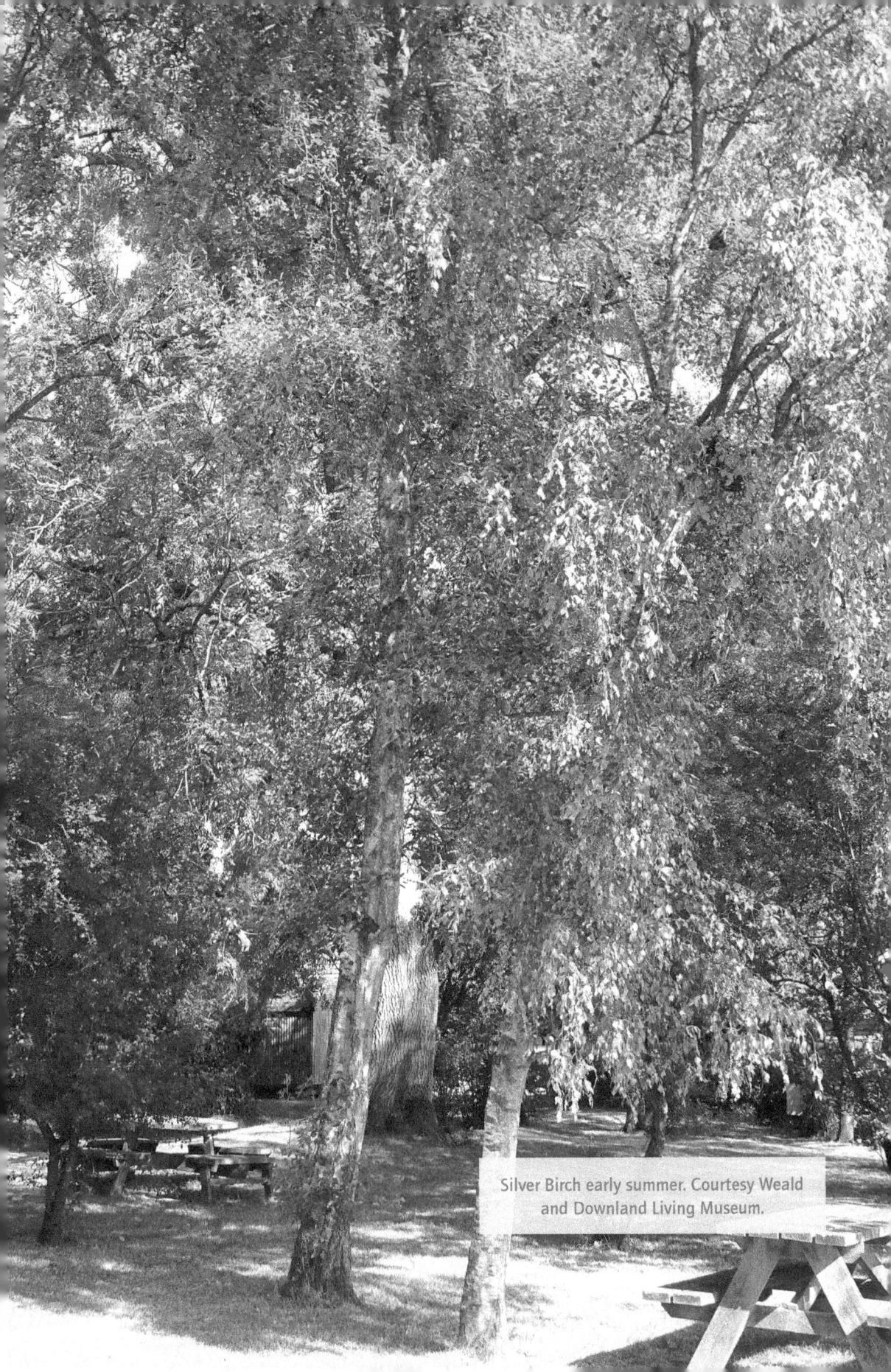

Silver Birch early summer. Courtesy Weald and Downland Living Museum.

Birch

Betula alba, B – lenta – Silver Birch – Betulaceae

SILVER BIRCH – Usefulness – The leaves, buds, twigs, bark and sap are used in herbal medicine. Birch tar has also been used in mainstream medicine. The sap may be made into ales or wine. The bark has provided material for waterproof flooring, roofing and containers. Birch bark was flattened to make sheets for writing on. In North America birch bark has been used to make wigwams and canoes. Birch tar from the tree provides strong glue. The bark can be lit as a torch. Birch sap, twigs and leaves have cosmetic uses. Twigs are bound as birch brooms. The leaves give a dye and act to fix fungal dyes.

Dangers – The tree produces a prolific amount of pollen. The grains are very small and scatter in the wind over a wide area. Many people unfortunately have allergic reactions to it.

Getting to Know the Silver Birch Tree – Many years ago I was given a young sapling of silver birch, only about seventy centimetres (two feet) tall. I planted it near the bottom of our third of an acre garden and watched it grow. I was delighted to give the tree a home as birch trees feed a variety of insects as well as birds, such as the siskin.

The bark, at first comparatively smooth, becomes split by irregular dark patches standing out against the silver surround. It is an interesting tree to draw in pen and ink, observing the varied patterns formed.

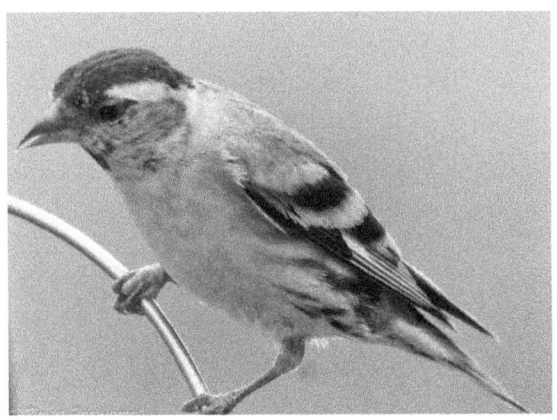
Siskin. Photo David Papworth.

The male catkins on the birch are familiar to most people as they hang on the tree all through winter, having formed in autumn. In April they hang down as decorative yellow tails, rather more open than those on the hazel. What fascinated me was the discovery of the female catkins. These are much smaller, curling upwards and while the male are on the ends of the branches, the female catkins are a little higher up, for better protection. These are followed by a small winged nutlet ready in summer, containing one seed. Seed dispersal is in early autumn.

On a visit to relatives in Canada I went in search of members of the first nation to ask for information about their use of herbs. On that first trip I was directed to Jeff Beaver, whose grandfather had been the tribal medicine man. On my second visit Jeff kindly took me to the cluster of wigwams he had made from birch bark to demonstrate traditional ways to schoolchildren. He was also making a birch-bark canoe and explained the processes involved in harvesting the bark which he stripped sustainably from much larger birch than the trees in Britain, the roots he used for stitching and so on. It was a fascinating day and inspired me to take up bark basketry which I later enjoyed.

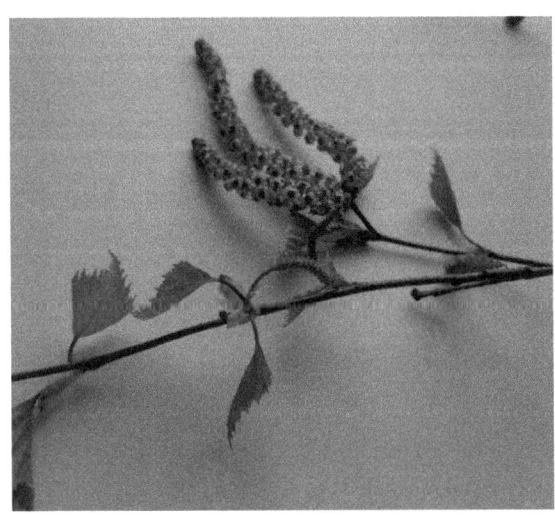
Male and smaller female birch flowers.

Silver birch is a fast growing tree with a possible height of ten to twenty-five metres (thirty-three to eighty-two feet) and a relatively short life compared to other trees, of a possible hundred but probable eighty years. Twenty years later my tree had grown to maturity, standing tall, and with sufficient girth for me to tap it in February for the sap. It is amazing to appreciate how swiftly the sap powers up the tree in spring, in preparation for forming and opening the leaves. I had a tap which was designed for this purpose given to me by my Canadian cousin. She could also offer guidance, as she and her husband tapped the maple trees on their farm each year.

My husband drilled the hole at shoulder height and inserted the tap which would take a half gallon wine demijohn on the hook beneath to catch the sap. This filled in a couple of hours and I very soon had plenty for my needs. Once finished it is important to seal the hole as tightly as possible. We managed to do this using a piece of a small branch from the same tree. Some of the sap was for wine-making and some I mixed with honey into syrup. The sap itself was not quite as sweet as I had expected, but still pleasant to drink. However, in Finland a sweetener, xylitol has been extracted from birch sap, this is also used in chewing gums. In 1916 it was noted that the juice could be evaporated off to leave a deposit of sweet crystals.[1]

Another useful harvest can be gathered just after the sap rises, when the buds and developing new leaves are covered by protective oily exudates of resin. At this stage they can be boiled to produce a soapy shampoo. Simple warming of the buds encourages more to exude, and this can be applied to polish leather shoes.

In the history of the tree I have also mentioned evidence of some of the many uses of birch bark in prehistoric Britain. Today the best known uses are probably from seeing and sweeping leaves with birch besom brooms, or hearing stories of children being punished with "the birch" made from the whippy branches. These, however are only the tip of the iceberg when we consider the whole picture both past and present. At the turn of the seventeenth century the wood was used for making ox-yokes and turned into smaller items.[2] Fascinating descriptions can be found of fishermen in Northumberland putting bark into a cleft stick and lighting it so that they could see to spear fish at night.[3]

Birch wood can be used for smoking fish. In the Highlands the bark was soaked for tanning leather and making ropes. The wood is recorded in the nineteenth century as making the best charcoal and the soot from burning it was recognised as good lamp-black for printers' ink.[4] The high tannin content of the pliable birch bark meant it was suitable for wrapping foods to keep them fresh and in Scotland the branches have been used as a fuel for distilling whisky.[5]

In Russia not only were house tiles made from the waterproof bark, the birch tar was added to Russian leather which gave an added distinctive aroma. It has also been highly thought of as a medicine there. The black birch, *Betula lenta*, gives sweet birch oil containing large amounts of methyl salicylate and has been used in dentistry products and perfumes. Wintergreen oil is now almost entirely distilled from the bark of the black birch in America, the chemical components coming together during distillation to produce oil almost identical with wintergreen oil from the wintergreen plant, although this form did not exist in the original tree.[6]

Legends and folklore. In many traditions in America a birch was planted on the grave of relatives to help them as a ladder to climb to heaven.[7] In Wales, Celtic tradition associates the White Goddess with the silver birch, viewing it as the tree of Arianrhod who is in charge of the silver wheel of the heavens.[8] In Scotland it was used to avert the evil eye and hung over doors and even signposts on Midsummer Eve.[9]

Notes

1. Teetgen A.B. *Profitable Herb-Growing and Collecting.* (London. 1916). 169.
2. Miller P. F.R.S. *Gardener's Dictionary.* (London. 1771).
3. Warren P. *British Native Trees, past and present uses.* (Wildeye. 2006). 34.
4. Green T. *Universal Herbal or Botanical Dictionary.* 2 vols, (Caxton. London. 2nd edition. 1824). Vol. 1. 169.
5. Freethy R. *From Agar to Zenry.* (Crowood Press. 1985). 67.
6. Mills S. *Out of this Earth.* (Viking. Penguin. 1991). 495.
7. Buhner S.H. *Sacred and Herbal Healing Beers.* (Siris Books. 1998). 249.
8. Gifford J. *The Celtic Wisdom of Trees.* (Godsfield Press. 2000). 12/13.
9. Phillips R. *Wild Food.* (Pan Books. 1983). 13.

BIRCH – History of Medicinal Use

We know that birch trees were valued by prehistoric man, firstly for the multitude of uses of easily detachable bark. This highly adaptable tree quickly colonised the areas that had been tundra in the Ice Ages. Birch has the ability to grow at a high altitude, together with a wide tolerance of soil types and high pollen productivity at an early age. These qualities made birch readily available over a wide area. Use of birch bark was clear at Star Carr Mesolithic site, where many birch-bark rolls were excavated.[1]

With the bark providing everything from waterproof flooring to containers and hats, that alone would make birch a necessity. Secondly, tar from the tree was widely used to cement flint arrowheads and spearheads in place. Finally, archaeology has also revealed that fruits of a parasitic fungus of birch were collected and could have been used for wound dressings. This fungus, *Fomes fomentarius* found with the bronze age, "Ice Man" when a glacier retreated in the Alps, contains an antibiotic substance, polyporic acid, which is highly active against certain mycobacteria.[2] This same fungus is common on birch trees in Britain.

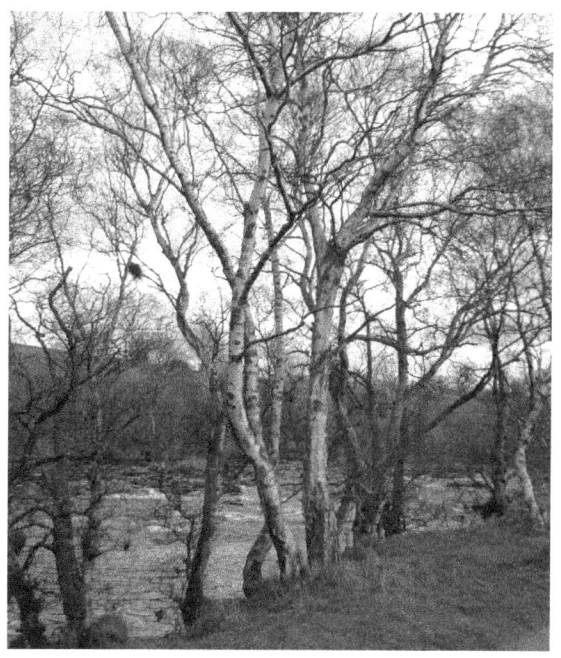

Silver Birch by the River Tees in winter.

In the Anglo-Saxon Leechbook of *Bald*, written in Winchester in the tenth century, bark from the birch is used, together with barks of other trees. They are pounded and boiled in whey before applying where a "burrowing worm" (p.395) had entered the skin.[3] Two hundred years later, Hildegard of Bingen also recommends applying birch roots to worms in the skin, as well as eruptive skin conditions. She classes the tree as more hot than cold in action.[4]

Although we do not have evidence for the very early times, it is unlikely the sap would not have been used. Fermented birch sap was popular in the medieval period and onwards, it was commonly prepared as ale with a small amount of malt added, or a country wine. Knowledge of this and other uses of birch stood the early settlers of America in good stead. There they tapped the black birch along with the maple trees.[5] In 1603, Sir Hugh Plat takes up the thread of a medicinal use for birch sap for clearing spots from the skin. He also remarks that he has the rare knowledge of the sap being able to dissolve pearls.[6]

It appears from Gerard's Herbal no record could be found of medicinal use for birch in the classical writers, but Culpeper, who does not give his source, recommends the distilled sap as a drink for breaking up kidney and bladder stones. This is interesting in light of Sir Hugh Plat's claim and makes one wonder whether they are connected. Culpeper classes the birch as a tree of Venus.[7]

We now have classifications of birch as being both hot and cold. Coles, writing a few years after Culpeper, makes a finer distinction. He relates that the leaves are thought to be cooling, but the bark and catkins are hot. This, of course, applies to their medicinal action on the body. Coles quotes Crollius, who travelled Eastern Europe as a physician and wrote what was to become the standard scientific work on iatrochemistry, *Basilica Chymica* (published in 1609). He was interested in the doctrine of signatures, and it is this observation that is repeated by Coles. The inner bark, he quotes, 'hath the signature of the Matrix with the bloudy veines thereof.' (p.594).[8] This last statement led to the presumption that a decoction would provoke menstruation and expel the afterbirth. This use has never been confirmed. Coles agrees with Culpeper on use of the distilled sap for the kidneys.[8]

In 1694, Pechey is enthusiastic on the subject of the sap in medicine. He refers to it as a sweet and potulent juice that shepherds drink. He quotes several sources for proof of efficacy with kidney stones and inflammation, adding a commendation for treating jaundice and removing spots when applied as a wash. He adds reported cures of scorbutick consumption with birch sap, wine and honey by Dr. Needham.[9]

A hundred years later the surgeon Meyrick gives a full description of tapping the tree for sap for wine-making or distilling. He writes this juice is an excellent medicine against scurvy, promotes urine, and taken in quantity will be laxative. The leaves and bark he tells us "resolve, cleanse, and resist putrefaction." (p.44).[10] He recommends a decoction of them for bathing skin eruptions or taking for dropsy.[10] In 1822 Waller goes even further, with both enthusiasm and detail. He writes that the sap is preferable to any other part of the tree and quotes Vauhelmont in describing the best source of sap to be from a branch not thicker than three inches (seven and a half centimetres). He instructs readers on preserving the sap by pouring a little olive oil on the surface in the container, as the air corrupts it.[11]

There is no mention of any part of the birch being used medicinally in the 1905 *National Botanic Pharmacopoeia*, issued by the National Association of Herbalists, however, use of birch has returned in modern herbal medicine – see Herbalists' Reference.

Summary. The birch tree has supplied many needs from prehistoric times through to the last century. Among these has been the use of fermented sap in ales and wines. Ales, wines and other ways of preserving the sap, which otherwise would not keep once exposed to the air, have been used for medicine. The sap has been consistently recommended for treating the urinary system, specifically kidney and bladder stones, and for clearing the skin when applied topically. A decoction of the leaves and twigs has also been used for this. There are brief mentions for treating jaundice, dropsy and scorbutick consumption, but the main emphasis for the sap has been on the urinary system and skin. We find enthusiasm for the leaves and twigs in the nineteenth century for resolving and cleansing, but in that century enthusiasm seems to die away only to return with renewed and more widespread uses, adopted from Eastern Europe in the twentieth century.

Recipe

Extracted from The Compleat Housewife. 1739. "To make Birch Wine. In *March* bore a hole in a tree, and put in a faucet, and it will run two or three days together without hurting the tree; then put in a pin to stop it, and the next year you may draw as much from the same hole; put to every gallon of the liquor a quart of good honey, and stir it well together, boil it an hour, scum it well, and put in a few cloves, and a piece of lemon-peel; when it is almost cold, put to it so much ale-yeast as will make it work like new ale; and when the yeast begins to settle, put it in a runlet that will just hold it; so let it stand 6 weeks, or longer if you please; then bottle it, and in a month you may drink it; it will keep a year or two; you may make it with sugar, two pounds to a gallon, or something more, if you keep it long; this is admirably wholesome, as well as pleasant, an opener of obstructions, good against the phthisick, and good against the spleen and scurvy, a remedy for the stone; it will abate heat in a fever or thrush, and has been given with good success." (pp.217/8).[12]

Notes

1. Godwin Sir H. *History of the British Flora.* (Cambridge University Press. 2nd edition. 1975).
2. Spindler K. *The Man in the Ice.* (Weidenfeld & Nicolson. 1994). 118.
3. Pollington S. *Leechcraft.* (Anglo Saxon Books. 2000). 395, *Bald* 39.
4. Throop P. (trans), *Hildegard von Bingen's Physica.* (Healing Arts Press. 1998). 125/6.
5. Buhner S.H. *Sacred and Herbal Healing Beers.* (Siris Books. 1998). 245.
6. Plat Sir H. *Delights for Ladies.* (1609). (Crosby Lockwood. 1948). 90.
7. Culpeper N. *Culpeper's Complete Herbal and English Physician enlarged.* (1652). (London. 1815 edition). 24.
8. Coles W. *The Paradise of Plants.* (London. 1657). 594.
9. Pechey J. *The English Herbal of Physical Plants.* (London. 1694). 19/20.
10. Meyrick R. *The New Family Herbal.* (Birmingham. 1790). 44.
11. Waller J. *Waller's New British Domestic Herbal.* Cox & Son. (London. 1822). 30.
12. Smith E. *The Compleat Housewife.* (London. 1739). 217/8.

BETULA LENTA, B. ALBA – Herbalists' Reference

The Parts of Silver Birch Used for Medicine – The sap, tapped from mature trees in February or March. The bark should also be stripped from branches in early spring. The buds and leaves are gathered in late spring into summer.

Dosage and Forms – Tea—Doses of birch leaf tea vary considerably from one herbalist to another. From one teaspoon of dried leaves per cup of boiling water three times daily to two tablespoonsful. The buds may be steeped in cold water in the fridge overnight, or gently decocted for five minutes. Bark decoction should still be carried out for twenty minutes. Again tincture doses vary from 1–5ml per day. Birch juice is commercially available and experience with this form has been positive.

Constituents – The volatile oil contains camphoraceous betulin, this is present in the bark with resin and tannins. The buds contain sugar,

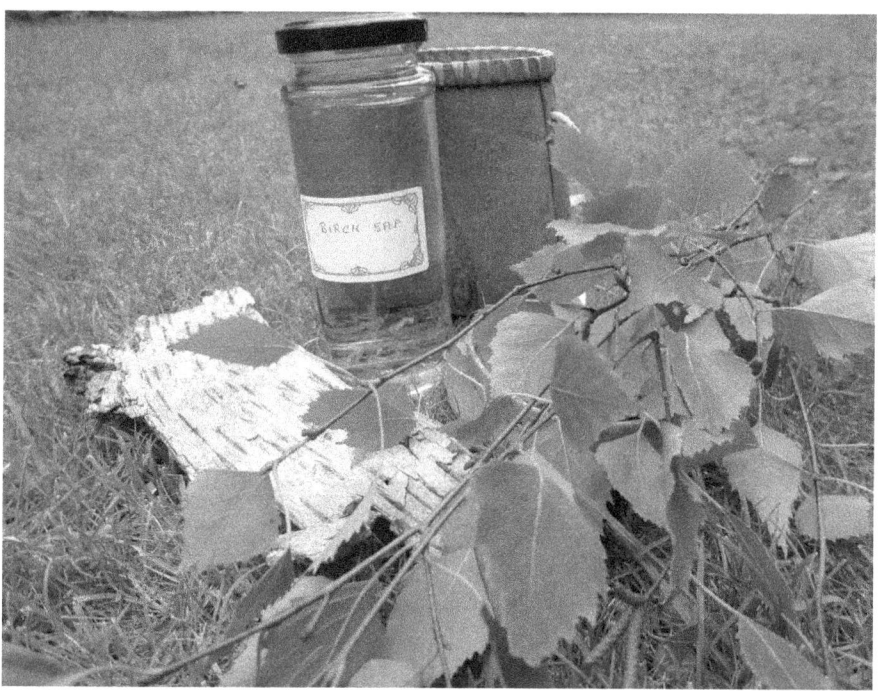

Birch sap with bark, bark container, twigs and leaves.

betulorentic acid, saponins and tannin. The leaves in addition contain phytocides, which are effective germicides. Salicylic acid methylester, hyperosides, bitters, procyanidins, and minerals are other active constituents. Of the minerals, the potassium has a ratio of 150 to one of sodium.

Actions and Uses – Teas of the leaves or buds, or decoctions of the bark are preferred by some herbalists who maintain these are more effective than alcoholic extractions. Native American tribes used the bark and leaf together as the most effective treatment. Birch is most valued for treating rheumatic diseases. The leaves and bark contain salicylates, which relieve pain. In addition the diuretic effects, which are stronger in the leaf, are appreciated in draining congested fluids and promoting detoxification to relieve eczema and other skin conditions. The buds may be given to reduce congestion and swelling in lymph glands.[1]

Diuresis is accompanied by action as a urinary antiseptic and silver birch is believed to improve uric acid excretion. Gout may respond well. Birch leaf tea has a positive recommendation from the German Commission E for treating bacterial and inflammatory disease of the efferent urinary passages, renal gravel, and rheumatic complaints.[2] Birch juice is a useful adjuvant in treating patients with fibromyalgia. The bark is naturally more astringent and has a stronger action on the liver, stimulating bile flow and relieving constipation. The saponins may add an anti-inflammatory effect.

Betulorentic acid occurs in the fruits of *Betula alba*, and has shown promise in activity against melanoma cells. We wait to see whether use may be made of this in future.[3]

Topical Applications – The fresh wet inner bark can be moulded to the skin to ease muscular or rheumatic pain. Dried bark is readily re-hydrated simply by pulling it through water to restore flexibility. Healing poultices, compresses, ointments or liniments can be prepared from all parts of the tree. The leaves may be mixed with nettle and burdock in oil applications to stimulate hair growth in alopecia.[2] Birch tar is used to treat scabies and skin infections.[4]

Precautions and Contraindications. Not to be used where there is oedema due to cardiac or renal insufficiency. The essential oil is toxic and easily absorbed through the skin.[5] Wintergreen oil is distilled from the bark of *B. lenta*, the salicylates forming during the distillation process.[6] Do not prescribe if there is salicylate allergy.

Notes

1. Holmes P. *The Energetics of Western Herbs*. Vols 1&2 (Snow Press. Boulder. Revised 3rd edition. 1989). 714.
2. Weiss R.F. M.D. *Herbal Medicine* (Thieme. 2nd edition. Revised and expanded. 2000). 410, 307.
3. Sumner J. *The Natural History of Medicinal Plants*. (Timber Press. 2000). 167.
4. Kelly W.J. (ed. Director). *Nursing Herbal Medicine Handbook*. (Springhouse Corporation. 2001). 55, 56.
5. Duke J.A. *Handbook of Medicinal Herbs* (CRC Press LLC. 2nd edition 2002). 76.
6. Mills S. *Out of the Earth*. (Viking Arcana. 1991). 495.

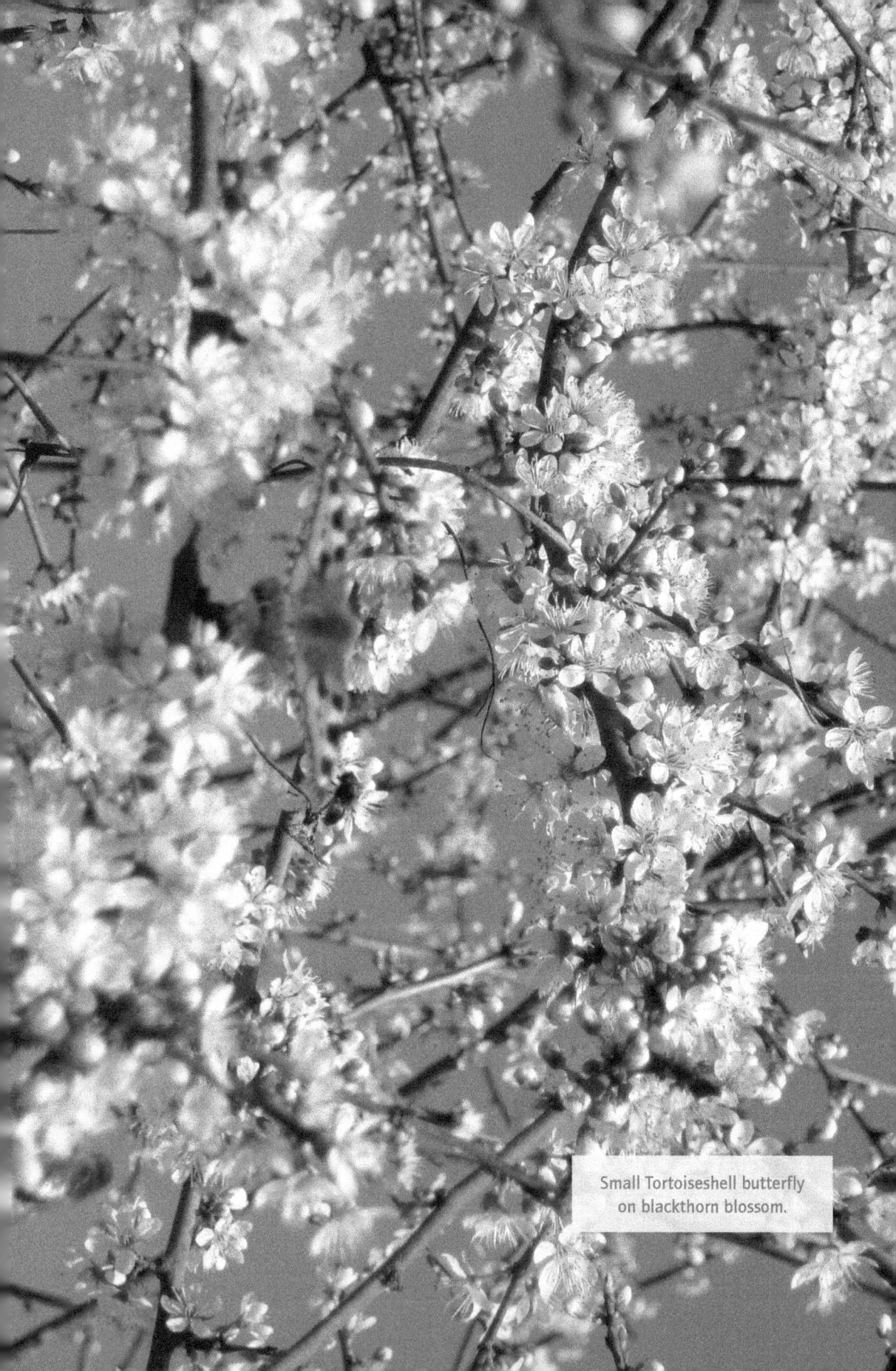

Small Tortoiseshell butterfly on blackthorn blossom.

Blackthorn

Prunus spinosa – Sloe, Blackthorn – Rosaceae

BLACKTHORN – Usefulness – Sloe fruits can be used in cookery but are better known in wine-making and liqueurs. Parts of the tree supply herbal medicine. The distilled water and fruits also have cosmetic uses. The juice of the fruits gives both a dye and ink, and the wood can be carved or turned. The tree supports butterflies, bees, other insects, and birds. Some mammals, such as foxes and badgers, enjoy the fruits.

Dangers – When harvesting flowers or fruits from the tree, gloves should be worn as the thorns on the tree are very sharp. The seeds contain amygdalin, which is toxic in large amounts.

Getting to Know the Blackthorn Tree – One of the first native trees to burst into blossom in March, blackthorn decorates the stark lines of bare trees at the field edges with lacy hangings, appearing as great sweeps of bright whiteness in places. The sight lifts the heart, even though rather than being a trustworthy harbinger of spring, blackthorn blossom can instead herald what has been referred to for centuries as the blackthorn winter. This is a period of sudden sharp frosts amongst bright, sunny days when you had hoped the frosts were over.

Standing beside a blackthorn in full blossom on a sunny, spring day can be magical. To be joined by tortoiseshell butterflies in addition to the many bees humming incessantly over the delicately scented flowers is an added treat. If you are very fortunate and live in Southern England, your sloes may attract the rare brown hairstreak butterfly. From Oxfordshire to Northamptonshire, there is again a chance of drawing the equally rare, black hairstreak butterfly. The leaves are the main food for the larvae of both species.

The flowers, growing in clusters, resemble smaller versions of simple white roses with their five petals, which are almost the badge of the rose family. At the centre of each flower are circles of at least twelve long, pretty, golden tipped anthers. The flowers appear on short lateral spikes from the branches of the tree before the leaves open, but some may remain after the leaves appear. At this point the long thorny spikes, which occur on the older branches between the flowering shoots, will identify the tree as a blackthorn, rather than the wild plum that also has white blossom at this time. I distil the flowers making aromatic water, a good skin toner for greasy skin. They can also be made into laxative syrup for the medicine cabinet.[1]

Some years ago I had a large enough herb garden to be able to plant a blackthorn tree at the edge of our fruit orchard. Sloe was included in the lists of fruit trees in medieval orchards and I felt it deserved a place, but I also had a particular motive. Once I started teaching those around me to pick the sloes growing wild nearby, for making sloe gin, I found it difficult to get there before them. I decided I needed my own supply! Although a blackthorn is not a tall tree, generally growing to stand two to three metres (six to ten feet) tall, the branches have vicious thorns, and there is another reason it is not for every garden. The space it will occupy in the future has to be considered. The canopy of a single tree is not large, yet sloes spread not only by seed but by putting out runners and, if allowed, can produce a sizeable thicket. It is, however, a good tree to include in a deliberately thorny hedge designed to keep animals from pushing through. Together with hawthorn, wild rose, and bramble, sloe can complete a formidable barrier.

Evidence of field hedges like these has been found from as early as the Roman period.[2] Blackthorn and hawthorn, or blackthorn and briar were other hedgerow combinations. In Miller's *Gardeners' Dictionary* of 1771 he has this to say, "This is very common in the hedges almost everywhere; the chief use of this tree is to plant for hedges, as Whitethorn &c. and being of quick growth, is very proper for that purpose."

In my work exploring the history of herbs, with practical workshops on uses from the Bronze Age through to the Victorian period, I have encountered recipes with the blossom, young leaves and bark, as well as the fruits, and their juice. On Victorian days we have experimented with original tea substitute recipes. Sloe leaves were particularly recommended at this time and Green wrote in 1824 of the tender young leaves being dried and sold fraudulently as real East India tea.[3]

For many years I have gathered the fruits every autumn to make sloe gin, or use with other wild fruits in pies. There are some lovely Elizabethan recipes that involve cooking the sloes in honey first. Freezing the fruits beforehand helps to sweeten them. Today, this can

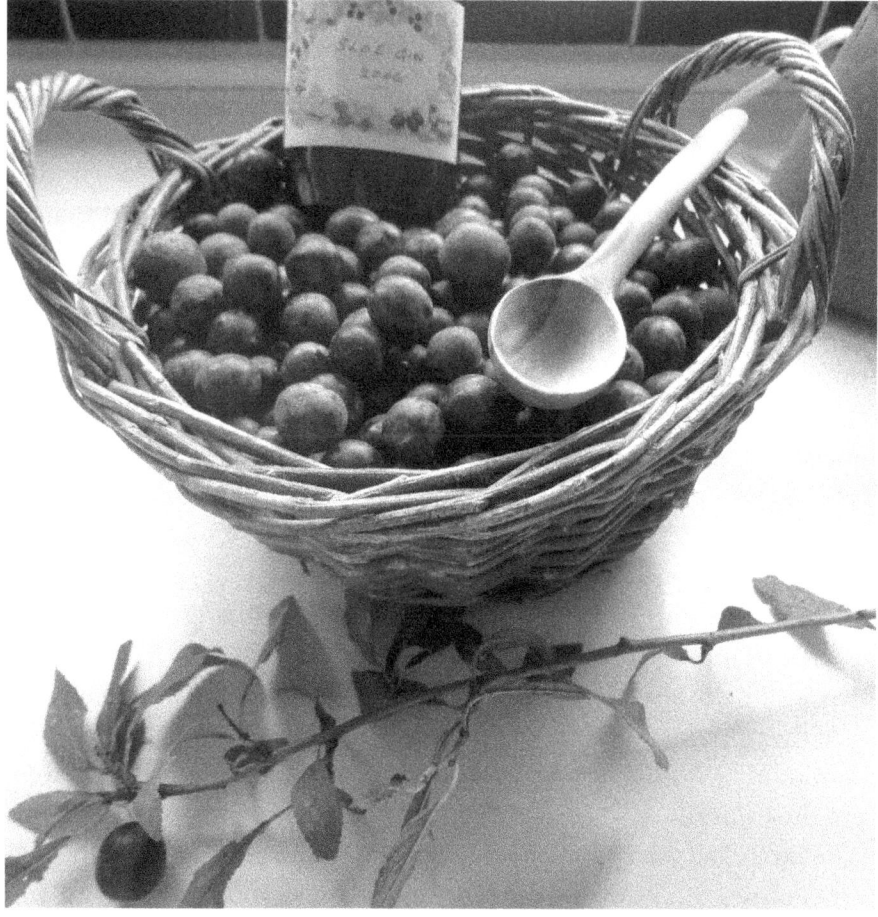

Sloes, sloe gin and a spoon of sloe wood.

be achieved by placing them in the freezer overnight. I have read that in the past gypsies used to bury them in shallow pits lined with straw for that purpose.[4] Sloe fruits come into their own in sweet jellies and jams; I like to mix sloe with blackberries and crab apple. Many hedgerow combinations can vary the store of goodness from one winter to another, making sloe and apple cheese or jam, wine, or autumn fruit syrups with blackberries.

Sloe gin is rich and syrupy, excellent for a sore throat and can be a welcome nightcap when suffering with a cold, or simply to soothe the throat. Sloe vodka can be just as successful. Sloe wine, which tends to be rather dry, is perfect for the red wine base when making spiced Christmas punch recipes. Indeed, dyed sloe leaves masquerading as East India tea has not been the only fraudulent use associated with this tree. In the late nineteenth century, *Brook's Herbal* tells us: "The juice of the sloe is much used by fraudulent wine merchants in adulterating port wine, for which purpose it is well adapted on account of its astringency, slight acidity, and deep red colour" …"It has been stated, that there is more port wine [so called] drunk in England alone, than is manufactured in Portugal". (p.148).[1]

My personal uses of the blackthorn have included both fruits and the bark as dyes, the unripe fruit juice as a linen marker and the ripe fruit juice and bark for making ink. The experiment with the unripe fruit juice happened because I found reference to it being used as an indelible marker on linen and was intrigued. Having tried it out, the difficulty of obtaining juice from an unripe fruit ensured it did not happen again. A friend has carved me a spoon out of blackthorn wood which shows the grain beautifully.

Legends and Folklore. Folklore declares that bringing white flowers into the house is unlucky. The blackthorn carries this warning in company with plants from snowdrops to hawthorn. Bringing them in, it has been thought, may foretell, or even result in death. I remember my own grandmother being very upset if anyone tried to bring white flowers into the house.

An old belief was that the magic of the hawthorn could undo the bad forces of the blackthorn. Fancy, twisted shapes on blackthorn walking sticks have long been popular. One was also given a ceremonial role as the badge of office of the mayor in Sandwich, Kent. This was reported by Vickery to be recorded from as early as 1301, and still to have been a part of the mayor making ceremony, passed from the retiring mayor to his successor in 1994. The blackthorn stick or wand was to keep evil away.[5]

Notes

1. Brook R. *Brook's Family Herbal*. (J.A. Brook, Richardson & Co. London. Revised edition. 1876). 148.
2. Rackham O. *The History of the Countryside*. (Phoenix Paperback. 1986). 184.
3. Green T. *Universal Herbal or Botanical Dictionary*. 2 vols, (Caxton, London. 2nd edition. 1824). Vol. 2. 416.
4. De Bairacli-Levy J. *The Illustrated Herbal Handbook for Everyone*. (Faber and Faber. London. 1991). 151.
5. Vickery R. *Oxford Dictionary of Plant-Lore*. (Oxford University Press. 1997). 37/8.

BLACKTHORN – History of Medicinal Use

Sloe is a native tree with a long history, stretching far back into interglacial periods. There are early finds of charcoal from cooking fires of sloe wood and finds of fruit stones indicate use either for food or possibly dyeing. The evidence of a wheelbarrow full of the stones found at the Iron Age Glastonbury Lake Village site could suggest either, or medicinal use.[1]

The earliest actual recipes come from the *Lacnunga* and other Anglo-Saxon Leechbooks. Then the astringency of the bark of the trunk or root of the tree was exploited in washes and poultices. Tannin rich herbs are indeed very protective and helpful in the case of an open, tender area of flesh. In a wash or ointment they can lay a film over the area to keep bacteria out, stop bleeding and discharges, and encourage healing. One complex recipe in *Bald's Leechbook* is particularly interesting as it is listed for palsy and may describe treatment for a stroke victim.[2]

In the twelfth century Hildegard of Bingen takes up the aspect of blackthorn against parasites. This time specified as "crabs" [genital lice]. (p.132).[3] The blackthorn and wild plum trees are closely related. The kernels of both contain hydrocyanic acid, which gives us good reason to think this recipe could well have been effective.

Over a period of 200 years, we find references to the interesting use of sloe juice in providing a substitute for the expensive juice of the Acacia from Egypt. This substitution was possible due to the astringency of the sloe, which made it valued for stopping all manner of discharges, from diarrhoea to excessive menstrual bleeding. William Coles records this use but states a personal preference for sumacs as the substitute. He then gives us a much wider picture of various preparations from

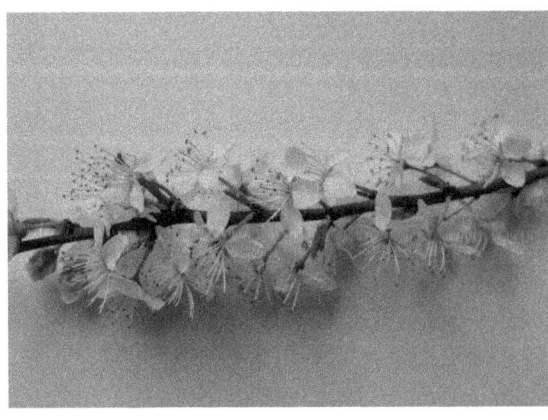

Blackthorn blossom.

blackthorn. He writes that the conserve is very much of use for pains in the sides, bowels and guts. Coles prescribes the distilled water of the flowers to ease griping pains, or pounded sloes with new ale, this, "helpeth the pain of the breast, and the decoction of the Bark in water being drunk, is good against pissing in Bed. The Bark boyled in water till it be black and thick with Rye meal and Honey added thereunto, is available to consume the dead flesh" (p.20).[4] He adds that "it cureth the Cankers". He gives us lotions prepared from the leaves for gargles or a mouthwash, which it has been suggested might also be helpful as an eyewash.[4]

Miller in 1722 and Quincy in his *A Complete Dispensatory* twenty years later, both record the practice of reducing the unripe sloe fruit juice until it resembled the Egyptian *Acacia germanica.* It was sold in the apothecary shops at this time as a cheaper substitute, a common theme with the produce from this tree it seems. Miller goes so far in his botanic herbal to give the name *Acacia Germanica* beside *Pruna sylvestra,* the sloe. The true *Acacia germanica officinalis* Miller writes is put into all the great compositions, being dark on the outside and "reddish within" (p.360).[5]

In 1746, a *Collection of Recipes for cookery and Physick* was published. One recipe is for blackthorn bark with red rose petals, boiled until reduced to one third in diluted claret wine. This decoction made an astringent base for the added orange peel, scurvy-grass and powdered myrrh, which complete the mouthwash. The desired effect of regular use was to fasten loose teeth in scurvy.[6]

At the end of the century, the surgeon William Meyrick in his herbal quotes the more renowned William Withering on the use of powdered bark in curing "some agues" or fevers. The tea of the flowers, he writes, "is a safe and easy purge".(p.421).[7] Use of the boiled down conserve of the juice as *Acacia Germanica* continued into the nineteenth century. In 1822 William Waller reports that it is, however, seldom used in medicine. Although he lists the leaves, bark and fruits all as astringent and cooling, he has serious reservations about using them, because of their acidity. He recommends only the fruit juice, or a decoction of leaves and bark to stop nosebleeds.[8]

Summary. From the earliest recipes in the Anglo-Saxon period onwards, it is ever the astringency of the sloe flowers, leaves, bark or fruits that is appreciated. All parts of the tree, even including the kernels within the fruits have been used. The practice of boiling down sloe fruit juice to make a thick, sharp tasting conserve, which kept all year, brought most interest in the tree. This became a well-known and frequently included constituent in popular preparations in the apothecary shops for 200 years. It replaced the juice of *Acacia germanica*, which came from Egypt and was therefore expensive.

While the conserve of sloes treated griping pains in the bowel, decoctions of the bark were recommended to stop incontinence, or prepared in a much stronger recipe with rye meal and honey to eat away dead flesh. A gentle distilled water of the flowers also eased pains, and lotions were prepared from the leaves. Mouth and eyewashes took advantage of the astringency of the herb. The popularity of the blackthorn wanes as the nineteenth century progresses and less tart remedies are preferred. See Herbalists' Reference for more modern uses, including for skin problems.

Recipe

Extracted from Thornton's Family Herbal 1810. "Conserva Pruni Sylvestris. Put the sloes in water upon the fire, that they may soften, taking care that they be not broken; then take them out of the water, press out the pulp, and mix it with three times its weight of double refined sugar into a conserve.

The preparation is a gentle astringent, and may be given as such in the dose of two or three drachms. It is used also for a gargle with considerable advantage, especially where the uvula is found to be relaxed" (p.483).[9]

Comment from *Quincy's English Dispensatory*—"We have in the Shops a Conserve made with them; which with care is a very good one. For this purpose they are to be gather'd before they begin to wither and mellow upon the Trees; for after they are frost-bit, as the Country People call it, and made fit for eating, they are not so rough; and consequently not so suitable for this Intention in Medicine" (p.101).[10]

Notes

1. Coles J. & Minitt S. *Industrious and Fairly Civilized.* (Somerset Levels Project. 1995). 193.
2. Pollington S. *Leechcraft.* (Anglo Saxon Books. 2000). 399. (*Bald* 47),
3. Throop P. (trans), *Hildegard von Bingen's Physica.* (Healing Arts Press. 1998). 131.
4. Coles W. *The Paradise of Plants.* (London. 1657). 20.
5. Miller J. *Botanicum officinale.* Bell. (London. 1722). 360.
6. Anon. *A Collection of Receipts.* (Printed for the Executrix of Mary Kettilby. 1746). 149.
7. Meyrick W. *The New Family Herbal.* (Birmingham. 1790). 421.
8. Waller J. *Waller's New British Domestic Herbal.* Cox & Son. (London. 1822). 319.
9. Thornton R.J. *A New Family Herbal.* (London. 1810). 483.
10. Quincy J. MD. A Complete Dispensatory. (10th edition. 1736). 101.

PRUNUS SPINOSA – Herbalists' Reference

The Parts of Blackthorn Used for Medicine – The newly opened flowers, leaves and bark are gathered in spring. Unripe fruit should be gathered in late summer.

Dosage and Forms – Tea of flowers, one to two cups daily, dose one to two teaspoons per cup. Tea of dried fruits is made as for the flowers. Syrup of the flowers may be given. Decoction of bark—add one tablespoon of fine bark shavings to 0.25 litre (1/2 pint) of cold water. Bring to the boil, simmer five minutes, then leave steeping for four hours, sweeten with honey, dose one tablespoon three times daily before meals. Medicinal wine, dose a glass in the evening. Sloe gin—fifteen to twenty ml, at night as necessary.

Constituents – The flowers and seeds contain cyanogenic glycosides, as in hawthorn. Tannins, flavonoids, essential oil, and amygdalin in the kernel.

Actions and Uses – The astringent leaves, bark and fruits are given to relieve constipation, colic, dysmenorrhoea and menorrhagia. They may reduce or stop bleeding and discharges. The bark has been given as a febrifuge. The flower syrup is expectorant, and in larger doses, laxative. The flowers are diuretic and depurative making them suitable as a tea for treating eruptive skin conditions. They have been traditionally associated with treating teenage acne in particular. The bark is antispasmodic, astringent, and sedative. It may be given in nervous disorders. Preparations of the flowers may be helpful for a range of conditions from colds to bladder problems. Marmalade may be made from the fruits, as a remedy for dyspepsia.[1] The fruits are

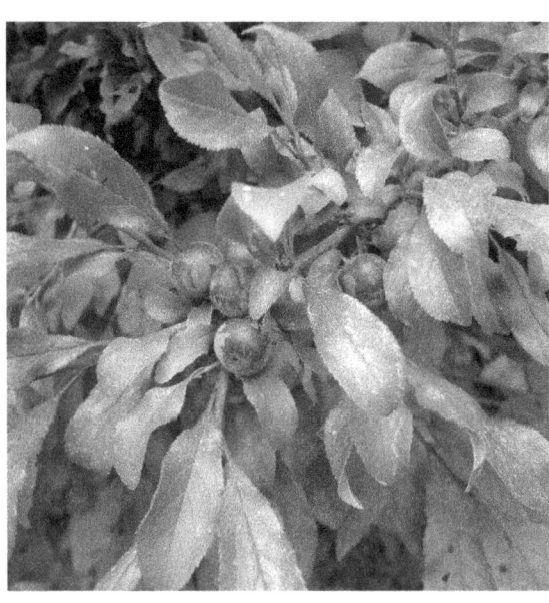
Ripe sloes.

astringent from their tannins and soothe mucous membrane inflammation in mouthwashes and gargles. Blackthorn flowers are active against intestinal worms.[2] Sloe wine can be taken as a laxative and to encourage sweating.

Topical Application – Tea of the flowers and leaves, or a decoction of the bark, has been suggested in the past as a healing wash for wounds.

Contraindications and Precautions – Breast feeding. Blackthorn is not for long term use. Do not exceed recommended dose.[3]

Notes

1. Kelly W.J. (ed. director). *Nursing Herbal Medicine Handbook.* (Springhouse Corporation. 2001). 66/7.
2. De Bairacli-Levy J. *The Illustrated Herbal Handbook for Everyone.* (Faber and Faber. London. 1991). 151.
3. Duke J.A. *Handbook of Medicinal Herbs* (CRC Press LLC. 2nd edition. 2002). 676.

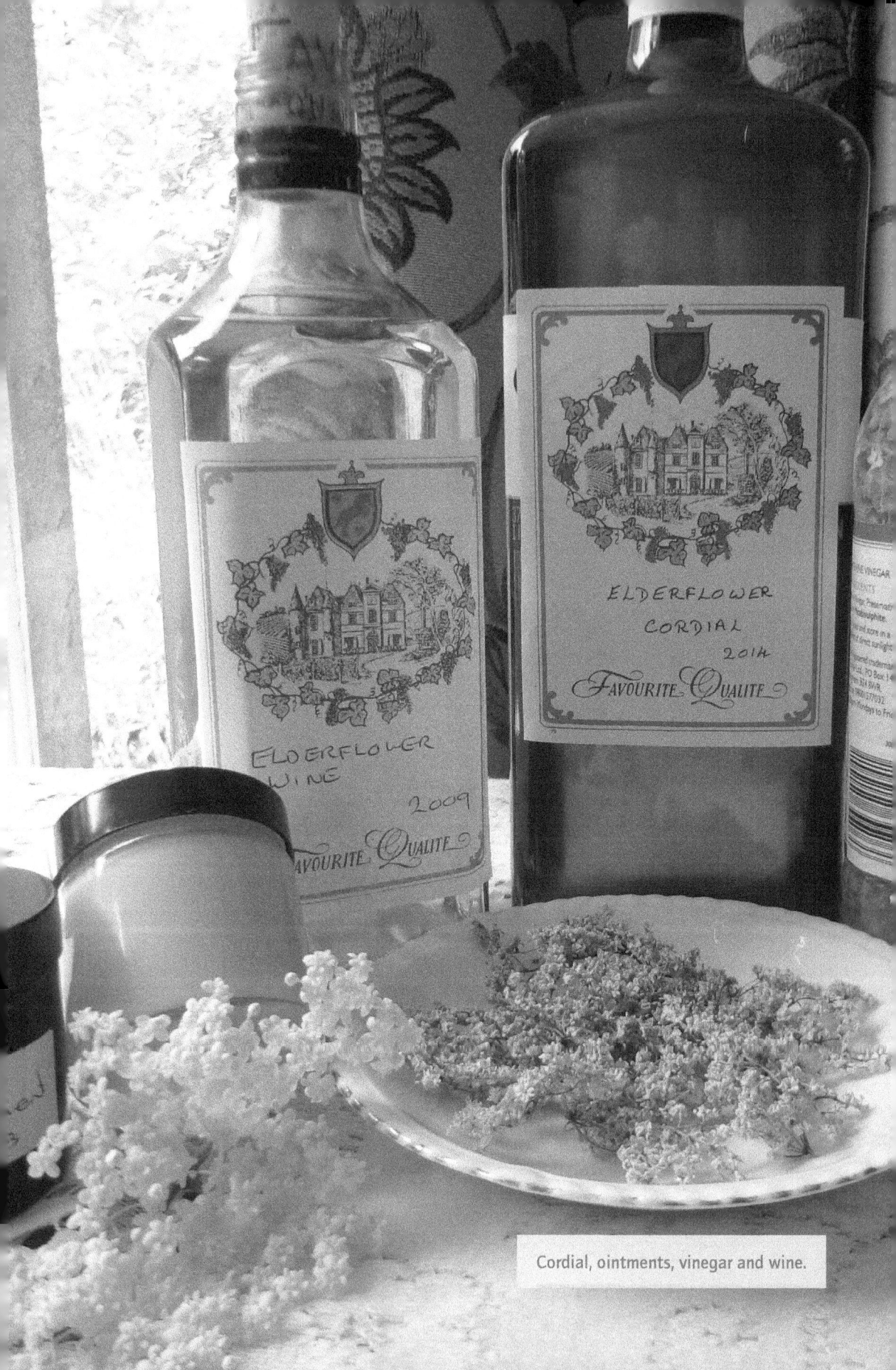

Cordial, ointments, vinegar and wine.

Elderflower

Sambucus nigra – Elderflower – Caprifoliaceae

ELDERFLOWER – Usefulness – The flowers have a place in cookery. They are valued in herbal medicine. Elderflowers can be made into wine and cordials. They have cosmetic uses. They also give an impressive gold dye on silk.

Dangers – The flowers are rich in pollen, however elderflower tea is used to treat hay fever and so the treatment is always at hand.

Getting to Know the Elder Tree – In my childhood I played beneath an elder tree in the garden of a friend. The heavy scent of elder has been part of my experience ever since and so I feel I have always been close to the tree. It has a very distinct character, which came to me most strongly when I first harvested the inner bark of a branch from a tree in my garden. I found it an intense experience to slip my hand inside the incision, opening the branch to part the bark from the wood. This must be done in spring when the sap is thin and both layers are slippery against your fingers. Every other tree I have opened for bark has simply smelled to me of cucumber. The elder gave out its own unmistakeable odour, a powerful marker of identity.

The elder has been variously described as a tree or shrub of the under-storey in woodlands, as it does not usually grow to any great height. However, when we moved into a large Victorian house, a very old elder in the front garden had reached up to the high guttering. The tallest elders can be fifteen metres (forty-nine feet), making it an impressive tree. In that garden, as in the previous one, I grew common elders, the very pretty purple elder with pink-tinged flowers and the variegated leafed elder. The flowers from each are good in cookery. There are several more varieties, but only the common elder is used in medicine.

The young leaves are soothing and cooling when included in cosmetic and medicinal creams, lotions and ointments, and when decocted they can provide an insecticidal liquor. Bunches of the leaves used to be tied to the bridles on horses to keep flies away. The *Booke of Secrets* 1588 mentions them specifically against flies.[1] The leaves are not for internal use. In the garden elder leaves put down into mole tunnels may discourage them, elder leaf tea can be used cold to water plants against greenfly and the flowers may be sprinkled amongst green vegetable leaves such as lettuces and cabbages to discourage caterpillars.

As with many white flowers, they are difficult to dry to perfection and should be laid out on muslin or on a hanging net herb dryer with a good free-flow of air around them in a steady, fairly low temperature. Sunlight should be excluded from the area. They can also be frozen on the umbels in freezer bags, for use later to be cooked with gooseberries or other fruits. Putting the flowers into white wine vinegar, filling the bottle and leaving it to stand without added heat or sun for four days will produce fragrant and tasty vinegar. Once strained, it can be used in salad dressings. When it is made in cider vinegar this preparation will be suitable for cosmetic use or to take as a home remedy for hay fever. Elderflower vinegar has been popular for centuries.

The profusion of delicate flowers has always tempted me to make many recipes, although I am ever careful to leave two thirds of the flowers on the branches; one third to become berries and be picked later, leaving another third on the upper branches for the birds. I have only once seen birds eating the flowers. This was a very unwelcome sight in my garden as a pigeon stripped whole branches of leaves and umbels. She was producing milk for feeding her babies at the time and I wondered whether the elder provided a constituent she instinctively knew her young needed. Pigeons are one of only three birds which produce milk for their young. It has not happened again, despite the pigeons nesting in the elder itself the following season.

My harvesting is more careful. The best umbels are plucked from the tree, with all the florets on the umbel open and perfect. Those that look right from below but when cut have some flowers that have passed their best, or have too many buds, I put into my dye pan for dyeing silk. With a mordant of alum the golden colour is fast and beautiful. Examining the umbels I never cease to marvel at the delicate beauty of the flowers that appear as if crafted from white china, their golden tipped stamens yielding pollen. They can be used to make an excellent ointment; a home remedy for the grazes suffered when picking gooseberries and may be equally helpful with itchy skin conditions, such as eczema. I have known this to provide great relief for animals too. In the First World War an appeal was launched for elderflowers to be made into ointment for the horses at the fighting front.[2]

Elderflowers have been used in the past to thicken sauces and are found in Anglo-Saxon and Anglo-Norman cookery recipes. In order to render the flowers easier to remove from the umbels, leave them in a bowl in the fridge overnight and then they will fall away readily. Elderflowers were made into a sugar conserve in the seventeenth century, using a half volume of flowers to sugar and beating or grinding them together. Dried in a just-warm oven or the sun this conserve can be kept in sealed jars to use in cookery, as well as for medicine. The flavour of elderflowers is sufficiently strong for it to be enough to add a little of the sugar for flavour to a jam, or even to place a bunch of the flowers in the jam for a minute or two at the end of cooking as it cools slightly before pouring into jars.

Early summer is always accompanied in my kitchen by a large bowl filled with elderflowers and lemon slices steeping in the sweetened liquor, to make elderflower cordial. Elderflower champagne has provided family anecdotes of fun and disasters, even exploding the thick glass of used cider bottles resulting in sticky liquid pouring down behind the freezer or into the cupboard under the stairs. This is always a danger in years when the natural yeasts are particularly lively. Elderflower wine is likely to have been made for several hundred years, a recipe in a published collection of the eighteenth century is for twelve gallons, a fact that supports its popularity.[3] Reference is made in several books to elderflower wine as Frontiniac or Frontignan, which also contained gooseberries.[4] I have tried numerous combinations of elderflowers and fruits in wines. Elderflower and kiwi has been the favourite. Elderflower beer has also been popular since the seventeenth century.[5]

Elderflowers have been distilled to produce elderflower aromatic water for centuries. As early as 1603, washing with water distilled from elder leaves in May was recommended to take away freckles.[6] The water remains a valued ingredient in recipes for cleansing lotions and softening creams for the skin and eye lotions. In the past, elder milk for the skin and elder oil for the hair have been made commercially.[7] The many elderflower recipes gave the tree the title of "cosmetic tree of the countryside".

Legends and Folklore. Few trees have attracted more legends than the elder. Many, however, refer to the berries, which will be described with their uses in the Summer section of this book. The belief that it is unlucky to cut down an elder tree still survives and may have begun in early times when the elder was worshipped and it was believed that Freya the Scandinavian goddess lived in the tree.

Protective amulets have been popular in the past. The *Anatomy of the Elder Tree* gives us instructions for making a "singular Amulet" from the elder growing on a Sallow (p.52).[8] This is to be done in October, a little before full moon. A twig of the elder must be cut between two of its knots into nine pieces, which are to be bound in a linen cloth and hung by a thread around the neck so that they lie over the heart. Another length of linen is then tied around the body to hold it in place. It is left until the thread breaks and then taken without touching it with bare hands and buried to ensure no-one else touches it.

Notes

1. Warde W. & Anglosse R. (trans), *The Secretes of Maister Alexis of Piemont.* (Atenar. 2000). 81.
2. Teetgen A.B. *Profitable Herb-Growing and Collecting.* (London. 1916). 170.

3. Anon. *A Collection of Receipts.* (Printed for the Executrix of Mary Kettilby. 1746). 93.
4. Smith E. *The Compleat Housewife.* (London. 1739). 227.
5. Buhner S.H. *Sacred and Herbal Healing Beers.* (Siris Books. 1998). 330.
6. Plat. Sir H. *Delights for Ladies.* (1609). (Crosby Lockwood.1948). 95.
7. Piesse S.G. W. *The Art of Perfumery.* (1855). (Echo Library. 2007). 18.
8. Blochwich M. M.D. *Anatomy of the Elder Tree.* (London. 1677). 52/3.

ELDERFLOWER – History of Medicinal Use

Elder is a common tree in Britain, the only exception being the northern-most Scottish isles. Archaeological finds of elder seeds, wood, and charcoal leave no doubt it is native, and the common association with human settlements is not surprising. The elder thrives on phosphate-rich soil, which is provided by bones from domestic rubbish heaps and buried bodies. As time passed, people are also likely to have encouraged elder nearby as it is a source of food. Finds were so common on Roman sites that it has been presumed the berries were eaten regularly.

In the Anglo-Saxon period the elder has numerous mentions in the Leechdoms, providing food and possibly wine. Medicinal uses throughout written history involve several parts of the tree. Medieval recipes include juice taken from the middle rind, or other parts of the tree, such as the leaves. Leaves and flowers might be used together, although to have the leaves at their best, flowering time is quite late. A manuscript of the fourteenth century (Harleian, 2378)[1] contains many herbal recipes for treating a wide variety of conditions. These include the anaesthetic drink called dwale containing very powerful herbs. One of the recipes includes the middle bark of elder prepared in wine with numerous other herbs, to treat dropsy. These can be found in Henslow, *Medical Works of the Fourteenth Century*.[1]

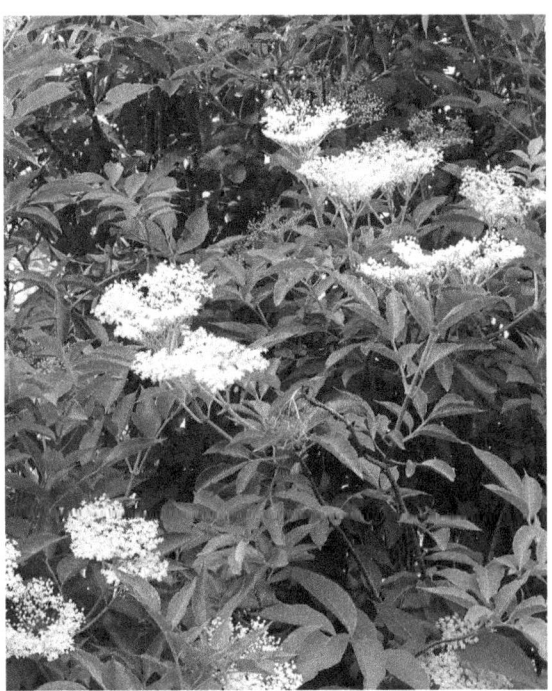

Elderflowers ready for harvest.

Culpeper set the elder under the dominion of Venus. He recommended gathering the leaves and flowers to be distilled in May, and using this water to wash ulcers and sores on the legs. His instructions include waters as an eye-wash for bloodshot eyes and to give a morning and evening hand-wash to help palsy and trembling hands.[2]

Coles repeats using elder to treat dropsy, gives the juice of the green leaves as anti-inflammatory for the eyes, and recommends the boiled leaves mixed with barley meal for applying to inflammations, burns, scalds, and fistulous ulcers. Also, the pounded leaves boiled with the tallow of a bull or goat was then laid onto the part affected, to ease pain in gout. In complete opposition to Hildegard centuries before, he writes with enthusiasm of the many diseases cured by the elder and states that he considers no part of the tree to be without medicinal use. He lists the leaves, berries, seeds, roots, bark, flowers, young shoots, and pith for medicine. Finally, he records the wood for making skewers for meat.[3]

In 1677, a newly published book written by Dr. Martin Blochwich, was recommended by the Royal Society. This details the uses and possible forms of medicine of every part of the tree, as well as "Specifick Remedies for most and chiefest Maladies".[4] It includes a conserve of the flowers with sugar, syrup, and honey of the flowers, the distilled water, and spirit, oil, vinegar, and oxymel. In the oxymel, honey, elderflower vinegar, and elderflower aromatic water are heated together.

The buds of the elder leaves were also to be powdered and kept alone or mixed with sugar over a slow fire. The juice from the buds was made into syrup with sugar, cinnamon and cloves. Distilled waters were prepared of the leaves and occasionally of the roots and pith of the tree. Syrup was also made of the juice of the middle bark, or roots. This was considered kinder to the stomach than the fresh juice, although slightly less cathartic.

Oil and liniments of the bark were made either from the bark and leaves together or green bark alone. Lastly, the salt was prepared from the flowers and leaves using the remaining solids left in the still after distillation, or solids left after the juice had been pressed from the leaves.[4]

In 1694, John Pechey refers to some of the recipes mentioned above and writes "Vinegar, wherein the Flowers have been infus'd, is very agreeable to the Stomach, and excites Appetite.." (p.72).[5] He quotes his father making an ointment for burns.[5] In the following century, a collections of recipes contain some for piles using elder flowers and buds with pilewort in suppositories and the rind in a laxative glister.

The leaves and buds are ingredients in ointments. The use of the leaves and flowers as anti-inflammatory applications continues, and the leaves are described as an excellent, cooling emollient by Meyrick.

By 1810, due to the strongly purgative properties of young leaf buds the green bark in wine was preferred. The distilled water, tea, wine, tincture, or ointment of the flowers comes highly recommended by Robert Thornton.[6]

Summary. The elder has been associated with human settlements from the earliest times and no doubt served well providing both food and medicine. Harvests may have also been used as ingredients for early cosmetic recipes. There are numerous mentions in the Anglo-Saxon Leechbooks. Juice of the inner bark was used in addition to the more obvious parts of the tree in the fourteenth and fifteenth centuries. William Coles echoed Culpeper's enthusiasm for the anti-inflammatory and healing properties of elder leaves for burns, ulcers and painful conditions. However, *The Anatomy of the Elder* published in 1677 provided the ultimate guide to use of all parts of the tree in every conceivable preparation.[4] Although the use of the leaf buds was discontinued in the nineteenth century,[6] the elder remains respected in herbal medicine.

Recipes

Extracted from Anatomy of the Elder. 1677. "The *Oximel* of the Elder, which *Quercetan. in Pharm. Dogm. restit. lib. 1.c.*10. mentioneth is thus prepared. *Take of Honey scummed well* lib. 1. *Of Elder Vinegar* lib. 5. *Of Simple water, or water of Elder Flowers* lib.1. Being mixt, put them in a Cucurbit, and let them be boyled in Balneo to a fit consistence. You may use here the simple Vinegar, either of the flowers, or that which is by the infusion of the berries of a purple die, as it shall please the phancy of the Physician or his Patient." (p.22).[4]

N.B. "lib." stands for pound weight. "in Balneo" means in a water bath.

Extracted from Anatomy of the Elder. 1677. "*The SYRUP and HONEY.* Take of the recent Flowers *lib.*1. let them macerate 12 hours in *lib.*6. of warm fountain water; having exprest and strained the liquor, put in again recent flowers, yea do it the third time. Add four ounces of the whitest Sugar to each five ounces of the liquor that is last strained, boyle them up to a Syrup according to art.

But if in place of the Sugar you add the same quantity of Honey and boyle it to a fitting consistence, you have *Mel Sambucinum*, which is commended by some." (pp.18/19).[4]

Notes

1. Henslow G. Rev. Prof. M.A. *Medical Works of the Fourteenth Century*. (Burt Franklin. New York. 1972). 92.
2. Culpeper N. *Culpeper's Complete Herbal and English Physician enlarged*. (1652). (London. 1815 edition). 68.
3. Coles W. *The Paradise of Plants*. (London. 1657). 296.
4. Blochwich M. M.D. *Anatomy of the Elder Tree*. (London. 1677). 18–33.
5. Pechey J. *The English Herbal of Physical Plants*. (London. 1694). 72.
6. Thornton R.J. *A New Family Herbal*. (London. 1810). 324–6.

SAMBUCUS NIGRA – Herbalists' Reference

The Parts of the Elder Tree Used for Medicine – Flowers, leaves, bark. (For uses of the berries see Elder in Summer).

Dosage and Forms – Tea—one to two teaspoons of flowers per cup of boiling water, infuse for five minutes. Fluid extract in 25% alcohol 2–4ml three times daily. Tincture of 1:2, 15–40ml per week.

Constituents – The flowers contain triterpenes and free sterols. The flavonoids include rutin, kaempferol, and quercetin. Phenolic acids are also present. The leaves contain triterpenes as in the flowers, cyanogenic glycosides, flavonoids, and tannins. The bark contains phytohaemagglutinins.

Actions and Uses – The flowers are diaphoretic and warming, possibly from the flavonoids and phenolic acids. This action is much used for colds and fevers. The flavonoids and triterpenes appear to be the main active ingredients also in providing some anti-viral action, which offers pertinent treatment for influenza. The diaphoresis is produced by drinking the hot infusion. A cold infusion works more strongly as a diuretic and depurative against skin eruptions and infections, or liver disorders.

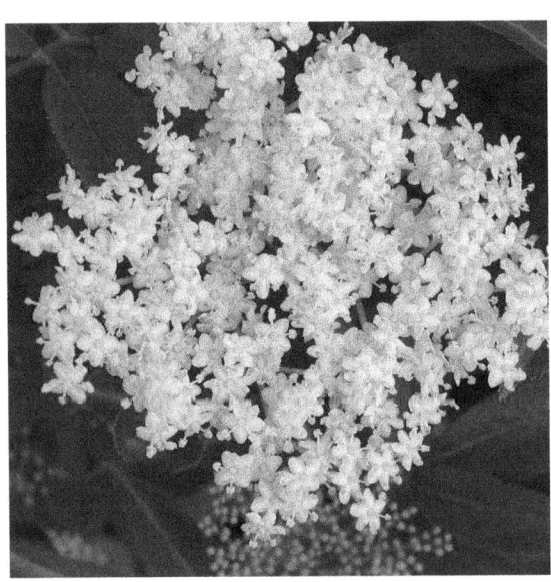
Elder florets at their best.

Elderflower tea may be made from the fresh flowers, using the pollen to treat hay fever and allergic rhinitis, and fresh or dried flowers in blended teas for asthma. The bark has been used, but is better limited to external application.[1]

Combinations – The flowers are anti-catarrhal and regularly teamed with *Plantago lanceolata* and *Euphrasia* to treat hay fever. A further herbal combination for sinusitis could be with *Solidago virgurea*, adding *Glechoma hederacea* if the ears were affected.

Topical Application – The flowers and/or leaves can be applied as compresses, or used as ingredients in creams, lotions and ointments to cool and soothe allergic reactions, skin conditions such as eczema and psoriasis, eruptive rashes, burns, or sprains. The distilled Aromatic Water of elderflower can be used as eyewash. Soaked pads of cotton wool are laid on the eyelids while resting lying down for fifteen minutes, for eyestrain and inflammation from hay fever.

Contraindications and Precautions – None are known for external use of the leaves. Caution would be required for use of the inner bark, which is for external use only.[1] No contraindications are needed for the flowers on present evidence.[2]

Notes

1. Barker J. *The Medicinal Flora of Britain and Northwestern Europe.* (Winter Press. 2001). (375).
2. Mills S. & Bone K. *The Essential Guide to Herbal Safety.* (Elsevier Churchill Livingstone. 2005). 376.

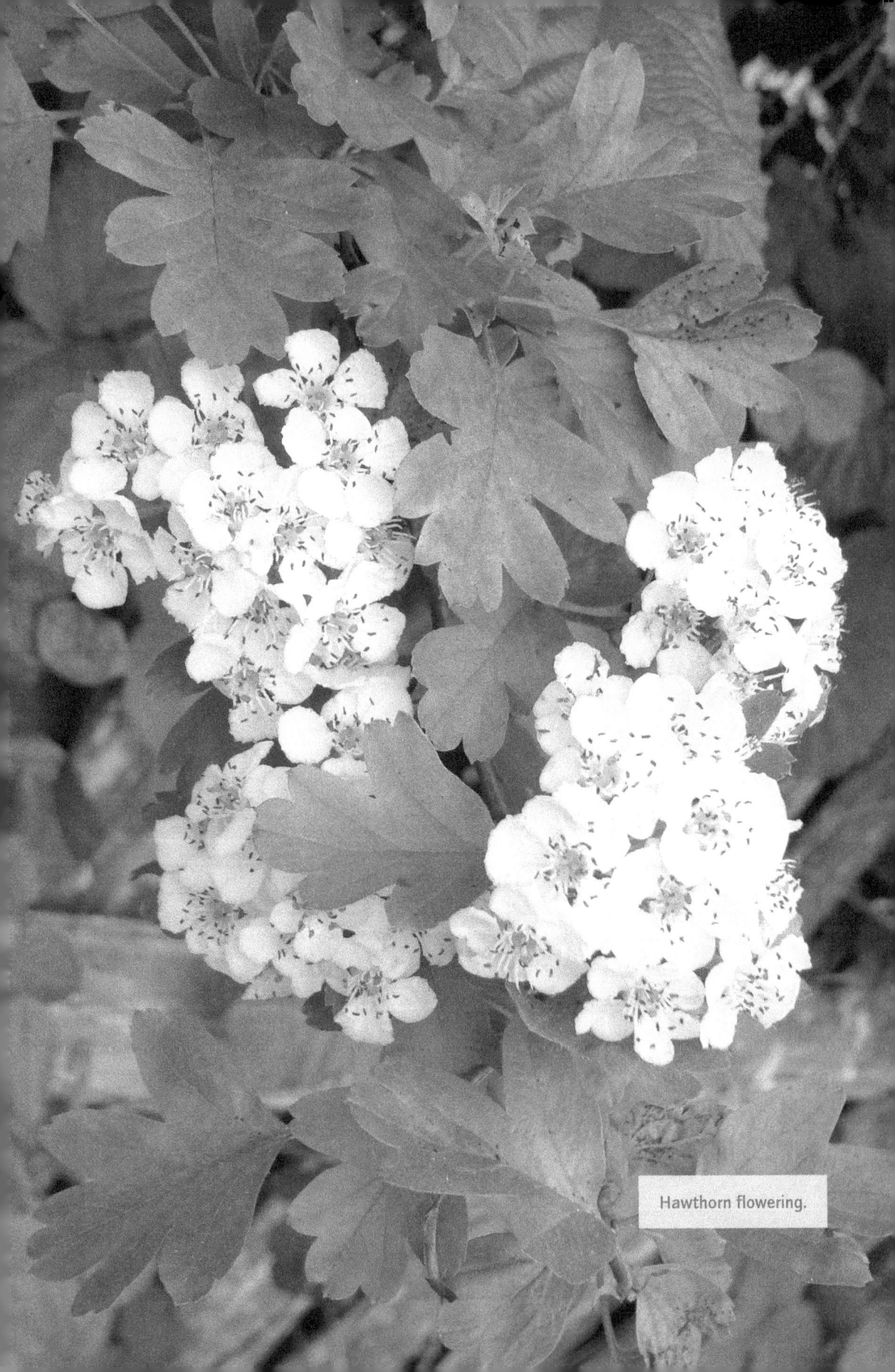
Hawthorn flowering.

Hawthorn

Crataegus oxyacantha, C. monogyna – Hawthorn – Rosaceae

HAWTHORN – Usefulness – The tree provides nutritious fruits for autumn preserves of jams, jellies, ketchup and wines. The flowers, leaves, and fruits are supportive to the heart and circulation in herbal medicine. The young trees can be trained into a thick hedge, valued as an ornamental yet effective thorny barrier, which supports wildlife. The root wood can be turned to make elegant and useful objects. The wood of the trunk can also be turned or used as a source of charcoal, as it burns fiercely. Flowering branches make attractive Easter wreaths. Both the flowers and wood provide dyes.[1] Medlars and pears are grafted onto a hawthorn stock.

Dangers – Thorns on the hawthorn are sharp and should be removed quickly if they pierce the skin.

Getting to Know the hawthorn Tree – The common hawthorn, native to Britain, is the *Crataegus oxyacantha*, also named *C. monogyna* as it has only one seed within the berry. This tree grows throughout Europe as far as Afghanistan and has leaves with deep-cut lobes. *Crataegus laevigata*, also known as the midland hawthorn, is widespread in western and central Europe but is not as common in Britain. It prefers heavier soils and shady woodland, and the leaves are not as conspicuously lobed as those of the common hawthorn. *C. laevigata* has two seeds within the fruit. A variety of *laevigata*, "Paul's scarlet" has the beautiful deep pink may blossom and is grown as an ornamental tree.[2] Although it is an important medicinal herb today, in the past the ornamental possibilities seem to have gained more attention. In the eighteenth century double-flowering hawthorns were for sale at one shilling each.[3] In the ornamental gardens at Hatfield House where Princess Elizabeth later to be Elizabeth I spent much of her childhood, an occasional hawthorn has been allowed to grow above the hedge and trimmed as a standard to stunning effect. The common hawthorn hybridises readily with other *Crataegus* species, heights varying between ten to fifteen metres (thirty to forty-nine feet). While Miller, in his *Gardener's Dictionary* of 1771, gives us ten species of hawthorn, Green, writing in 1824, names twenty-three.

The often rounded, red, false fruits are an important food for birds and it is a real treat to see a flock of field fares descend on a tree in late autumn. The naturalist Gilbert White, who recorded all manner of nature around him in the eighteenth century in Hampshire, quoted John Ray's description of great flocks of German silk-tails appearing in England, feeding on haws in the winter of 1685.[4] These birds are known to us as waxwings, appearing unpredictably and are worth watching out for. One is illustrated in the Autumn section with the rowan. Perhaps because it is so popular with birds, hawthorn is a frequent host for mistletoe. Voles and mice also eat haws, but a small thorny branch can be used to deter moles by placing it in their tunnel. The tree provides food for numerous species of moths, including the Lappet Moth which has a distinctive snout and wings which resemble folded brown leaves. One moth—the *Scythropia crataegella* takes its name from the source of its food, the hawthorn tree. In addition to moths, the hawthorn shield bug (*Acanthosoma haemorrhoidale*) feeds mostly on the leaves and berries.[2]

Since planting the hedge for our first house, I have continued to choose hawthorn. It has been found and recommended as a hedging plant throughout British history with good reason. Not only does it quickly become a strong, thorny barrier, but this thorny thicket soon recommends it to nesting birds. If you are fortunate, thrushes may move in. In the garden the blossom gives valuable food for the hoverflies early in the year. The hawthorn tree in my Hampshire garden soon grew to over four and a half metres (fifteen feet) tall. It was the end bush of a line of hedging and gave harvests of flowers and fruits for many years. Early in the year the newly opened leaves may be picked and eaten as a garnish with salads. They have a delicious, nutty flavour which is short-lived however. I look upon this as an annual treat to enjoy for the few days before the tree starts producing more tannin to protect the foliage. Once this happens they become too bitter for human food.

Hawthorn has dual aspects. On one hand it has been beloved as the blossom is associated with May Day celebrations and bringing in summer. Unlike the blackthorn, hawthorn has a reputation for flowering just before a spell of really warm weather. On the other hand, as a white flower it has been shunned as an indoor decoration, signalling death. The smell of the flowers is not always pleasant and has been likened to the smell of plague and death in the past. This is produced by the content of trimethylamine in the flowers. It does not stop them giving a pleasant flavour and mild, pleasant scent when used in recipes. The flowers are dried for medicine together with the young leaves. They may alternatively be made into a white medium dry wine, or can be steeped in brandy to add flavour in cakes. At woodland herb workshops, I have supervised making hawthorn flower syrup as a useful country preserve, which has become almost forgotten. This can be appreciated in drinks, to flavour ice cream or desserts. On medieval workshops days, it has been a pleasure to add ground hawthorn flowers to flavour puddings made with almond milk and ground rice.

The five small, white petals cup the golden nectar, ready for the eager bees, within a circle of red-tipped stamens. When the blossom is more mature it becomes suitable for dyeing silk, but requires a long period of boiling for good colour. A decoction of the bark can also produce a yellow dye and more importantly, together with iron has been used in the Highlands in the eighteenth century to give a black dye[5] Later in the year, the abundance of the attractive fruits has given rise to many descriptive local names for the tree, such as cuckoo beads, pig-berry and pixie pears. I prefer the Anglo-Saxon name of hart bramble.

In autumn I enjoy making haw, crab apple and rosemary jelly, as a food medicine for the heart and circulation. Haws go together well with other hedgerow fruits in preserves also. Wine of the berries can be so packed with natural yeast that it overflows the demi-john and using

Campden tablets to kill the natural yeast before adding bakers or wine yeast can be wise in some years. The resulting wine has been a favourite in my family as it is similar to a good sherry, with a rich colour.

Legends and Folklore. The saying "Ne'er cast a clout till May be out" refers to waiting for May blossom before setting aside winter clothes. With the strong associations of May Day and the Green Man, it is not surprising that hawthorn was also linked in love allegories with carnal rather than spiritual love. On May Day in Ireland, whitethorn (hawthorn) was sprinkled with holy water and set in the fields to stop fairies stealing the crops.[6] The legendary Glastonbury thorn, is supposedly a descendant of the staff planted there by Joseph of Arimathea who had been sent by the apostle, Phillip, with a group of disciples to the island of the Britons. It was believed that the wooden staff was cut from the same tree as the crown of thorns. Joseph of Arimathea had supervised the burial of Jesus. The Glastonbury thorn traditionally flowers twice, at Christmas and again at Easter. Culpeper wrote that other hawthorn trees in the midlands also flowered at those times.[7]

Notes

1. Green T. *Universal Herbal or Botanical Dictionary.* 2 vols, (Caxton, London. 2nd edition. 1824). Vol. 1. 381.
2. Sterry P. *Collins Complete Guide to British Trees.* (Harper Collins. 2007). 234–6.
3. Harvey J. *Early Gardening Catalogues.* (Phillimore & Co. 1972). 31.
4. White G. Rev. M.A. The *Natural History and Antiquities of Selborne.* (1778). (Swan Sonnenschein & Co. 1911). 43.
5. Grierson. S. *The Colour Cauldron.* (Su Grierson. 1986). 116.
6. Vickery R. *Oxford Dictionary of Plant-Lore.* (Oxford University Press. 1997). 170.
7. Culpeper N. *Culpeper's Complete Herbal and English Physician enlarged.* (1652). (London. 1815 edition). 90.

HAWTHORN – History of Medicinal Use

Interglacial and post-glacial records are a testament to the native status of the hawthorn *Crataegus monogyna* in Britain. The large amount of hawthorn charcoal that has been found affirmed that the wood was being gathered in these early times, and it may be presumed that haws were eaten as a food. Francis Pryor reported archaeological evidence of Neolithic hedging with hawthorn from Etton in East Anglia. He believed this to be the earliest discovered at the time, dated to around 3,500BC.[1]

The Anglo-Saxon references in the *Leechbook of Bald* and the *Lacnunga* reveal the early reverence for hawthorn; It has long been associated with the beginning of summer and the Green Man. In the book of *Bald* we find hawthorn with a commonly used trio of magical herbs, lupin, fennel and betony, to guard against the work of the devil.[2]

Culpeper classes the tree as under the dominion of Mars. He tells us something mentioned by Gerard, that the seeds in the berries pounded to a powder and taken in wine are believed to be effective against kidney stones. He adds to this that they may be used to relieve dropsy. This is the earliest mention I have found of a use related to the failing heart. Distilled water of the flowers, meanwhile, is given an astringent use against discharges, or applied with a sponge to draw out splinters. Strained wine in which the cleaned and bruised seed has been boiled he writes is then drunk for "inward tormenting pains" (p.90).[3]

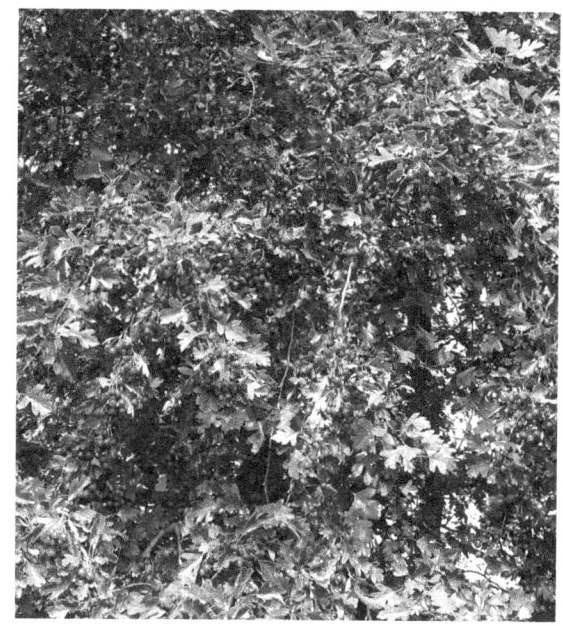

Haws ripe for preserves.

Coles agrees with these uses and adds that if the flowers are steeped in wine for three days and then this is distilled, it is not only used to remove thorns, but also as a "Sovereign Remedy" (p. 367), for pleurisy.[4] As an alternative to the distilled water of the flowers for removing thorns, Coles uses hawthorn bark pounded with red wine and then fried in the grease from a male pig, to be applied hot as a poultice.[4]

In 1722, Miller includes the hawthorn in his herbal and supports the use of flowers and fruits as diuretic, for kidney stone, urinary gravel and pleurisy, mentioned before. Haw, or whitethorn as it was also known, continued to be associated with treatments for kidney or bladder stones.[5] A published collection of recipes from 1746 has no fewer than three hawthorn recipes in which the herb is given to ease the pain caused by these conditions.[6] See recipes.

In the tenth edition of Quincy's English Dispensatory [1736], a guide to dispensing used by apothecaries, we find an interesting comment that may explain the impending reversal of opinion on hawthorn for treating urinary problems. It is recorded that little use is made of hawthorn in medicine, yet haws have a great reputation for treating stone and gravel, and being very diuretic. It goes on "The mighty *nephritic Water*, so much in the good Opinion of the late Dr. *Ratcliffe*, was made from the Flowers.... But whether this will be able to hold its Credit by its own Merit, now its great Promoter is gone, may very much be question'd." (p.164). The recipe for "Nephritick Water" for the kidneys follows, with haw blossom being distilled with nutmeg in sherry and water.[7]

By the end of the eighteenth century the doubts on efficacy expressed in Quincy's Dispensatory had been proven, for hawthorn seems to have fallen out of favour. Herbs for treating the urinary system are many and hawthorn was not, after all, destined to be a lasting herb of choice for treating kidney stones. Sir John Hill states it baldly, writing the flowers and fruit are "good in gravel, and all complaints of that kind; but there are so many better things for the same purpose at hand, that these are not much regarded" (p.163).[8]

Neither Meyrick nor Woodville include hawthorn in their herbals, and the same applies to Thornton and Waller writing in the early nineteenth century. In 1825, Green quotes Hill, also dismissing use of hawthorn in medicine. The *National Botanic Pharmacopoeia* of 1905 published by the National Association of Medical Herbalists did not include hawthorn. It is not until 1916 when war with Germany had cut off the imports of herbs, that a guide for collecting them was published to aid the war effort.

This book lists the gathering of haws amongst other tree herbs, for use as a cardiac tonic.[9] I have not found an identifiable source for this view of hawthorn in England at the turn of the century. Looking to America it appears that Dr. Thomas Reilly, professor of applied therapeutics, had read a paper on hawthorn for treating angina to the American Medical Association in 1909. The physician who first introduced use of hawthorn in this way was Dr. Greene of Ennis, County Clare who gained a high reputation for treating heart disease with a secret recipe. On his death in 1894, his daughter revealed the secret to be tincture of hawthorn. This was subsequently taken up and publicised.[10]

Summary. Before the sixteenth century medicinal use of hawthorn had depended upon its astringency for stopping bleeding and drawing out thorns. In the Anglo-Saxon Leechbooks this was repeated, along with inclusion in recipes against the devil, suggesting an early magical reputation in spell medicine. Hawthorn was not, however, widely used in history.

Culpeper uses hawthorn for urinary stones and adds that the seeds may be taken in wine to treat dropsy. This may be the first mention of a heart related condition being treated with hawthorn. Coles increases use for the distilled water of the flowers for pleurisy, but the main emphasis remains on the reputation of the distilled water of the flowers for treating urinary problems.

Dr. Ratcliffe was a strong promoter of this use. Following his death, hawthorn loses popularity and is absent from many herbals after 1750. In 1916, haws reappear as necessary for medicine in a book on gathering herbs to replace the loss of imports from Germany. The herb is then classed as a cardiac tonic. It appears this new use was found by Dr. Greene in Ireland and made public after his death in 1894. See Herbalists' Reference for more.

Recipes

Extracted from A Collection of Receipts. 1746. "*An excellent* Water *for the* Stone-Cholick. Put four Pounds of Haw-berries bruis'd, into four Quarts of strong White-wine; let it steep twenty-four Hours; then draw off, in a cold still, two Quarts of very strong; and what runs after, keep by itself. A quarter of a Pint of the Strongest has given Ease in very bad

Fits at once taking; but if it comes up, you must repeat it, 'till it does stay" (p.160).⁶

Extracted from A Collection of Receipts. 1746. "*Another for the* Stone. Dry and powder the Haw-thorn Berries, and take as much as will lie on a Shilling, in a Glass of White-wine: This has done great Cures, by constant taking; it may be taken in Ale, if you cannot have Wine: The Virtue is in the Berry and has been experience'd, to the great Ease of many poor people, in Ale as well as Wine; but the last is best; and a Posset-Drink turn'd with White-wine, is a proper Vehicle for it; taking it fasting, or when in Pain" (p.148).⁶

Notes

1. Pryor F. *Seahenge.* Harper. (Collins. 2001). 147/148.
2. Pollington S. *Leechcraft.* (Anglo Saxon Books. 2000). 405. *Bald* (64).
3. Culpeper N. *Culpeper's Complete Herbal and English Physician enlarged.* (1652). (London. 1815 edition). 90.
4. Coles W. *The Paradise of Plants.* (London. 1657). 367.
5. Miller J. *Botanicum officinale.* Bell. (London. 1722). 423.
6. Anon. *A Collection of Receipts.* (Printed for the Executrix of Mary Kettilby. 1746). 103, 148, 160.
7. Quincy J. MD. *A Complete Dispensatory.* (10th edition. 1736). 164.
8. Hill Sir J. *The Family Herbal.* (Bungay edition). Brightly. 163.
9. Teetgen A.B. *Profitable Herb-Growing and Collecting.* (London. 1916). 177.
10. *Ellingwood's. therapeutist.* A Monthly Medical Journal. (1914). Vol. 8. 142. Available online at babel.hathitrust.org.

CRATAEGUS OXYCANTHOIDES, *C. MONOGYNA* – Herbalists' Reference

The Parts of Hawthorn Used for Medicine – Flowers, leaves, and fruit.

Dosage and Forms – Leaves and flowers 1–2 teaspoons per cup, infuse 5–10 minutes, dose 1 cup. Haws 1–2 heaped teaspoons per cup of water, simmer gently for 2 minutes, dose. ½–1 cup three times daily. Alternatively, leave in a flask overnight. Tincture 1:2 20–40ml per week.

Constituents – Oligomeric procyanidins (OPCs), glycosides, including flavonoids, saponins, aesculin, trimethylamine, hyperoside, and phenolic acids. The levels vary with the species and the plant part. The flowers contain the highest level of flavonoids, their distinctive and unpleasant smell is due to the presence of trimethylamine. It is assumed

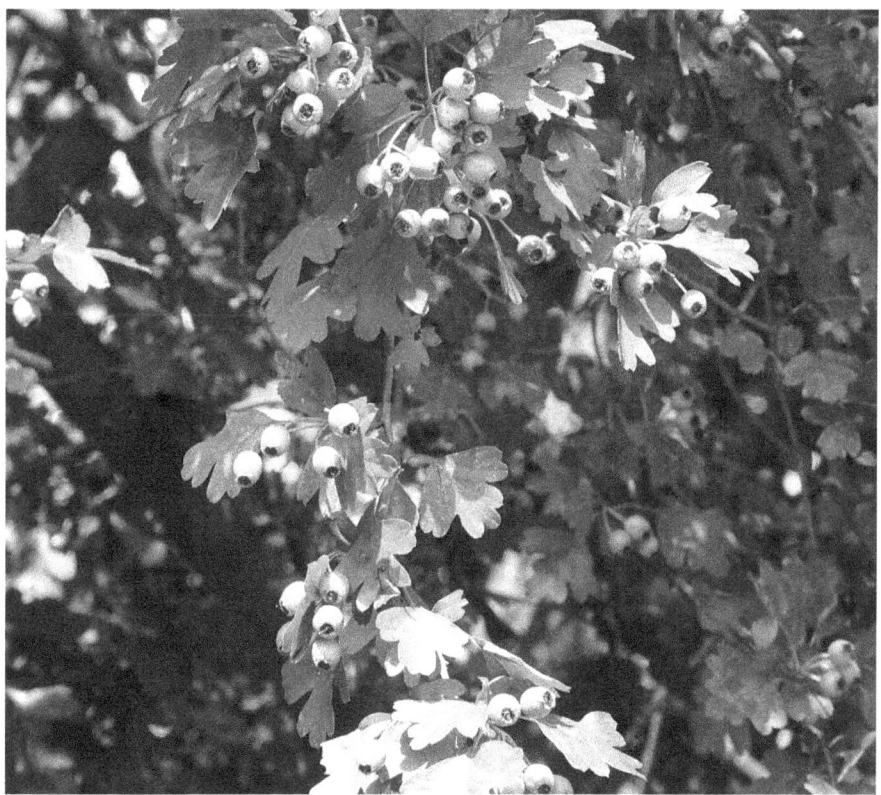

Haws for medicine.

that the leaf is more active than the berry. The leaves contain the highest level of OPCs. The berries contain both flavonoids and OPCs in smaller amounts.

Actions and Uses – Hawthorn produces numerous actions that support the cardiovascular system. While increasing coronary blood flow by dilating the blood vessels, it increases cardiac output, strengthening the action of the heart muscle with reduced oxygen consumption. A number of supportive studies are given in Schultz, *Rational Phytotherapy*.[1]

Hawthorn has a gradual action. It is assumed that unlike digitalis, hawthorn does not act on the contractile system of the myocardium, but improves the myocardial energy metabolism. While hawthorn aids in lowering high blood pressure, it can raise low blood pressure if this is specifically due to weakness of the heart muscle. Hawthorn is therefore indicated for the aging or failing heart, which does not, as yet, need digitalis.[2]

Decreased performance, angina complaints, and arrhythmias, including mild bradyarrhythmia, may respond to hawthorn. While supporting heart action in arterio-sclerosis, hawthorn is indicated particularly in cerebral sclerosis due to latent underlying cardiac insufficiency. Hawthorn is anti-aggregant, hypocholesterolaemic and anti-inflammatory. The presence of oleanolic and ursolic acids which are COX-2 inhibitors, may be significant in treating Alzheimers, arthrosis and cancer.[3]

Austrian research shows hawthorn decreases fatty acids and lactic acid, indicating stimulation of digestive enzymes with decreased oxygen demands. Hawthorn is therefore prescribed for digestive enzyme deficiency with intestinal fermentation. It may be helpful with menopausal irritability and hot flushes.

Specific Indications – Hypertension with myocardial weakness. Angina pectoris.[4]

Interactions – Hawthorn inter-reacts positively with a number of diuretic drugs, giving an additive effect. Also with Doxorubicin and related anthracycline chemotherapy it is known to reduce the side-effect of the drugs that induce dose-related cumulative cardiotoxicity.[5]

Precautions and Contraindications. Not to be taken alongside other heart medications unless supervised by a qualified herbalist or physician.[6]

Notes

1. Schultz et al. *Rational Phytotherapy.* (Springer. 2004). 126–137.
2. Weiss R.F. M.D. *Herbal Medicine.* (Thieme. 2nd edition revised and expanded. 2000). 144.
3. Duke J.A. *Handbook of Medicinal Herbs* (CRC Press LLC. 2nd edition. 2002). 369.
4. *British Herbal Pharmacopoeia.* (British Herbal Medicine Association. 1983). 75.
5. Stargrove et al. *Herb, Nutrient and Drug Interactions.* (Mosby Elsevier. 2008). 102.
6. Mills S. & Bone K. *The Essential Guide to Herbal Safety.* (Elsevier Churchill Livingstone. 2005). 466.

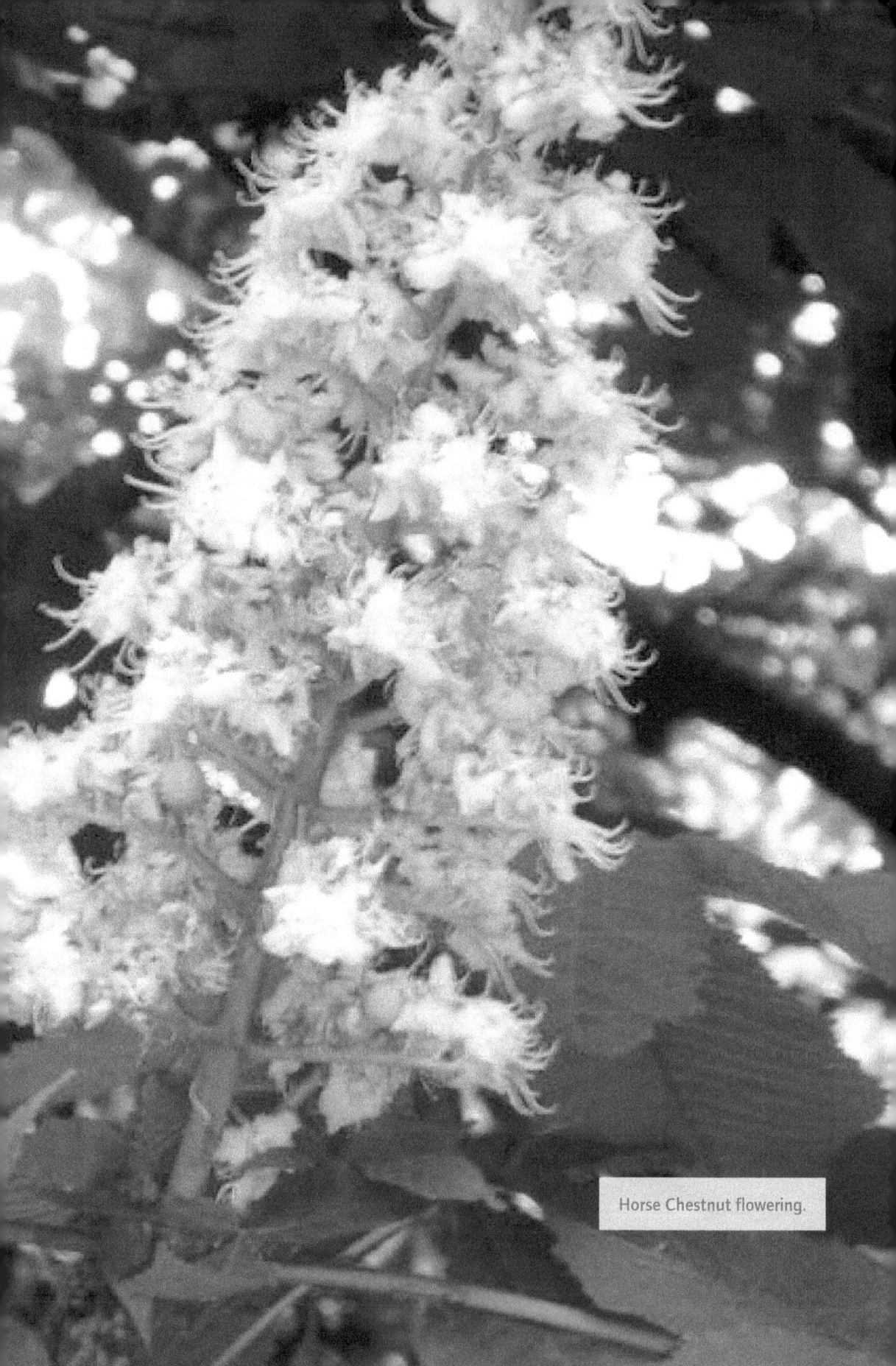
Horse Chestnut flowering.

Horse chestnut

Aesculus hippocastanum – Horse chestnut – Hippocastanae

HORSE CHESTNUT – *Usefulness* – A beautiful tree, it has been grown in parks for both the decorative qualities and harvests. The seeds, often known as fruits, the flowers, and bark are used medicinally. The seeds were once used to treat horses, hence the name. They have been mixed into food for several animals. Chestnut buds are the source of a Bach flower remedy for those who are slow to learn from experience. Saponins in the fruits made them suitable for washing clothes in the past. In both World Wars they were a source of starch, which was used to make acetone. Horse chestnuts are also known as "conkers", famously pitted against the other players' fruits in a tremendously popular childhood game, which has only recently fallen into comparative disuse. Both fruits and bark provide strong dyes.

Dangers – Handling or being near the fruits can cause allergic reactions and bring on asthma attacks in sensitive people. The fruits in overdose are mildly toxic.[1]

Getting to Know the Horse Chestnut Tree – Although it is an unlikely garden tree, due to fast growth to a considerable size, the horse chestnut has been popular as an ornamental tree in parks since its arrival in this country in the early seventeenth century. The horse chestnut grows wild from the Balkans to the Himalayas. Later, in the Victorian era it became fashionable to plant horse chestnuts, along with Turkey oaks across the countryside, even at the edges of some farmland on estates. The opening of the tightly closed leaf buds comes quickly. All that is needed is a spell of warm weather to melt the resin that binds the protective scales covering the leaf bud against frost, releasing the new growth. The leaves are strikingly large, generally with five to seven almost fully divided leaflets giving them the appearance of a hand with long, pale green fingers with serrated edges. Aesculetin, extracted from the bark and leaves, has been included in sun-tan preparations because it absorbs short-wave UV radiation that is damaging to skin while allowing transmission of long-wave UV radiation, necessary to produce the appearance of a tan.[2]

The flowers follow rapidly. The upper ones on the pyramid are usually male, while the lower ones are female. A large horse chestnut, fully in blossom in May, as if ablaze with so many tall candles, is a magnificent sight. One such, which overhung my daughter's garden, provided an abundant crop of fruits for my use for several years. I look forward each spring to gathering the flowers for making pain-relieving massage treatments. Their elegance is accentuated as they lie steeping, suspended in the oil.

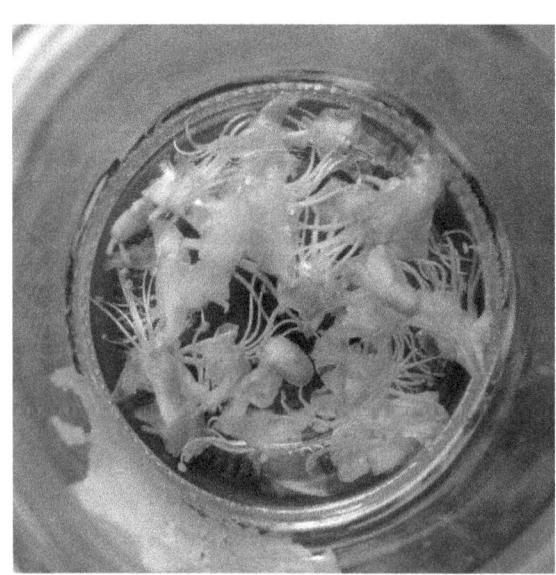
Horse Chestnut flowers steeping in olive oil.

The buds are also gathered to make the white chestnut Bach Flower remedy which is indicated for persistent worrying thoughts and mental arguments.[3] Although the fruits are not eaten in the same way as those of the sweet chestnut, they bear a strong resemblance to the edible chestnut and so carry the same common name. Horse chestnuts have been leached of their tannins to make tolerably good flour, or roasted to make coffee in times of shortage, but are not a food of choice. In too large an amount they are toxic to both the liver and kidneys. No serious cases of poisoning have been reported in the twentieth century.[4]

In my childhood, the playground game of conkers involved all sorts of measures to harden your conker so that the opponent's conker could not break it to win. They were part-baked or steeped in liquids, such as vinegar or even urine. The World Conker Championships were started in Northants in 1965.[5] Years later, when my son was at school the game of conkers was still played frequently. Another generation on and the number of children who are allergic to many natural substances, including horse chestnuts, and possible injury from enthusiastic play, has seen a rapid decline due to health and safety considerations.

A magic trick with bark from some twigs and a glass of water is perhaps more attractive today. The bark is soaked in the water and then a light is shone through the liquid. With light the colour of the water appears to change to blue. A change brought about by a fluorescent substance in the bark.[6]

Legends and Folklore. Perhaps due to the late arrival of the tree in Europe, there do not seem to be any legends of particular note. I know of the idea that keeping a conker in your pocket will keep rheumatism away. This belief may relate originally to the use of the flowers or seed to treat rheumatic pain. As a spinner I have also often heard that keeping conkers with wool will deter moths and spiders. I tried this but it did not work against moths. Whether it works against spiders I could not tell, but it did attract mice to eat the conkers!

Notes

1. Burlando B. et al. *Herbal principles in Cosmetics.* (CRC Press. 2010). 33.
2. Samuelsson G. *Drugs of Natural Origin.* (Apotekarsocieteten.1999). 155/6.
3. Weeks N. & Bullen V. *The Bach Flower Remedies.* (C. W. Daniel & Co. Ltd. 1990). 68.
4. Fröhne D. Pfander H. *A Colour Atlas of Poisonous Plants.* (Wolf Science. 1983). 135.
5. Vickery R. *Oxford Dictionary of Plant-Lore.* (Oxford University Press. 1997). 193.
6. Campbell-Culver M. *The Origin of Plants.* (Headline Book Publishing. 2001). 123.

HORSE CHESTNUT – History of Medicinal Use

The horse chestnut tree is native to the Balkan peninsula and grows in Macedonia and Albania. The trees were introduced to Western Europe around 1550 A.D. and sent to Vienna about 1558. It was called *Castanea* from the shape of the fruit and *Equini* as the ground seed was a good food for horses. Andrea Mattioli [1501–1577] imported the tree into Italy from Constantinople using it as an astringent for the vascular system, although it became better known as a fever treatment.[1] Doctor and naturalist, he is cited as the first to have described the horse chestnut. This was in his *Compendium of Plants* published in 1586.

On reaching England, it was cultivated by John Tradescant in 1633 in his botanical garden.[2] Shortly after this date the trees were chosen to be planted in parks for their ornamental value. In addition they provided considerable shade after only twelve to fourteen years of growth. John Evelyn in his *Elysium Britannicum* writes about trees that are suitable for planting at the sides of great walks in parks. He writes of "tall & goodly Trees," including the "Horsechessnut" (p.127)[3] amongst them. He recommends *Castanea equina* to be raised from suckers, as when it is old it will bear beautiful flowers.[3]

The flowers are the glory of horse chestnuts, appearing in May on the end of new shoots which are up to eighteen inches long, and have grown in less than three weeks since the leaf buds opened. The flowers have also been used in medicine. In the seventeenth century William Coles included the tree in his herbal, writing about the plentiful horse chestnut trees in Turkey

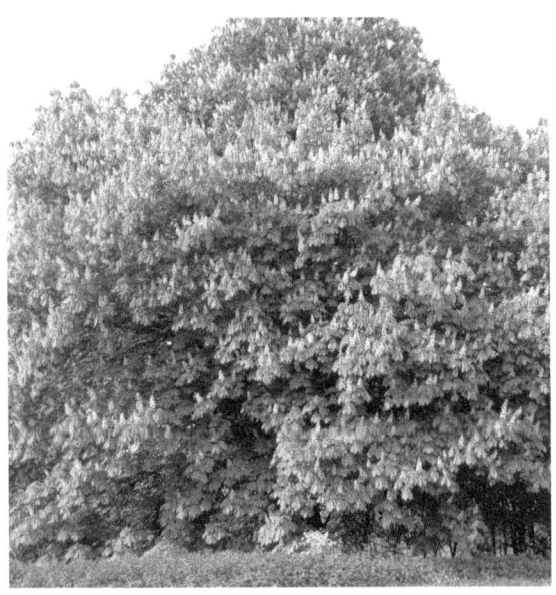
An old, vigorous horse chestnut tree.

and Eastern countries, where the seeds were given to horses to cure them of shortness of breath and other diseases.[4]

In 1771, Miller refers to the tree as *Aesculus hippocastanum*. He also explains the earlier Latin name of *Castanea Equini*. After this date the tree is to be found in herbals as Aesculus. In 1790, William Woodville refers to the entrance of the powdered seed into the Edinburgh College Materia Medica as a sternutatory; that is to say it was taken as a snuff or drawn into the nostrils in the form of an infusion or decoction to bring on sneezing, which might be necessary to clear the head. It was prescribed for complaints of the head and eyes. Meanwhile, on the Continent use of the bark for treating fevers gained support from several authorities, ranking it alongside Peruvian bark (*Cinchona*) for its effects.

Thornton writes about many successful experiments with the bark being given internally to treat typhus fever, and applied externally as a lotion, to treat gangrene. The bark of the horse chestnut was described as rarely disagreeing with the stomach, but that the astringency might require a follow-up of a laxative. Thornton is aware that in 1810 chemistry is young when it comes to identifying constituents of plants, yet he notes the evident tannin in horse chestnut bark can hardly be compared to cinchonin which he knows to be the predominant and probably active constituent of Peruvian bark.[5]

By 1829 an American Materia Medica records that numerous experiments have proved that horse chestnut cannot successfully be substituted for Cinchona. However, at that point the seeds had also been investigated chemically, and along with starch Joshua Canzoneri had identified a substance he called "esculin".[6] In nineteenth century France, Aesculus was used to treat fevers and haemorrhoids.[1]

In 1916 in Britain, however, the bark and fruits of the horse chestnut are listed to be gathered for homoeopathic medicine. There is no mention of allopathic or herbal use here at that date.[7] In the 1930s Dr. Edward Bach perfected his system of flower remedies for treating disease. One of the remedies, (white chestnut), is made from the buds containing leaves and flowers of the horse chestnut.[8] In 1932, The *National Botanic Pharmacopoeia* published by the National Association of Medical Herbalists does not mention Aesculus. Two years after this date Mrs. Grieve records treatments for rheumatism and neuralgia using the seeds, treating fevers with the bark and an external application for ulcers.[9]

In the 1960s Lorenz and Marck conducted studies in an animal model, which showed the aescin content made horse chestnut 100 times more effective than horse chestnut with this constituent removed.[10] Medical research and observational studies continued in Germany and led to approval of horse chestnut extracts for treating varicose veins and related conditions.

Summary. The horse chestnut is native to the Balkan Peninsula. It was introduced into Europe in 1550 and first grown in England in 1633 by John Tradescant in his botanical garden. Initially it was named *Castanaea Equina,* and the beauty of the tree soon made it a popular planting in parks. Formerly noted by Coles in the seventeenth century as a medicine for horses, the seed entered British medicine in powdered form as a sternutatory snuff used to provoke sneezing to clear the head and benefit the eyes. It already had a history of use for treating fevers and vascular conditions on the Continent however. In England, after unsuccessful attempts to use the bark as a substitute for Cinchona in treating fevers, by 1916 the fruits were gathered for homoeopathic medicine only. It was not until the twentieth century that the real value of the seeds for treating vascular conditions was fully appreciated. See Herbalist's Reference.

Recipe

Extracted from Thornton's Family Herbal. 1810. (Aesculus). Peruvian bark substitute in Intermittent Fever. "A solution of a drachm of the extract in an ounce of cinnamon water, of which sixty drops are to be given every three hours." Preference of Buchholtz. (p.368).[5]

Notes

1. Burlando B. et al. *Herbal principles in Cosmetics.* (CRC Press. 2010). 33.
2. Woodville W. *Medical Botany.* 3 vols + Supplement. (London. 1790). Vol. 2. 350

3. Evelyn J. *Elysium Britannicum.* [1650–1700]. (University of Pennsylvania Press. 2001). 127.
4. Coles W. *The Paradise of Plants.* (London. 1657). 43.
5. Thornton R.J. *A New Family Herbal.* (London. 1810). 368.
6. Togno J. Durand E. (trans) *A Manual of Materia Medica and Pharmacy.* (Philadelphia. 1829). 148.
7. Teetgen A.B. *Profitable Herb-Growing and Collecting.* (London. 1916). 178.
8. Weeks N. & Bullen V. *The Bach Flower Remedies.* (C. W. Daniel & Co. Ltd. 1990). 21.
9. Grieve. M. *A Modern Herbal.* (1st published 1934 Jonathan Cape. Saavas. 1984). 193.
10. Schultz et al. *Rational Phytotherapy.* (Springer. 2004). 179.

AESCULUS HIPPOCASTANUM – Herbalists' Reference

The Parts of Horse Chestnut Used for Medicine – Flowers harvested in May, extracts from bark and seeds from within the prickly hard coat harvested in September.

Dosage and Forms – Tincture of flowers dose 10–15 drops. Decoction of seeds 3–6g in 500ml of water. Tincture of the seeds 1:2 Dose 2–5ml per day, 15–30ml per week. Tea ½ teaspoon powdered dried chestnut to each cup of boiling water, infuse 15 minutes, dose ¼–½ cup, three times daily. Aescin is fairly soluble in water but poorly soluble in lipid solvents. Orally administered aescin is either sparingly absorbed or undergoes a substantial first-pass effect. Average elimination half life twenty hours for single dose 100mg aescin.

Constituents – Saponins, including aescin, flavonoids, coumarin aesculetin, scopoletin glycoside, and tannins.

Actions and Uses – Aesculus is an astringent, anti-inflammatory vasodilator, which tones and protects blood vessel walls. In preventing collagen breakdown it enables capillaries to work more efficiently as they retain flexibility and larger pore size, aiding blood supply to surrounding tissue. The herb is restorative and anticoagulant.

Aescin is an acidic saponin in two types: beta-aescin is less water soluble, so that only about 5% of the dose is absorbed; alpha-escin has twice the absorption rate and a longer elimination time in the body.[1] Both aescins show greater action on capillaries than on veins and venules. The herb is therefore antiexudative, anti-oedematous, and useful in removing congestion and restoring blood-vessels.

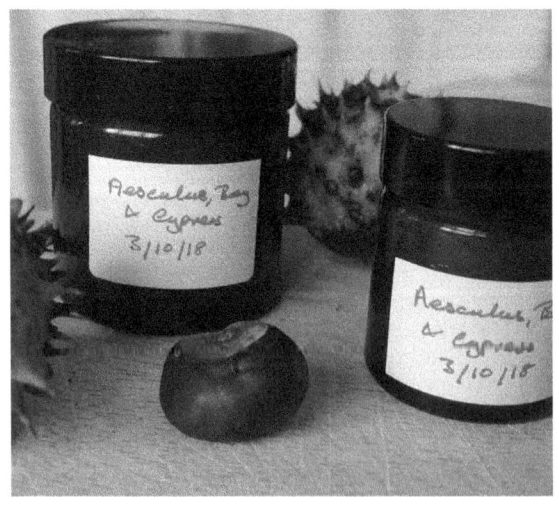
Ointment for treating varicose veins.

Aesculus is indicated for moderating menstruation, enhancing the portal circulation, relieving abdominal bloating, water retention, benefitting the prostate and relieving symptoms from haemorrhoids. Heavy legs and swelling or varicose veins in the legs, are accepted indications, as well as varicocele, phlebitis, and congestive dysmenorrhoea. A huge amount of research is available on this herb.

Topical Application – The flowers may be added to hand or footbaths. Alternatively they can be added as an infusion to a full bath to treat rheumatic or neuralgic pain. Flowers can be steeped in oil to include in liniments.[2]

Contraindications and Precautions – Do not prescribe where there is severe renal or hepatic impairment, or to patients who are taking anticoagulants. Not to be given in pregnancy and when breast feeding. Aescin binds to plasma protein and may affect binding of other drugs.[3]

Notes

1. Weiss R.F. M.D. *Herbal Medicine*. (Thieme. 2nd edition revised and expanded. 2000). 178.
2. Holmes P. *The Energetics of Western Herbs*. Vol. 1&2. (Snow Press. Boulder. Revised 3rd edition. 1989). Vol. 2. 742.
3. Barnes J. et al. *Herbal Medicines*. (Pharmaceutical Press. 2nd edition. 2002). 298.

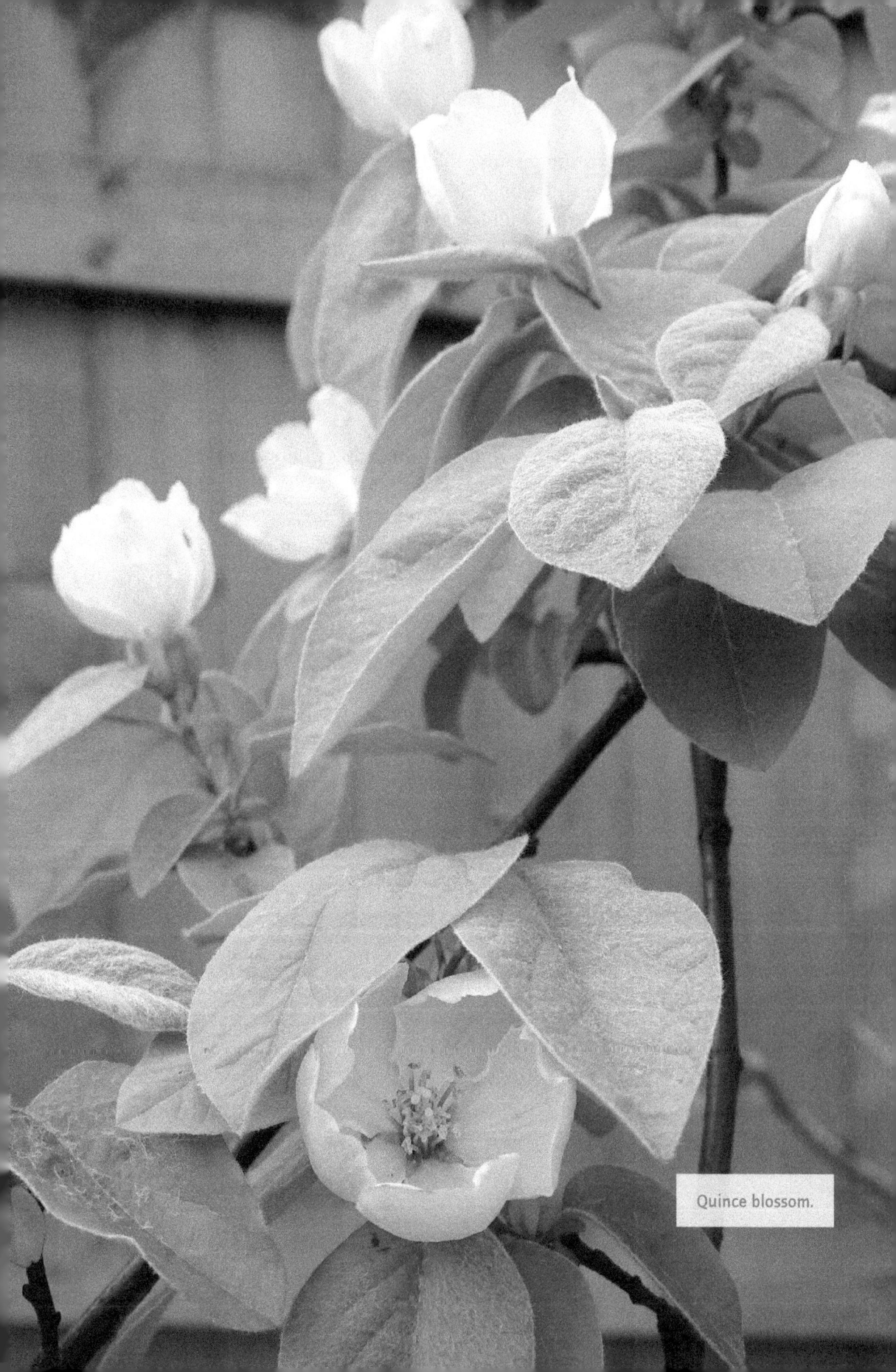

Quince blossom.

Quince

Cydonia vulgaris – Quince – Rosaceae

QUINCE – Usefulness – The fruit can be enjoyed in cookery, and in wine and liqueurs. Both fruit and the seeds have medicinal properties.

Dangers – None known.

Getting to Know the Quince Tree – After trying recipes made with fruits from the Japonica, or Japanese quince, I decided to grow my own quince tree. The true quince comes from south-west Asia and has been grown in the Mediterranean area for 2,000 years.[1] It likes a sunny position with plentiful water that drains away quickly, rich soil and protection from cold winds. *Cydonia vulgaris* is an attractive small tree—mine is expected to grow to four and a half metres (fifteen feet), others are available as semi-dwarf at three metres (nine feet). The spring leaves are pale, wonderfully soft, and furry to the touch. All quinces are self-fertile and so I did not have to worry about buying a companion tree. The blossom is quite beautiful, opening after the leaves, in late April. The five cupped petals resemble white roses and are a popular draw for the bees. The calyx behind the flower is formed of one leaf divided into five oval, notched segments, just as the later core of the fruit will have five cells containing many oval seeds.

Even a young tree will give a good crop of fruits, which are the size of a grapefruit and either apple or pear-shaped, depending on the variety. Those varieties, which have soft, downy skin on the fruits, give out a heady fragrance, and are traditionally set in a bowl in the house to sweeten the atmosphere as they ripen. The most famous use of the fruit is to make membrillo. This is imported from Spain in wooden boxes and can be found for sale on good cheese counters, where it is sold to accompany Manchego cheese in particular. This heavily sweetened, lemon-flavoured quince paste, is easy to make at home from your own fruits. Quince marmalade is another treat to enjoy.

When Eleanor of Castile married Edward I, she was familiar with the taste of mermelada. This is now eaten as membrillo or quince cheese. Membrillo was the original marmalade, which was only later made with oranges. In early times, it was sliced and placed in round boxes, then sweetened with sugar to give the appearance of segments of an orange. On the King's return from the Crusades the garden at the Tower of London was planted with quince trees and there were more at Westminster bought in 1292.[2]

In making historical recipes, I have found some delicious ideas among the fifteenth century collections. At that time, quinces were often cooked with ginger and other spices and covered in pastry, or the quince was first roasted and then peeled and the flesh sweetened and mixed with spices. Quynade was made by first cooking the quinces in rosewater. Almond milk was then boiled with white wine vinegar to curdle it and the curds, quinces and cream together, flavoured with spices and saffron. (p.27).[3] The popularity of quince is evident from a remark made by William Coles in 1657, that "the Marmalade of Quinces is toothsom, as well as wholesom, and therefore I cannot blame such Gentlewomen, which are seldom without it in their Closets" (p.29).[4]

In the seventeenth century there were various ways of preserving them aside from membrillo. The fruits might be put straight from the tree into a barrel and covered in ale before being sealed, or they could be dried in slices.[5] The stillroom *Receipt Book of Lady Anne Blencowe* has a superb recipe for "quince chipps" (p.19).[6] These "chipps"

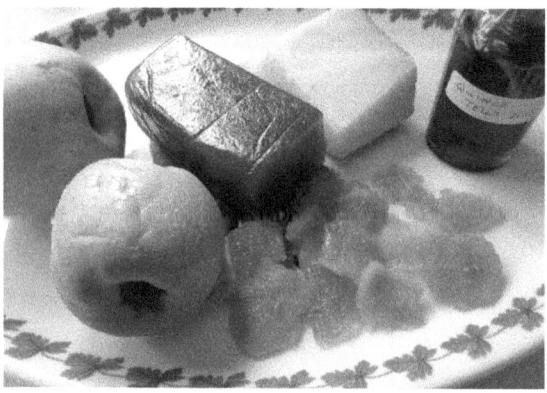

The fruit, membrillo, and quince chipps.

as dessert treats are candied slices of quince, dried and packed into boxes. They are a delicious favourite of mine.

There are many recipes for quince wine and in later times, ratafia. Quince is also used to flavour gin. When you have prepared the quinces for any of these recipes you will be left with a number of three-sided mahogany brown coated seeds which will feel greasy. As soon as the seeds become wet, the cell walls of the outer skin of the seeds swell and dissolve releasing large amounts of sticky mucilage, which is capable of thickening forty times their weight of liquid. This has given them medicinal use both in applications for skin problems and in soothing eye washes for removing foreign objects and moistening the eyes. Within the mahogany coloured skins, the kernels taste and smell of bitter almonds as they contain a little amygdalin in common with almonds, which are of the same Rose family.[7]

The hairy nature of the fruit peel was seen in the past as suggesting the peel would be good as a hair restorer. We find this use has continued for the past 2,000 years. Juliette de Bairacli-Levy notes Spanish gypsies in the twentieth century using quince for hair growth.[8] Quince preparations have been used for the hair in many other countries. Quince seeds also have been an ingredient in hair-fixing lotions in recent years.[9]

Legends and Folklore. The quince has the good fortune of being considered an emblem of happiness and fertility and so decorated the Temples of Venus. It is possible that quinces are the real golden apples of the Hesperides. The name Cydonia refers to the town in Crete, Kydon.[7] An old tradition was to plant a mulberry tree to the south of a house and a quince to the north to give good luck and guard against lightning.[10]

Notes

1. A Virginia Farmer. (trans), *Roman Farm Management.* Treatises of Cato and Varro. (Macmillan. New York. 1916). 169.
2. Campbell-Culver M. *The Origin of Plants.* (Headline Book Publishing. 2001). 61.
3. Austin T. (ed), *Two Fifteenth Century Cookery Books.* (1888). (Oxford University Press. Reprint 1964). 27.
4. Coles W. *The Paradise of Plants.* (London. 1657). 29.

5. Plat Sir H. *Delights for Ladies.* (1609). (Crosby Lockwood.1948). 51, 33.
6. Stapley C. (ed), *The Receipt Book of Lady Anne Blencowe. 1694.* (Heartsease Books. 2004). 19.
7. Flückiger & Hanbury. *A History of Drugs.* (Macmillan & Co. 2nd edition. 1879). 270, 269.
8. De Bairacli-Levy J. *The Illustrated Herbal Handbook for Everyone.* (Faber and Faber. London. 1991). 133.
9. Trease & Evans W.C. *Pharmacognosy.* (W.B.Saunders. 14th edition. 1999). 216.
10. DeCleene M. & Lejeune M.C. *Compendium of Symbolic and Ritual Plants in Europe.* (Man and Culture Publishers, Ghent. Belgium. 2003). 428.

QUINCE – History of Medicinal Use

A native of south-west Asia, the quince was well known to the Romans in the first century AD. Cato in his book on farming gives instructions for keeping the fruit in cold, dry fruit houses, laid on straw.[1] Pliny points out that when cooked, although more pleasant to eat, they lose their astringency, which was valued against bleeding and diarrhoea. It seems all possible uses, including treating carbuncles with the down from the fruit skin, were investigated.[2]

In another section on perfumes, Pliny lists a quince blossom unguent called melinum, used to improve vision.[3] Dioscorides gives similar uses to Pliny, when treating the choleric patient, who might be spitting purulent matter, he recommends the roasted fruit as milder.[4] Medieval surgeon Henri de Mondeville also classes the quince as a styptic, cool, and dry in the second degree.[5]

In the Women's Book published in 1540, an infant with poor digestion is prescribed neat quince juice as an anti-emetic. Another recipe with spiced and sweetened quince sounds more acceptable.[6]

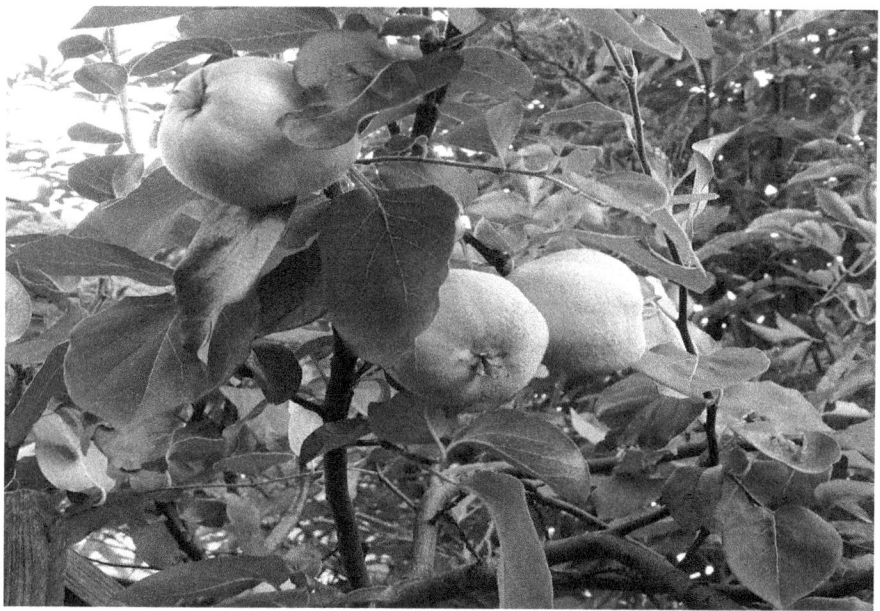

Quinces.

Enthusiasm for their culinary use was more evident in England, while the Arab physicians practised Galen's idea, using the properties of the quince to provide a vehicle for administering the strong purgative scammony safely. The scammony herb was placed inside a quince and the fruit boiled. Once cooked, the scammony was removed, and the pulp of the fruit, which had absorbed some of the drug, was then given to the patient mixed with the bulk laxative psyllium seeds of the Plantain family.[7]

Culpeper translated recipes from the 1618 *Pharmacopoeia Londinensis*, including the *Trochisci Bechici nigri* from Rhasis using the mucilage from the seeds with liquorice, sugar, gum tragacanth and sweet almonds mixed with rose water for sore throats. The *Trochisci Gordonii* contains the 4 greater cold seeds with those of the quince, gums and sweet almonds for ulcers of the bladder. Also, the recipe for a pastill from Galen, *Pastilli Adronis* which was for treating wounds. His last prescription is for oil of quinces which takes weeks to make. In his herbal, he tells us that old Saturn owns the tree.[8]

Coles supports Pliny's cure for baldness using the down on the fruit, giving it a contemporary feel by using it to treat the problem of falling hair from the French pox (syphilis). He then gives the instruction to boil the down in wine to apply to plague-sores. Both of these conditions were of great concern in the seventeenth century. His detail of the indications for taking the syrup, and manner of taking it, is enlightening. "The Syrup of the Juyce of Quinces strengthens the heart and stomach, stayes loosness and vomiting, relieves languishing Nature: for loosness, take a spoonful of it before meat, for vomiting after meat; for others purposes it is to be taken in the morning, and may be then taken for these also. It helpeth the Liver also, when it is opprest, that it cannot perfect digestion, and correcteth Choler and Flegme" (p.29).[9]

Pechey in 1694 gives a gargle for fevers, which he recommends as excellent, although a modern patient would have qualms about it. In this the mucilage of the seeds is extracted with "Spawn of Frog's water" (p.155). He gives recipes for both the marmalade and syrup of quinces with a dosage for the syrup of one ounce in water. This could be given for spitting blood, the bloody flux and other discharges.[10]

Miller, in 1722 after recognizing the usefulness of the fruit for the digestion, returns our attention to the seed. This he describes as "balsamic and mollifying, tempering the Acrimony of the Humours, and serviceable against sore Mouths and Throats, and a Thrush; for which a Mucilage made of them is frequently prescribed. The same outwardly used is very healing to sore chap'd Nipples" (p.169).[11]

A 1746 recipe gives us mucilage decocted from the seed in rose or plantain water, then egg white added and the whole sweetened with syrup of mulberrries. This was for a sore throat. Perhaps my favourite from this collection on quince is "A *pretty* Medicine *for* Sore Nipples. Infuse Quince-seeds in White Rose-Water, till it is a Jelly; strain it thro' a Muslin, and wash the Sore Part often with it" (p.258).[12] White rose would be more suitable than red as it is less astringent.

1790 saw Meyrick's *Family Herbal* giving a new recipe for the syrup. He also recommends the jelly and the seed mucilage. By 1791, the fifth edition of the revised and improved Pharmacopoeia, the formerly officinal syrup and electuary are omitted. However, quince fruit and seed remained in the Materia Medica section. Mucilage of the seed continued with the proportions of one dram of seed to eight ounces of distilled water.[13] In 1792, Woodville wrote that this was recommended in ulcerations of the mouth and throat. He classes it as a more pleasant application than simple gums but feels they would be more effective.[14] Although it is still in the dispensatory thirty years later, Thornton has little good to say about the mucilage, *Seminum cydoniorum* complaining that it quickly goes mouldy. He prefers the preparation of the seed with sliced liquorice root for treating kidney stones.[15]

Summary. All possible uses of the quince, taking advantage of the astringent properties of the fruit and profuse mucilage of the seeds, date back at least 2,000 years to Pliny. In the 1879 *History of Drugs*, it is noted that use of the quince seeds originated in Arabic medicine.[16] Those uses which continue over centuries for the fruit refer to digestion, as an anti-emetic, for the liver, and the urinary system. The mucilage from the seeds has constant application for burns, soothing sore throats, healing wounds, and particularly tender places on the body, such as chapped nipples. Inclusion in eye applications was common and the belief in the fruit acting as a hair restorer is persistent.

In 1879, a decoction of the seeds is occasionally used externally, as a soothing application for skin complaints and in eye lotions. In India, still part of the British Empire in that year, the seeds were imported from the Persian Gulf and seen as a demulcent tonic and restorative. Europeans in India found the seed mucilage helpful in treating dysentery. Use in India was still included in the extra Pharmacopoeia of 1967 using the unripe or half-ripe Bengal quince.[17] The decoction of the seeds is listed as a base ingredient for lotions and creams and the mucilage of *Cydonia* prepared in cold water as a useful suspending agent with added preservative. See Herbalists' Reference for the present uses.

Recipe

Extracted from The New Family Herbal. [1790] "A grateful cordial, and lightly restringent syrup, is made by digesting three pints of the clarified juice, with a dram of cinnamon, half a dram of ginger, and the same quantity of cloves, in warm ashes, for the space of six hours, then adding a pint of red port, and dissolving nine pounds of fine sugar in the liquor, after straining it" (p.388).[15]

Notes

1. A Virginia Farmer. (trans), *Roman Farm Management*. Treatises of Cato and Varro. (Macmillan. New York. 1916). 169.
2. Jones W.H.S. (trans), *Pliny Natural History* VI Books XX-XXIII. (Loeb Classical Library. 1989). 481.
3. Stewart S. *Cosmetics & Perfumes in the Roman World*. (Tempus. 2007). 11. 59.
4. Gunther R.T. (ed), *Dioscorides Greek Herbal*. (Hafner. 1968). 83.
5. Rosenman Leonard D. MD. *A Medieval Surgical Pharmacopoeia and Formulary*. 1170–1325. (San Francisco. 1999). 57, 85, 157.
6. Hobby E. (ed), *The Birth of Mankind*. (1560). (Ashgate. 2009). 176.
7. Griggs B. 1981. *Green Pharmacy*. (Jill Norman and Hobhouse. 1981). 28.
8. Culpeper N. *Culpeper's Complete Herbal and English Physician enlarged*. (1652). (London. 1815 edition). 347/8, 354, 351, 148.
9. Coles W. *The Paradise of Plants*. (London. 1657). 28.
10. Pechey J. *The English Herbal of Physical Plants*. (London. 1694). 155.
11. Miller J. *Botanicum officinale*. Bell. (London. 1722). 169.
12. Anon. *A Collection of Receipts*. (Printed for the Executrix of Mary Kettilby. 1746). 152, 258.

13. Healde T. M.D. F.R.S. *The Pharmacopoeia of the R.C.P. of London.* (1791). 25, 216.
14. Woodville W. *Medical Botany.* 3 vols + Supplement. (London. 1790). Vol. 2. 222.
15. Thornton R.J. *A New Family Herbal.* (London. 1810). 493/4.
16. Flückiger & Hanbury. *A History of Drugs.* (Macmillan & Co. 2nd edition. 1879). 269.
17. Todd R.G. (ed), *Extra Pharmacopoeia Martindale.* (Pharmaceutical Press. 25th edition. 1967). 1415. 80.

CYDONIA VULGARIS – Herbalists' Reference

The Parts of the Quince Tree Used for Medicine – The seeds and fruit pulp.

Dosage and Forms – Tea—soak the seeds in water for three to five hours. The dose is as much as needed three times daily. Tincture 1–2ml three times daily or as needed. Expressed juice or fruit pulp can be given for mouth and throat inflammations. Raw fruit is best for treating diarrhoea. Syrup of the fruit may be prescribed.

Constituents – The fruit contains generous amounts of ascorbic acid, as well as protein, carbohydrates, sugars, vitamins, iron, and pectin. The seeds contain about 20% mucilage, fixed oil, a small amount of cyanogenic glucoside and an enzyme that affects its hydrolysis.[1]

Actions and Uses – As a demulcent to the whole of the digestive tract, quince has clear use for treating inflammation from the mouth and throat, the oesophagus, stomach and gut. It is also carminative and the fresh fruit or syrup is astringent. Quince is considered to be helpful to the liver and spleen. The herb has been included in treatments for diarrhoea, dysentery and dysmenorrhoea. As a diuretic, it addresses water retention. Quince has a reputation for being antialcoholic and so suitable for treating alcoholism, also for acting as a pectoral and cardiac tonic. Quince seeds are especially demulcent and can act as an emulsifying agent in preparations.[1]

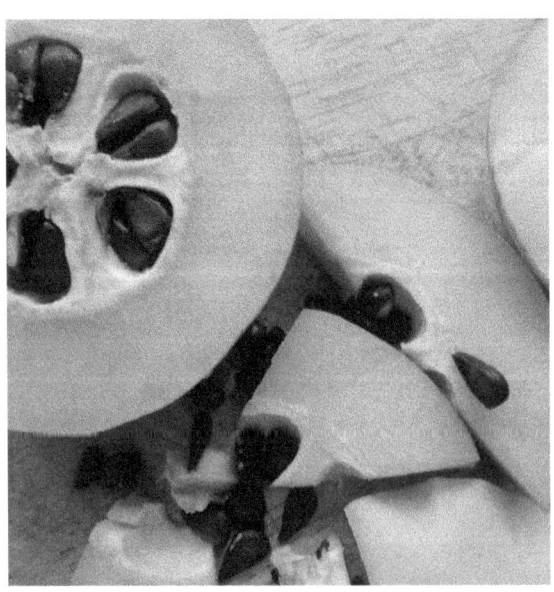
Seeds in the core chambers.

Topical Application – Mucilage which has accumulated over several hours through soaking the seeds in water can be applied to minor burns, inflamed joints, irritated skin or wounds, to soothe pain and encourage healing. A poultice could also be made by crushing the soaked seeds. A decoction is made by boiling two drams of seed in one pint (about 7g in 600ml) of water in a pan with a tight-fitting lid for ten minutes. Strain before use.[2]

Contraindications and Precautions – Prescribe this herb cautiously for patients with peptic ulcers or immune disorders. Do not give in pregnancy as it is an emmenagogue.[2]

Notes

1. Trease & Evans W.C. *Pharmacognosy*. (W.B.Saunders. 14th edition. 1999). 216.
2. Kelly W.J. (ed. director). *Nursing Herbal Medicine Handbook*. (Springhouse Corporation. 2001). 358.

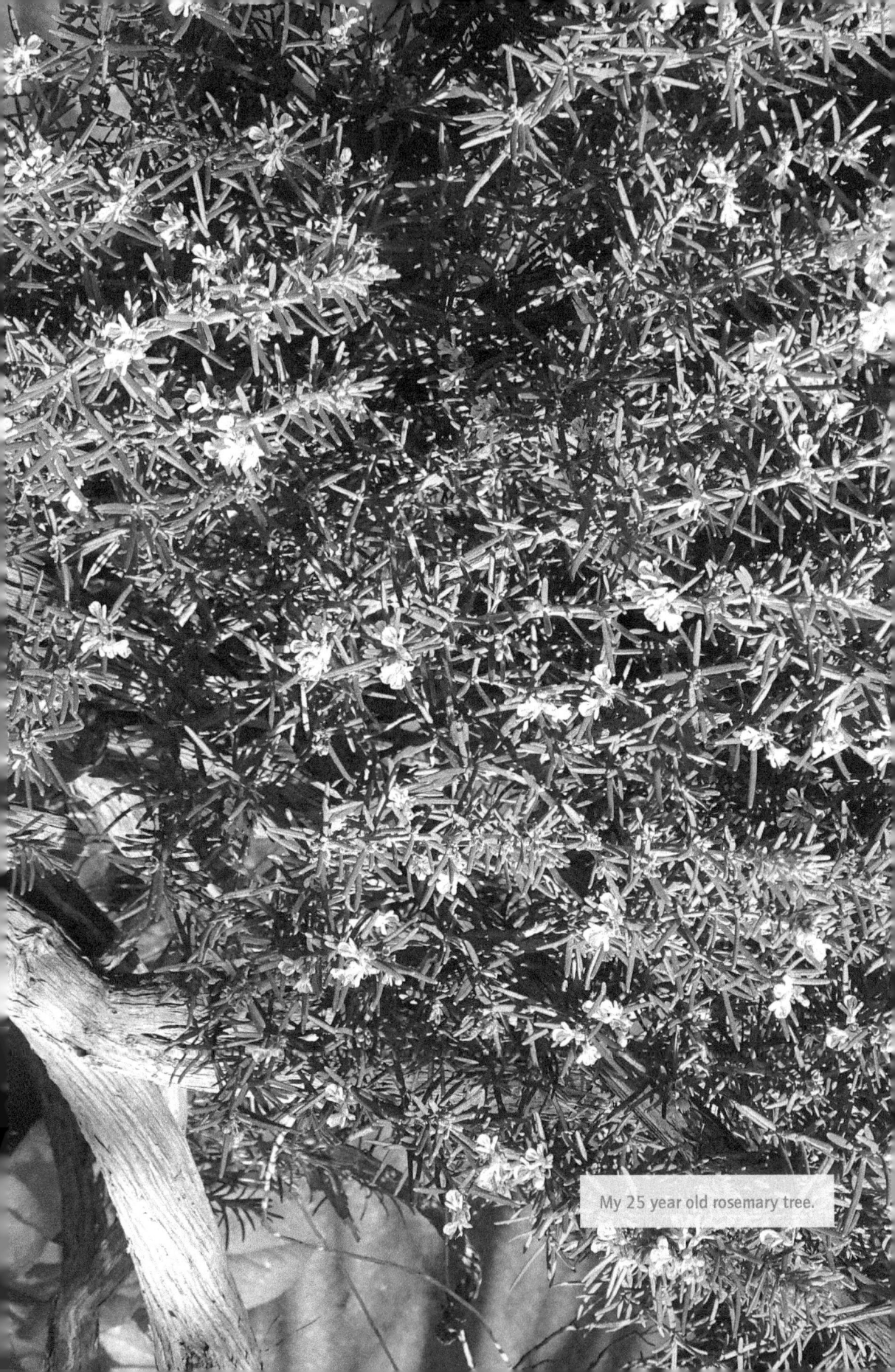
My 25 year old rosemary tree.

Rosemary

Rosmarinus officinalis – Rosemary – Lamiaceae

ROSEMARY – Usefulness – The leaves are a popular flavouring and digestive in cookery. Rosemary is an important ingredient in shampoos and conditioners for the hair and finds a place in cosmetics for the skin. Rosemary leaves, flowers and aromatic water are prescribed in herbal medicine. This herb adds strong fragrance to pot-pourri and herb pillows and has been used in perfumery. In the garden it is an ornamental evergreen and attracts bees.

Dangers – It is a powerful flavour, which requires discretion. It is reputed to be abortifacient.[1]

Getting to Know the Rosemary Tree – Rosemary originates in areas of France, Spain and Italy, which enjoy the Mediterranean climate and needs a sunny position with well-drained soil to thrive. Most people think of rosemary as a fairly small bush, but grown in the right conditions and trimmed twice a year it can mature as a small tree. After twenty-five to thirty years, rosemary can have developed a sturdy trunk with wood that can be turned to produce one or two boxes. Hence, strictly speaking it is a shrub, although in the past it has been referred to as the rosemary tree. I have often been asked if I could have only one herb what herb I would choose. My answer would have to be rosemary and so it has found a place among the trees in this book.

In Britain it is usual for rosemary to flower in the spring, possibly beginning in March or early April and flowering on until the end of May. Flowering depends on how quickly the temperature changes and whether the rosemary is planted to be south or north facing. The herb can be long-lived even on a north facing slope with sufficient shelter from cold winds. In some cases, when rosemary is really healthy it can flower almost all year round. The highest content of essential oil can be found in the calyx at the back of the flower and so the optimum time for harvesting is when the flowers are first open. The famed Queen of Hungary's Aromatic Water was distilled using just the flowering tops for concentrated effect. This water is supposed to have rejuvenated her and restored her beauty, so much so that she married again in old age. On the strength of the resulting good reputation it was sold to the crowned heads of Europe and the wealthy at a high price.

Flowering branches can be cut and dried on net in an airy room, out of sunlight. Take the dried branches outside to strip away the leaves and flowers to store. Carrying this task out in a closed room will give too strong a dose of the powerful perfume and make your nose and eyes run. Store the dried herb in dark glass jars for use in cookery, medicine, cosmetics or fragrances. It may be stored as whole leaves, or the dried leaves ground to a powder for culinary use. The flowers have long been preserved in sugar by pounding equal parts of the two together. The seeds are tiny and take patience to gather, four from each flower-head. The bush or tree will benefit from being trimmed back again when autumn approaches. Rosemary is a good companion with sage and rosemary and sage bushes can be kept low by trimming them twice a year to make an aromatic hedge in the garden. They then form a useful fragrant protection against pests in the vegetable patch.

Many cultivars have been bred from the original form, some short in growth, some not as hardy, and we can choose rosemary with all shades of blue, pink, or white flowers. I have also grown gilded rosemary with gold lines on the leaves, and a silver cultivar. These were status symbols in the past when some people who were unable to find the right plant actually painted leaves to imitate them. In general, these plants are not as hardy as the *officinalis*.

Rosemary is in one word a rejuvenator. It stimulates circulation to the scalp, which makes it an effective hair restorer and conditioner, and in doing the same for the skin it helps to retain a youthful complexion in age. Distilled aromatic water of rosemary makes a lovely addition to the water for washing your hands and face. It will be both antibacterial and stimulating for the health of the skin. From the medieval period we find bowls of herbal waters offered to guests to wash their hands before or during meals and some of these contain rosemary.[2]

Rosemary can be an important flavouring for food and is just as appropriate in sweet dishes, such as rhubarb puddings, biscuits, or fruit cakes as it is with chicken or fish. The ground herb can be used very effectively from the fresh or dried leaves and flowers. To infuse the flavour, scent, and properties into a bottle of wine, add four sprigs of rosemary, pounded slightly, then keep the bottle sealed for four days, tilting it each day. At this point the rosemary can be removed, leaving the infused wine. This can be enjoyed as a warming, stimulating medicinal wine, or used in cookery. Rosemary liqueurs are also recommended.[3]

In the house, the antibacterial properties of rosemary make it an ideal antiseptic support. The herb can be added to the water when washing floors or cleaning the sides in the kitchen. Rosemary is one of the few herbs that is still effective against moths and is a regular ingredient in my anti-moth blends, being perfect to hang in wardrobes or include in a carpet sprinkle.[4] I enjoy following an old custom by including sprays of the herb in my Christmas decorations. Rosemary is the only herb traditionally part of the decorations that does not have an earlier pagan association with the darkest, shortest days.

By stimulating circulation to the brain rosemary also aids memory. Having read that owning a box of rosemary wood, opening it and smelling it every day preserved your youth, I could not resist having one made. When my rosemary was thirty years old we moved house and since it was not in good health after being damaged by restoration on the house, I dug it out. Three years later I found a wood-turner who made two small precious boxes for me. His comment afterwards was that he was used to all wood having life but the rosemary wood had seemed to him to be alive. It had both jumped off his lathe and given out such a strong perfume it had really impressed him. This seemed to me to fit the reputation and properties of rosemary perfectly.

Legends and Folklore. The idea that smelling a box of rosemary every day would preserve your youth goes at least as far back as a herbal printed in 1525.[5] Putting rosemary leaves under the head of the bed against evil dreams comes from the same source. Rosemary has been seen as a protective herb against snakes, witches and evil in general for many centuries.

It is perhaps the link to memories that made it part of celebrations on Shakespeare's birthday, 23rd April. Vickery also quotes the story of Mary while fleeing from Herod's soldiers into Egypt carrying baby Jesus. On the journey, she washed her robe, hanging it to dry over a rosemary bush. After that the white rosemary flowers became blue.[6] Long ago I was told that rosemary never grows taller or older than Jesus was when he died. The longest lived rosemary I have grown was about 28 years old, by which time it had not reached my height, but I have seen a much taller one on the Isle of Wight in perfect growing conditions.

Notes

1. Barnes J. et al. *Herbal Medicines* (Pharmaceutical Press. 2nd edition. 2002). 406.
2. Power E. *The Goodman of Paris.* (original. 1393). (Folio Society. 1992). 196.
3. Stapley C. *Herbcraft Naturally.* (Heartsease Books. 1994). 85.
4. Stapley C. *Herb Sufficient.* (Heartsease Books. 1998). 24.
5. Larkey S.V. (ed), *An Herbal* (1525), (Scholars Facsimiles and Reprints, New York. 1941). 70.
6. Vickery R. *Oxford Dictionary of Plant-Lore.* (Oxford University Press. 1997). 318/9.

ROSEMARY – History of Medicinal Use

Rosemary may well have been brought to Britain by the Romans, Dioscorides classes it as warming and writes of it curing jaundice.[1] Pliny also mentioned Rosemary. If they did introduce the herb here, however, the plants do not seem to have survived the following centuries. There is an occasional reference to rosemary but these, e.g. "bothen" in the Anglo-Saxon Leechbooks (p.153),[2] can generally be interpreted as a confusion with wild rosemary, *Ledum palustre*, which was an entirely different plant, included in recipes for ales.

It is generally thought that rosemary was either introduced, or re-introduced around 1340, when Queen Philippa, wife of Edward III, received plants from her mother, Countess Joan of Valois. The *Agnus Castus* herbal text as we read it is from the end of the fourteenth century and gives us the medicinal applications for Rosmarinus. This seems straightforward, but the common name of field madder sows doubt as to the identification. It is described as having leaves like lavender and a great stalk with many boughs and flowers, which might be the right herb but again the idea of digging the root to be held between the teeth for toothache and mixing the juice of rosemary with honey and applying it for sore eyes, makes it seem unlikely.[3]

In the collection of medieval remedies of the physicians of Myddfai, there is a long entry for rosemary. Much of what is written can also be found in the 1525 herbal below, but several recipes are different. Rosemary is decocted, the flowers distilled in wine or the bark used. The herb is recommended for a wide range of conditions from urinary obstructions and impotence, to intolerable skin irritation from

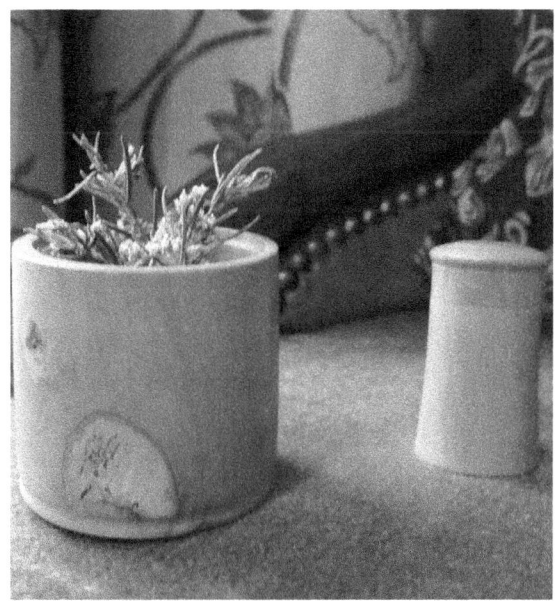

Boxes turned from rosemary wood.

a condition where clearly the kidneys are not functioning properly and toxins have built up in the blood. A lotion is also made to apply to the head for headache and insanity. The Welsh recipes appear to be slightly more elaborate and involve more internal remedies. Both have included the magical element, with rosemary as protector against evil dreams and this is extended to thunder and lightning by the physicians of Myddfai.[4]

Although the 1525 Herbal printed by Banckes usually follows the Agnus Castus both in the order of the herbs, and in much of what is said about them, with rosemary there is a big difference. The herb has one of the longest entries in Banckes, with initial emphasis on uses for the flowers. There are familiar ways of using rosemary. Then face wash and tooth powder are detailed. Rosemary is also prepared variously to treat coughs, gout, cankers, to regain a sense of smell, ease breathing, and act as a digestive. Not to mention the protection it could give against snakes and poisons. Here is rosemary in all its glory.[5]

Gerard writes of rosemary as we know it and names wild rosemary, which he says grows in Lancashire. Of rosemary he writes little compared to our last reference, emphasising the power of rosemary flowers to dry the brain, quicken the senses and memory, adding quotes on this from other sources, such as Serapio and the Arabian physicians.[6]

By Culpepers' day, 1652, he regards description of the plant as unnecessary for everyone knows it. He writes the sun claims the privilege of it and the herb is under the celestial Ram (Aries). He says it is very much used for inward and outward diseases to give warmth and comfort. This helped all cold diseases. Culpeper gives rosemary for dumb palsy, giddiness in the head, lethargy, and epilepsy. He also prescribes rosemary to aid the eyes, dim sight (eaten this time, not applied), weak memory, for problems with the stomach, spleen, bowels, and liver. He recommends the flowers and leaves for leucorrhoea in women and suggests smoking the leaves in a pipe in place of tobacco for coughs and consumption in the lungs. Lastly he refers to the chemical oil with a drop dosage, distilled from flowers and leaves.[7]

Rosemary is already appearing in every publication for the stillroom as well as the official Pharmacopoeias and was hugely popular in aromatic waters, especially after the high reputation of Queen of Hungary's Water made from the flowering tops became known. There is not space here to follow the many possible references. Having set the scene the history will now simply recount new information given.

Pechey repeats all the uses given by Culpeper in a very concise form, adding "The Herb burnt, corrects the Air, and renders it wholesome in the time of a Plague" (p.161). That the seed as well as the herb decocted, cures jaundice, and that "desperate and long Diarrhoea" (p.161) has been cured with rosemary wine.[8]

The *History of the Materia Medica* in 1751 points out that while rosemary conserve consists simply of rosemary petals and sugar, when making any other medicine with the herb, the term flower includes the calyx and young leaves immediately behind them. With another herb this would be classed as flowering tops. The conserve of the flowers, it states, is very proper for treating the head and it is an ingredient in a great many compositions in the (apothecary) shops. It is interesting that rosemary is listed under flowers in this work.

The antibacterial and aromatic power of rosemary took it in early times into use in vinegar. The vinegar of the four thieves who used it to cover their bodies as much inwardly and outwardly as possible to guard against plague as they robbed the houses of victims, contained rosemary. In later times, rosemary remained in aromatic vinegars, referred to as anti-putrid recipes and rosemary was an ingredient in smelling salts.[9]

Summary. The uses of rosemary have been remarkably consistent since the medieval period. The flowering tops in particular have been regarded as particularly effective in treating the head, brain, memory, and eyes. It has been seen as a warming, rejuvenating herb for treating all disease conditions coming from cold causes. Rosemary has been prescribed additionally to aid the digestive process, boosting circulation with effects on the stomach, liver, spleen, and bowel. The conserve of flower petals and sugar, rosemary wine, smoking the leaves, use of the distilled water and essential oil are some of the less usual ways the beneficial effects are gained. For the role of rosemary in modern herbal medicine, see Herbalists' Reference.

Recipe

Extracted from The Complete English Dispensatory. Quincy. 1736. "*Compound Powder of Rosemary Flowers.* Take of Rosemary Flowers, 1 ounce; of red

Roses and Liquorise, of each 6 drams, of Cloves, Spikenard, Nutmegs, Galangal, Cinnamon, Ginger, Zedoary, Mace, Aloes wood, the lesser Cardamoms, the Seeds of Dill, and Anise, of each 4 scruples, and make them into a Powder together."

This is originally ascribed to *Nicolaus* (of Salerno)... "It is certainly a very good Composition for all nervous Intentions... It is a great Strengthner of the Brain, and a good Preservative against those Distempers which Age is apt to bring upon it; as Apoplexies, Epilepsies, Palsies, Loss of memory, and the like. It greatly warms the Stomach and Bowels" (p.489).[10]

Notes

1. Gunther R.T. (ed), *Dioscorides Greek Herbal*. (Hafner. 1968). 321.
2. Pollington S. *Leechcraft*. (Anglo Saxon Books. 2000). 153.
3. Brodin G. *Agnus castus*. Upsala. (Harvard University Press. 1950). 201/02.
4. Pughe J. (trans), *The Herbal Remedies of the Physicians of Myddfai*. (Llanerch. 1989). 127–29.
5. Larkey S.V. (ed), *An Herbal* (1525), (Scholars Facsimiles and Reprints, New York. 1941). 69–71.
6. Johnson T. (ed), *The Herbal*. John Gerard. (1633 edition). (Dover Publications, New York. 1975). 1292–4.
7. Culpeper N. *Culpeper's Complete Herbal and English Physician enlarged*. (1652). (London. 1815 edition). 155/6.
8. Pechey J. *The English Herbal of Physical Plants*. (London. 1694). 160.
9. Piesse S.G. W. *The Art of Perfumery*. (1855). (Echo Library. 2007). 51–4.
10. Quincy J. MD. *A Complete Dispensatory*. (10th edition. 1736). 489.

ROSMARINUS OFFICINALIS – Herbalists' Reference

The Parts of Rosemary Used for Medicine – The flowers and leaves.

Dosage and Forms – Fluid extract. 1:1 in 45% alcohol. Dose 2–4ml three times daily. Tincture 1:2 15–30ml per week. Tea one teaspoon of dried herb per cup of boiling water, dose half to one cup. If using fresh herb, use one short terminal shoot, comparable to two teaspoons, pound it a little first to open the leaves. To make the wine. Two 10cm (4 inch) fresh terminal shoots of the herb steeped for four days in a bottle of white wine, half to one wineglass three times daily.

Constituents – The volatile oil contains 1.8 cineole, α-pinene, and camphor. Flavonoids include apigenin and diosmin. Phenols. Carvacrol, thymol and tannins. Salicylic acid.

Actions and Uses – Rosemary has multiple uses relating to its stimulant, circulatory tonic actions. In the digestive system, there are added benefits from the carminative and spasmolytic actions. Where a condition such as migraine produces headaches with a gastric origin, rosemary is able to address this, while as a nervine it also includes emotional factors. The herb is indicated in adrenal, spleen, and pancreatic deficiency (diabetes), and dyspeptic complaints. Rosemary aids the liver, since it is hepatoprotective and enhances phases I and II detoxification,[1] and may be helpful for patients suffering from gallstones through liver support and spasmolytic action.

The anti-inflammatory role is possibly due to the organic acids and apigenin. Strong anti-oxidant

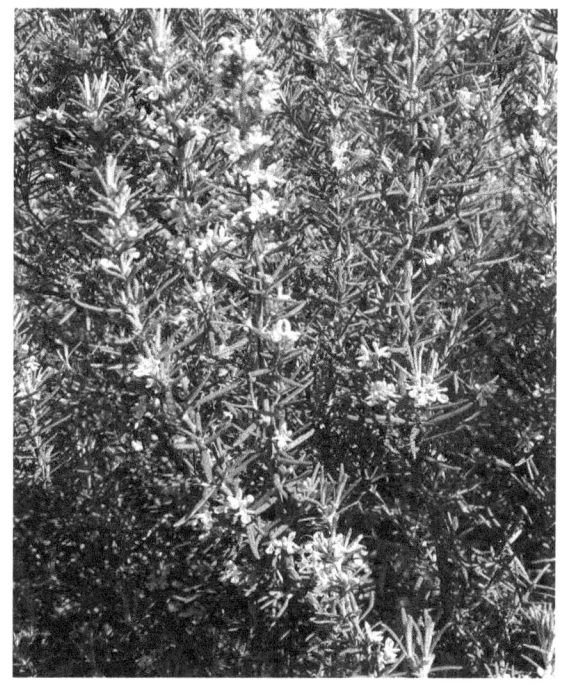

Flowers for harvest.

actions are attributed to phenolic diterpenes and rosmarinic acid. The herb is powerfully antibacterial and antifungal. The antibacterial and stimulant properties can be helpful in specific situations, such as where a limb is disabled by a stroke. For instance the patient's hand can be left as a closed fist that cannot be opened for washing. In an institutional environment the patient may be subjected to use of powerful antibacterials, even diluted bleach to clean the enclosed palm in such a situation. Rosemary introduced into the palm regularly is not only cleansing and antiseptic but encourages blood-flow in the affected part, with possible benefit in movement over time and is enjoyable for the patient.

Rosemary as a circulatory tonic in particular, is recommended for constitutional hypotension and has positive effects on coronary blood-flow, as well as circulation to the brain. It is valued for cardiac debility, fatigue, and chronic fatigue syndrome,[2] additionally increasing concentration and memory. The herb is regarded by numerous sources as possibly helpful in Alzheimers and mental depression. Rosemary contains diosmin as well as rosmarinic acid, and both have been linked to decreasing capillary permeability and fragility. It is indicated internally for varicose veins. Rosemary is used to treat oestrogen deficiency disorders and PMS with depression.[3] The stimulant action also applies to the uterine muscles.[4] Rosemary extract has shown promise in research for use in reversing multidrug resistance in mammary tumours and reducing the development of mammary cancer.[1]

Specific Indications – Depressive states with general debility and indications of cardiovascular weakness.[5]

Topical Applications – These may take several forms. Inhalations with other herbs for sinusitis or cautious use of the essential oil, which should never be applied neat to the skin. As a hand/footbath using a decoction of the herb or distilled aromatic water, in creams or ointments, to treat myalgia, sciatica, intercostal neuralgia, joint or muscular pain, palsy, and as an antiseptic for wound healing.

Interactions – There do not appear to be adverse effects or current drug interactions. Higher doses in an anti-cancer context may revise this.[6]

Precautions and Contraindications. Rosemary should not be prescribed in pregnancy and breast-feeding. Asthma and contact dermatitis have resulted from occupational exposure. Seizures have happened at high doses. Rosemary oil contains 20–50% camphor; given orally camphor readily causes convulsions when taken in sufficient quantity.[7] The herb, as well as the essential oil, is better avoided in inhalations and tea by epileptics and children subject to fitting.

Notes

1. Bone K. *A Clinical Guide to Blending Liquid Herbs*. (Churchill Livingstone. 2003). 391.
2. Bartram T. *Bartram's Encyclopedia of Herbal Medicine*. (Robinson. 1998). 376.
3. Holmes P. *The Energetics of Western Herbs*. Vol. 1&2.(Snow Press. Boulder. Revised 3rd edition. 1989). Vol. 1. 341.
4. Kelly W.J. (ed. director). *Nursing Herbal Medicine Handbook*. (Springhouse Corporation. 2001). 370.
5. *British Herbal Pharmacopoeia*. (British Herbal Medicine Association. 1983). 181.
6. Philp R.B. *Herbal-Drug Interactions and Adverse Effects*. (McGraw Hill. 2004). 218.
7. Barnes J. et al. *Herbal Medicines* (Pharmaceutical Press. 2nd edition. 2002). 406.

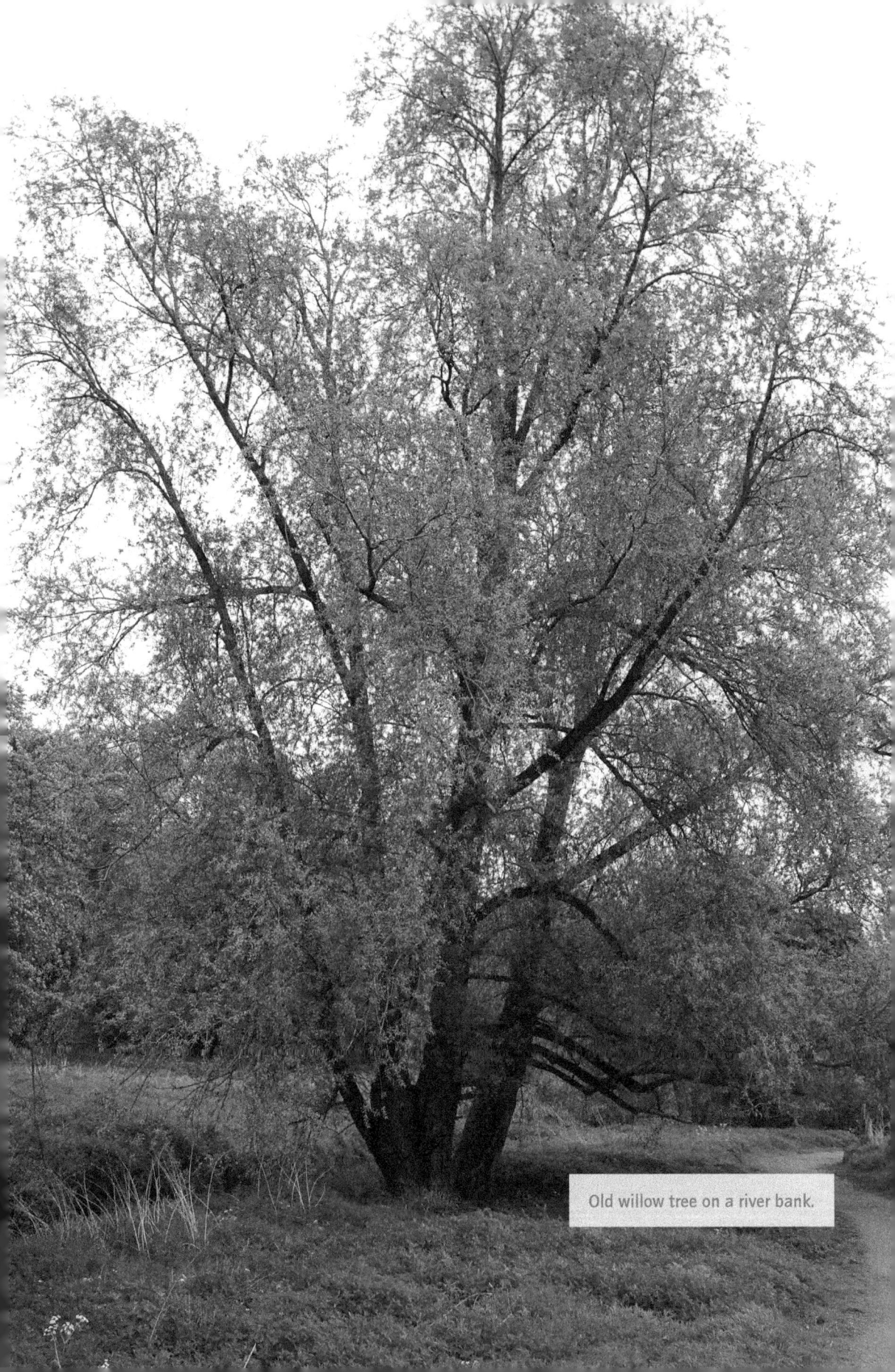

Old willow tree on a river bank.

Willow

Salix alba, *S. fragilis, S. Purpurea* – Willow – Salicaceae

WILLOW – Usefulness – Willow has been an important medicinal herb for treating pain and fevers since antiquity. A Bach flower remedy is made from yellow willow.[1] Growth hormone extract can be made from willow bark. The bark has also been used to tan leather and give a brown dye. Willow has supplied materials for sturdy baskets, especially those used beneath hot air balloons, coracle frames, hurdles, and wicker furniture throughout history. Garden structures are readily formed of the young growth. Timber of the white willow is used to make cricket bats. Willow wood supplies charcoal for medicine, burning perfumes and art.

Dangers – None known.

Getting to Know the Willow Tree – The name *Salix* comes from the Celtic *Sal-lis,* which means near water. This is certainly the perfect environment for willows and they are frequently found along river and canal banks. In these situations the white willow can become a sizeable tree with a potential height of twenty metres (sixty six feet), but is often seen leaning out over the water as the roots are compromised by proximity to the bank edge. It is a joy in April to see the new leaves and fluffy catkins appear. Male and female flowers are carried on the branches of separate trees. As is usual with trees, the female catkins are smaller. These have a nectar-producing gland, which draws in the bees and other insects.

S. fragilis is distinguished from the others by how readily the newest shoot breaks off, the other name for this variety being crack willow for the same reason. *S. purpurea* or the violet willow is a variety I was introduced to by my friend and colleague Anne Stobart at Holt Wood Medicinal forest. It is growing there in the valley bottom by water. She harvests bark for medicine from this willow as well as the *alba*. Violet willow had a special mention in the First World War instructions for gathering the bark for medicine. It was seen as especially helpful to collectors in remaining small enough to be more readily available for harvest.[2]

I learned basketry as a teenager going to classes with my mother. We each made baskets that are still in regular use half a century later. From the 1990s, I taught hedgerow basketry and planted a willow herbar in my garden to supply lengths both for stakes and weavers in the larger, heavy duty baskets. Although a herbar can mean a garden area planted with herbs, in the sixteenth century the term "upright herbar" was also applied to a covered alley. We used ours for playing Tudor skittles.

This project, based on instructions in Richard Mabey's edition of the earliest gardening book *The Gardener's Labyrinth* to use ashen or willow poles bound together with osiers to frame the herbar, proved the amazing resilience of this water-loving tree. The second-year growth poles, of *S. viminalis* brought from Somerset as the willow of choice for basketry, were planted to make the frame. These went into solid clay that was already quite dry. I wove younger willow lengths around the frame for about thirty-three centimetres (thirteen

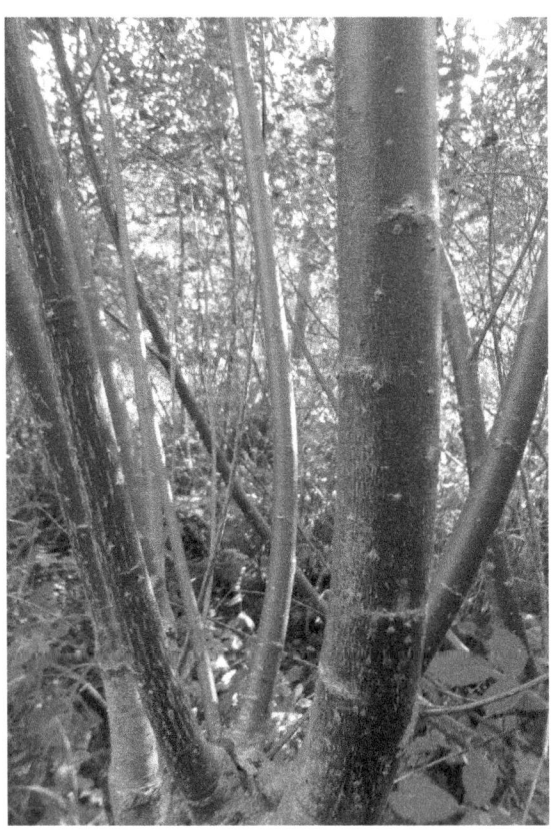

Violet willow. Photo courtesy Anne Stobart.

inches) at the base to give stability. It then did not rain for six weeks and I lost hope of my willow herbar coming to life. However after the first good shower the poles began to sprout leaves, and soon not only were there new shoots from the sides, but growth across the arched top, which took the height up another two and a half to three metres (eight to ten feet) each year. Instructions on building a similar herbar can be found in my earlier work, *Herb Sufficient*.

Not only did the herbar provide stakes and weavers for some forty baskets a year, but it gave a place to sit in welcome shade, which was two degrees cooler than on the lawn in summer. It was not altogether welcome that wasps also found this source of wood pulp handy for chewing to secrete material for their nests, but they generally kept to the outer shoots. Willow was the favourite food of the goat, who often looked on at basketry days at Butser Ancient Farm. She eagerly provided shredding services for any lengths left over at the end of the day, as fast as I could feed them into her mouth.

Other less ambitious garden structures are readily made of willow, but it should always be remembered that once in contact with the ground, willow will grow and grow. The seeds when they come from the fruits are tiny and seem almost superfluous when every stick of willow placed in the ground appears to shoot new growth almost immediately.

The best way to take a cutting of willow is to take it horizontally just below a bud. Willow has been grown as osiers to supply basketry and timber needs.

Talking to people coming round my teaching garden I learnt from a retired nurseryman that it is easy to take advantage of this hormonal growth drive in the willow. He instructed me in boiling willow bark and then simmering it until it was reduced down to one tenth of the former volume. A few drops can then be added to water in which cuttings are stood before planting,

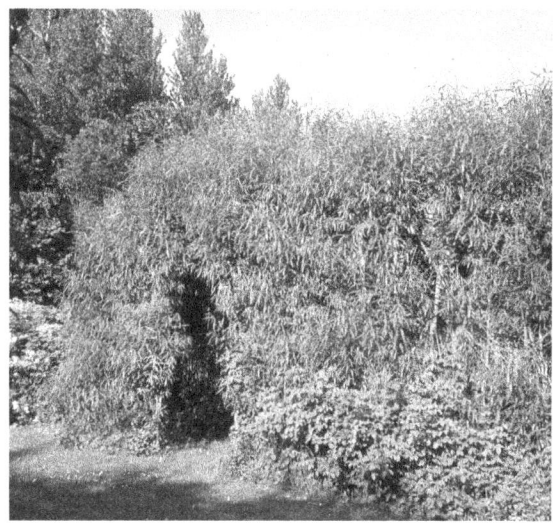

Willow herbar in my East Meon garden.

or used when watering young plants to encourage growth. I add a little essential oil of tea tree to the finished liquid as an antibacterial protection. Another gardening tip regarding willow comes from Sir Thomas Hanmer in the seventeenth century. He had evidently observed that when old willow trees begin to rot and break down, they provide fine compost for young tender seedlings. He recommended this mixed with sand for growing tulips, which were much valued at the time.

On historical workshops I have tutored we have used willow charcoal as an ingredient in pastilles for burning to perfume the air. The recipes have come both from the sixteenth and nineteenth centuries. Willow charcoal is preferred for medicinal purposes because it contains no harmful residues. It is absorbent and used not only internally for removing toxins from the system, but externally for dressing wounds. Willow bark also appears in old recipes for dandruff treatments and hair dyes. The hair dye was tested by willing participants on stillroom days.[3] This moderately successful experiment proved to be a great deal of fun. When dyeing with willow, the bark is the most popular material, although leaves and young branches of several varieties can be used, including goat willow. Different colours are achieved at different times of year. Bright purple dye from crack willow roots that often grow into the water has decorated Easter eggs in the past.

Legends and Folklore. Although willow has had an association with grief and mourning to my knowledge there is no original legend to account for this.

Notes

1. Weeks N. & Bullen V. *The Bach Flower Remedies.* (C. W. Daniel & Co. Ltd. 1990). 82.
2. Teetgen A.B. *Profitable Herb-Growing and Collecting.* (London.1916). 178.
3. Anon. *The Toilet of Flora.* (London. 1784). 10/11.

WILLOW – History of Medicinal Use

There is plentiful evidence of numerous species of willow being native to Britain, unfortunately identifying exactly which species is involved in the finds of charcoal or pollen is untrustworthy. Certainly a species of willow was used in building Iron Age dwellings at the Glastonbury Lake village.[1] The Ancient Egyptian records are a good source for early evidence of medicinal use. Willow leaves were used in several cooling, anti-inflammatory applications, together with other ingredients. The fruits of the willow were also included in an anti-inflammatory unguent.[2] Another example of an unidentified willow (*S. safsaf*) this time being given internally was in the Ebers Papyrus and was recommended "to cause the heart to receive bread"(p.158).[3]

The Greek writer Dioscorides writes of using the fruit, leaves, bark, and juice of Salix species in the first century. Egyptian recipes are echoed by a recipe for griefs of the ears, administering the warmed juice of the leaves and bark.[4]

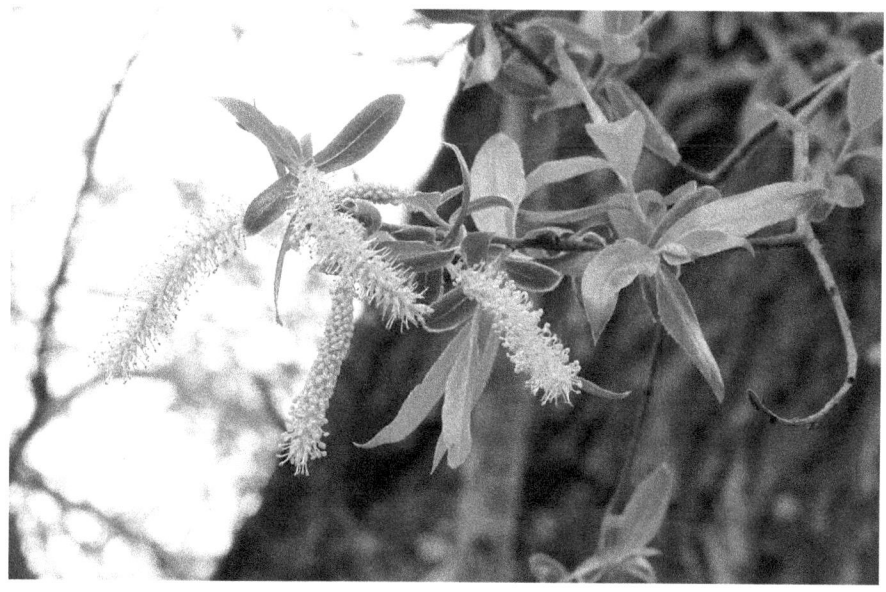

Flowering in spring.

In the Anglo-Saxon Leechbooks willow only appears twice, once in the *Lacnunga* and once in *Bald*. Both references are to treat pain, although in the first it is one of many ingredients. It would be tempting to make a connection with willow as a source of the building blocks of aspirin, but that is not necessarily valid here. Constantine, the African who translated Greek, Roman, and Arabic medicine and was associated with the School of Medicine in Salerno in the eleventh century, included a contraceptive recipe of willow leaf juice in his pharmacy. This had been adapted from an earlier Arabic recipe, and certainly willow leaves had appeared in contraceptive recipes several centuries earlier.[5]

Formularies of the continental medieval surgeons, Henri de Mondeville [1260–1320] and Jehan Yperman [1260–1330], used tree bark and flowers of *S. alba* and *S. niger*. Willow was classed as cleansing, repressive, and resolutive.[6] Gerard's Herbal takes the cooling aspect of willow to extreme, suggesting laying branches of willow around the sickbeds of fevered patients to cool the air. Culpeper continues the references to cooling by classifying willow as owned by the moon. He writes of several previous uses, staunching bleeding, sap for dim sight, bark to remove corns and warts and leaves or bark in wine against dandruff. Culpeper repeats Dioscorides recipe for the leaves in wine with pepper, as well as placing boughs of the tree in the sick chamber. He then adds, a drink made of the leaves boiled in wine "stays the heat of lust in man or woman, and quite extinguishes it, if it be long used" (p.192).[7]

Coles especially recommends the catkins for staunching blood, otherwise he gives mostly the same information seen in Culpeper a few years before. However, he adds another use from Dioscorides, this being that decoctions of the bark and leaves in wine are good for the sinews and to treat gout as well as to cleanse the head of scurf. Just fifty years later it seems the practice of laying boughs of trees around sickbeds has stopped, for Miller records simply that it was a practice of the "antients" (p.385). He recommends the sap once again for inflamed and bloodshot eyes.[8]

In America in 1785, Cutler shared an account from the *Transactions of the Royal Society. England. 1763*[9] by the Rev. Stone, of the great efficacy of white willow bark in curing intermittent fevers. The Rev.

Stone had gathered the bark in summer and dried it by gentle heat. He administered the powder every few hours. Cutler goes on to say that physicians in the United States have tried this, mainly using the bark of the roots.[9] Reaction to Rev. Stone's claims in England is given in Meyrick's herbal in 1790. He quotes Dr. William Withering who views this as a blessing since the current use of Peruvian bark for treating fevers was very high and this resulted in a high price and adulteration with other barks. Withering hoped this success would be proved on a larger scale.[10] William Woodville, writing five years later, does not seem particularly impressed by this account when he considers *S. fragilis*, and gives his opinion that *S. triandria* is more effective.[11]

In 1810 Thornton also writes of *S. fragilis*, quoting Woodville, but pointing out that several other willows, including *S. alba* have the same properties. He quotes Dr. Closs successfully using willow to treat fevers, and Haller as dipping weakly infants in a decoction of the bark with much success.[12] Twelve years later Waller repeats the astringent and febrifuge uses. This is followed by the interesting reference to the "antients" (p.357) use for destroying the ability to have children. He quotes Etmuller who he gathers believed that all procreative powers in either sex would be destroyed if use persisted. He then states although this belief has existed for such a long time, there does not appear to be the slightest foundation for it.[13]

Salicin was identified in 1828 by Buchnerin and in America in 1892 it was commented that salicin seemed to have a more thorough and effective action than the bark.[9] Salicin given alone at that time still caused serious side effects however. A safer form, aspirin, was not available to patients until 1899.[15] Still, willow bark was collected from half a dozen species of willows during the First World War for medicinal use.[15]

Summary. For much of the medicinal history of willow, the uses for relieving pain and fever that we associate with willow today were apparently not discovered, or little used. The astringency of the tannins to stop bleeding made willow a wound herb, and a marked cooling effect of the leaves in decoctions was appreciated in many treatments. The anti-inflammatory properties were used in ancient Egypt, but seem to appear later mostly in treatments for the eyes and ears. Treating dandruff, corns, and discussion of the contraceptive possibilities appear regularly over centuries. Prescribing for fevers begins around the 1760s and with the isolation of salicin and subsequent development of aspirin in the following century, willow is superseded by the drug. The herb is however still a valued herb in the herbalists' dispensary. See Herbalists' Reference.

Recipe

Extracted from A Leechbook of the XVth Century. "*441.* Hair, to make it grow. Sethe leaves of withy with oil and lay [it] where the hair is wanting." (p.149).

"1026. For ache that swelleth. Take the leaves of alder, the leaves of white willow, and the leaves of poplar, and boil them in running water a mileway.[1] Then take them out and grind them in a mortar, and fry it with swine's grease, and make thereof a plaster, and lay it all hot to the sore" (p.313).[16] 1. A mileway refers to the time taken to walk a mile at a brisk pace—20 minutes.

Notes

1. Coles J. & Minitt S. *Industrious and Fairly Civilized.* (Somerset Levels Project. 1995). 104.
2. Manniche L. *An Ancient Egyptian Herbal.* (British Museum Press. 1989). 70, 137, 145/6.
3. Nunn J.F. *Ancient Egyptian Medicine.* (British Museum Press. 2000). 152, 158.
4. Gunther R.T. (ed), *Dioscorides Greek Herbal.* (Hafner. 1968). 75.
5. Riddle J.M. *Eve's Herbs.* (Harvard University Press. 1997). 61.
6. Rosenman Leonard D. MD. *A Medieval Surgical Pharmacopoeia and Formulary.* 1170–1325. (San Francisco. 1999). 66.
7. Culpeper N. *Culpeper's Complete Herbal and English Physician enlarged.* (1652). (London. 1815 edition). 192.
8. Miller J. *Botanicum officinale.* Bell. (London. 1722). 386.
9. Erichson-Brown C. *Medicinal and other uses of North American Plants.* (Dover Publications. 1979). 92.
10. Meyrick W. *The New Family Herbal.* (Birmingham. 1790). 465.
11. Woodville W. *Medical Botany.* 3 vols + Supplement. (London. 1790). Vol.3. 543.

12. Thornton R.J. *A New Family Herbal.* (London. 1810). 830.
13. Waller J. *Waller's New British Domestic Herbal.* Cox & Son. (London. 1822). 357.
14. Sumner J. *The Natural History of Medicinal Plants.* (Timber Press. 2000). 135.
15. Teetgen A.B. *Profitable Herb-Growing and Collecting.* (London. 1916). 177/8.
16. Dawson W. (ed), *A Leechbook of the XVth Century.* (Macmillan & Co. 1934). 149. (441), 313. (1026).

SALIX ALBA & S.SPP. FRAGILIS, PURPUREA, NIGRA – Herbalists' Reference

The Parts of Willow Used for Medicine – Bark from trees two to three years old is collected in spring.[1] Leaves and young twigs gathered in spring.

Dosage and Forms – Decoction—2–3g finely chopped or coarsely powdered bark to 150–250ml cold water, simmering time 5 minutes. Give three to four times daily. Fluid extract 1:1 in 25% alcohol, dose 1–3ml three times daily. Tincture 1:5 25% 5–8ml three times daily. Syrup, medicinal wine.

Constituents – Salicylates calculated as salicin vary between species, *S. alba*, *S. fragilis*, *S. purpurea* and *S. daphnoides*. Salicin is a pro-drug that is metabolised to saligenin in the GI tract and to salicylic acid after absorption.[2] Flavonoids, lignin, tannins, resin.

Actions and Uses – The anti-inflammatory, antiprostaglandin, antiseptic, and analgesic properties from salicylic acid make Salix a herb of choice for treating inflammation, infection, and pain. The inhibition of cyclooxygenase (COX)[3] gives treatment usage ranging from headaches and earaches through sciatica and tendonitis to menstrual pain and migraines. Salix may be considered to have particular use as an antirheumatic for muscular rheumatism, osteoarthritis, and gout.

A mild diaphoretic and febrifuge, willow also helps to lower fevers, being valued in treating colds and influenza. The tannins give useful astringency aiding in healing ulcerations, burns, and wounds. It is stated that salicylic acid does not have the anti-platelet properties of aspirin, as the acetyl group in aspirin is not present in Salix. It is therefore not useful for cardiovascular patients to reduce the risk of heart attack.[4] Some

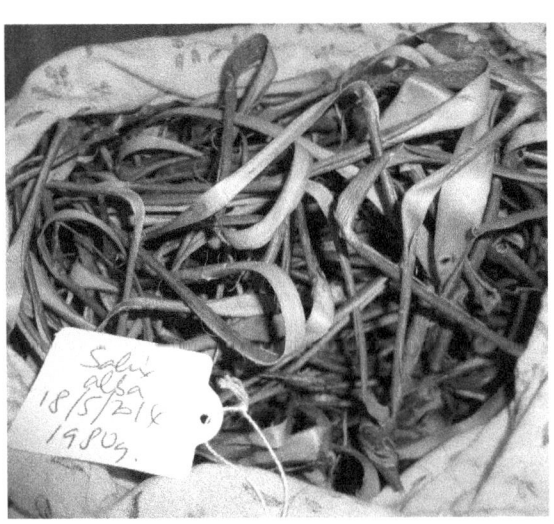

Harvested bark. Photo courtesy Anne Stobart.

herbalists suggest combining willow with other herbs for this but I have not seen clinical evidence of success.

Sedative properties of Salix are helpful for insomnia and it is also given to reduce sexual overstimulation. Historically the flowers or catkins were given for the last use, confirmed in the twentieth century.[5] White and black willows are apparently anaphrodisiac and may be considered contraceptive.

Specific Indications – Rheumatoid arthritis and inflammation in connective tissue disorders.[6]

Topical Applications – A decoction may be added to hot baths to relieve pain and fever. Bark that is first macerated in vinegar can be applied to remove corns and hard skin.[7]

Combinations – With Calendula and Boswellia or Guaiacum for severe rheumatic pain.

Interactions – There is the potential for enhancement of the effects of other NSAIDs, barbiturates and sedatives.

Side Effects – On theoretical grounds these are as for salicylates in aspirin.

Contraindications and Precautions – Care with patients who have salicylate sensitivity. – this may be more likely in asthma patients. Discouraged in breast-feeding as salicylates are transferred in breast milk.[8]

Notes

1. Stobart A. *The Medicinal Forest Garden Handbook*. (Permanent Publications. 2020). 210.
2. Barnes J. et al. *Herbal Medicines* (Pharmaceutical Press. 2nd edition. 2002). 485.
3. Philp R.B. *Herbal-Drug Interactions and Adverse Effects*. (McGraw Hill. 2004). (Phytother. Res. 2001;15:344. Quote). 256.
4. Mills S. & Bone K. *Principles & Practice of Phytotherapy*. (Churchill Livingstone. 2000). 25.
5. Holmes P. *The Energetics of Western Herbs*. Vol. 1&2.(Snow Press. Boulder. Revised 3rd edition. 1989). Vol. 2. 659.
6. *British Herbal Pharmacopoeia*. (British Herbal Medicine Association. 1983). 185.
7. Chiej R. *The Macdonald Encyclopedia of Medicinal Plants*. (Macdonald Publishing. London. 1984). (271).
8. Mills S. & Bone K. *The Essential Guide to Herbal Safety*. (Elsevier Churchill Livingstone. 2005). 627.

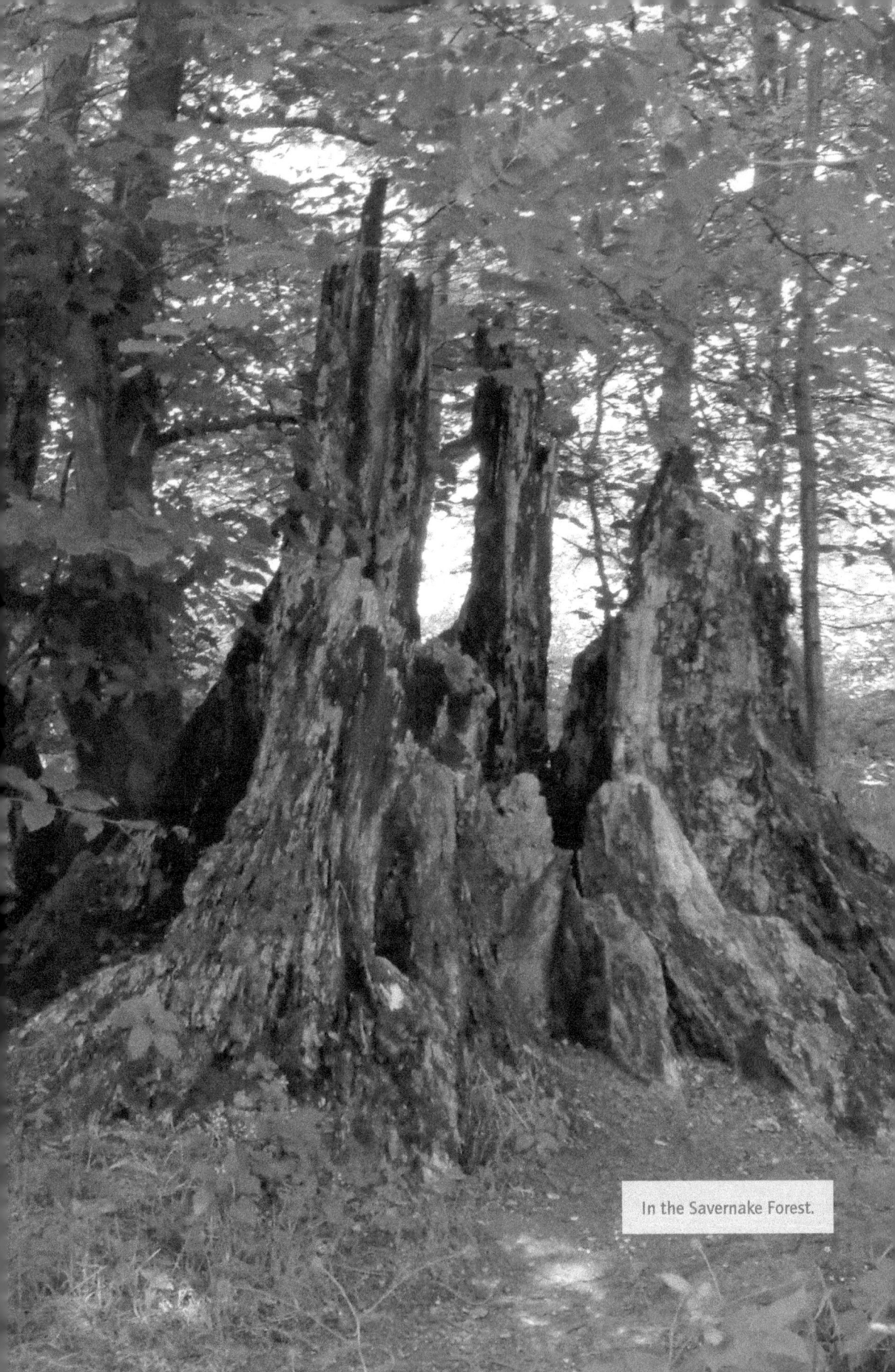
In the Savernake Forest.

SUMMER

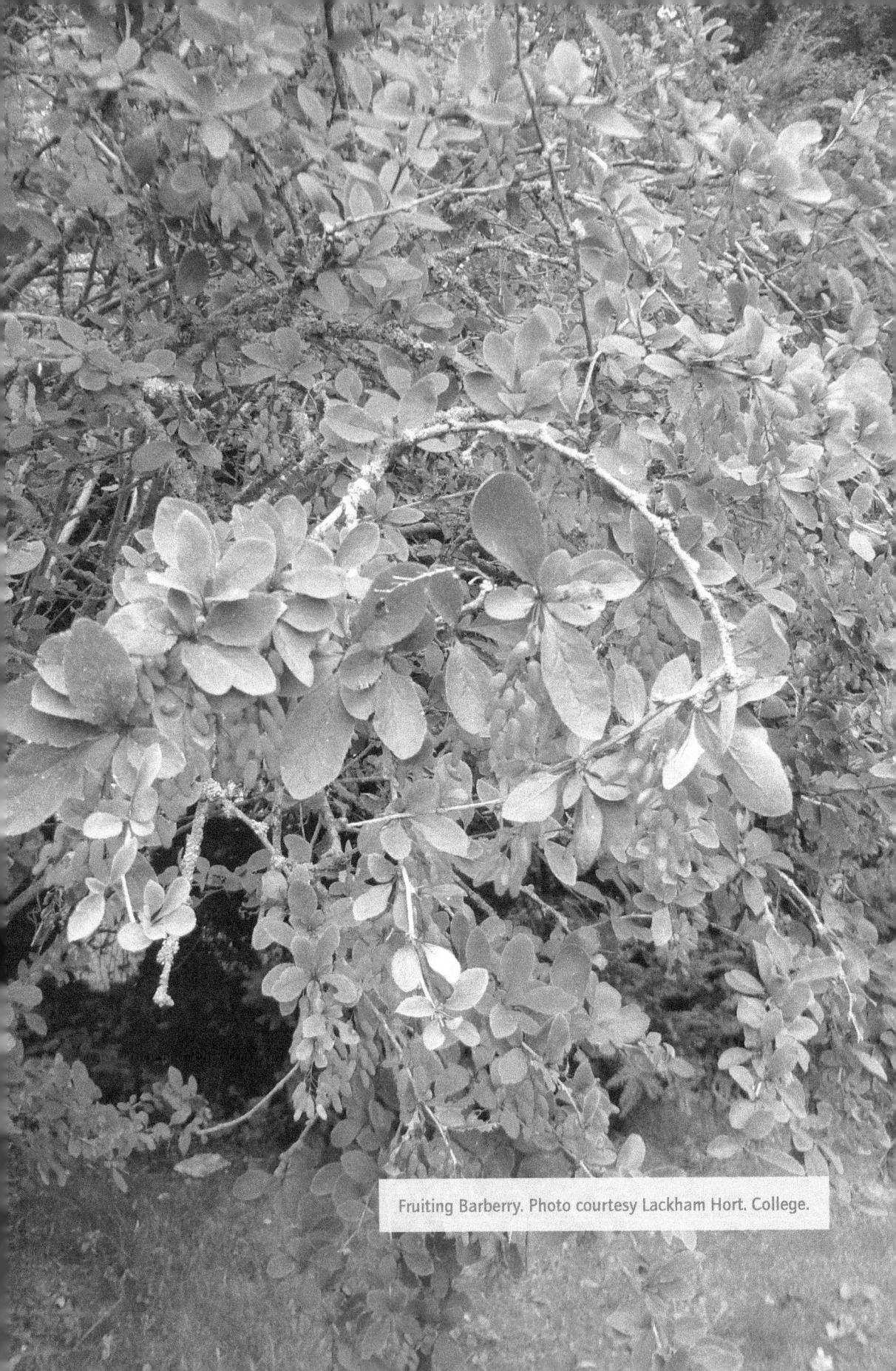

Fruiting Barberry. Photo courtesy Lackham Hort. College.

Barberry

Berberis vulgaris – Barberry – Berberidaceae

BARBERRY – Usefulness – Bark from the root or trunk is gathered in autumn and contains medicinally valuable berberine. The leaves, which also have medicinal properties, are gathered in summer. The leaves were used as a seasoning and the berries make a zingy preserve, syrup, and comfit sweets. Wine can be made from them. Roots and bark of the stem give an impressive bright yellow dye for fabrics and leather.

Dangers – While *Berberis vulgaris* has leaves, berries, and seeds free of alkaloids and harmless fruits rich in vitamin C, fruits of other *Berberis* species are presumed to contain the alkaloids, including berberine and are not safe to eat.[1]

Getting to Know the barberry Tree – The common barberry *Berberis vulgaris* is native to south-west Asia, northern Africa and much of Europe, including Britain. Years ago, having read so many recipes for barberry jellies, syrup, pickles, conserves, and sweets while researching historical recipes, I was surprised to find I had never seen a wild tree. It was clear from herbals and stillroom books that barberries were considered on a level of importance with raspberries, apricots, and other fruits in the past and yet they were nowhere to be seen.

In fact they were sufficiently important to have been one of the first fruit trees to be sent to the New World for settlers to use both for food and medicine. In 1759 the American barberry, *Berberis canadensis*, was shipped to Britain.[2] I have commonly seen Berberis shrubs covered in yellow berries in gardens, but these were clearly not the barberry trees I was reading about.

I could, and did, buy barberry bark both from dye and herbal suppliers and found dried barberries for sale in the supermarket, but the trees were almost nowhere to be seen in Hampshire or Wiltshire. A single tree gave me my first observations at the Chiltern Museum when I was taking workshops there. The reason for this mass disappearance from the countryside of a tree that once was familiar in the hedgerows was the reaction of farmers who suspected the barberry to be contributing to the ruin of their wheat if growing within a few hundred yards of it. They began taking action in the eighteenth century. William Woodville mentions this in his book *Medical Botany* in 1790. Then came the discovery in 1865 that barberry actually was host to the fungus *Puccinia graminis*, which caused a black stem rust on wheat.[3] Bushes were removed wholesale in wheat growing areas of England, and other countries.

Now that wheat has been grown to be resistant to the rust the barberry can be encouraged to return. This would also be helpful to the survival of the barberry carpet moth *Pareulype berberata*, as the caterpillars feed on the leaves. The barberry may still be found in certain areas of England, Wales and Scotland.

Although considered by some to be a shrub, the tree can be the same height as an elder but often has numerous stems rather than a thick trunk. The bark is grey with bright yellow colouring just below the surface, due to the content of berberine. The branches have thorn-like spines and tend to be brittle, meaning care needs to be taken when picking the fruit. Dorothy Hartley in *Food in England*[4] suggests helpfully that the clusters of berries, which hang together along the stem rather in the way of bunches of grapes, should be cut away with scissors and allowed to fall into a jar held below to catch them.[4] This works well. Advice to Elizabethan gardeners was to place the barberry in hedges with hawthorn and brambles to make a thickset thorny hedge to keep out animals and intruders.

The flowers are out in late April or early May and look rather like soft yellow balls, dangling in long, pretty but barely scented spikes. The stamens in the flowers are sensitive to touch, waiting as they must for a bee to arrive. At the slightest contact the anther strikes against the stigma, releasing pollen which then sticks to the female stigma. The oval pale green leaves are tooth-edged and grow in clusters often with groups of five, some larger than the others, rather as if someone had held them together and pinned them on as a decoration.

The fruit ripens in September, each berry containing two seeds. The long, red berries appear rather like capsules, which seems appropriate when they contain so much Vitamin C. The berries are extremely tart and so the birds generally leave them to eat other fruits first. Sufficiently sweetened, however they can be made into tasty preserves. As may be imagined from the nature of the whole tree, the leaves are also tart and have been eaten as a substitute for sorrel.

When editing and making recipes from Lady Anne Blencowe's Receipt Book dated 1694, I found her recipes for barberries produced elegantly presented preserves. She gives instructions to take bunches of them and boil them with sugar "till ye barberryes look very cleare & shine & look of pure scarlet colwer" (p.46).[5] Syrup made of more barberries is then poured over. She also makes drop jelly sweets of the pulp with sugar which could be set to decorate rich, sweet desserts.[5]

Recipes from other books that followed in the eighteenth century have a similar pattern and also give barberries covered with a white wine vinegar and salt pickle. "Barberrie wine" appears in another collection of recipes, in this five gallons of wine is made from ten pounds of sugar and ten quarts of barberries. There is a note below pointing out that the same recipe can be used for raspberries, which would need a pound less sugar than the barberries.[6]

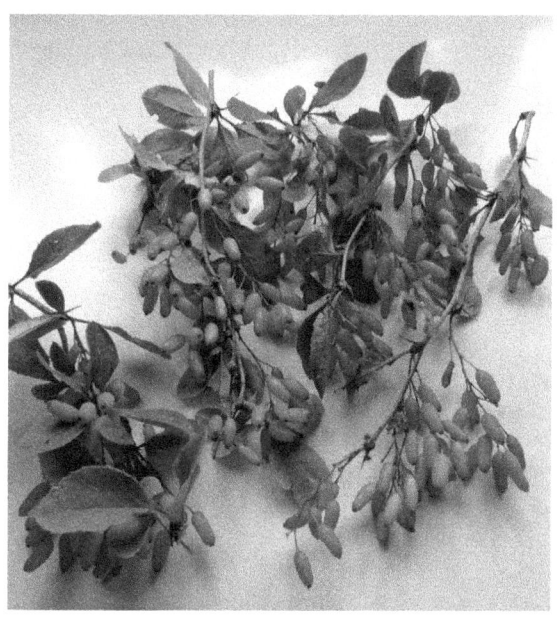

Ripe Barberry fruits.

Many barberry recipes come from an era when the wealthy ate a particularly sweet and fatty diet and the tartness of barberries was perfect to provide the sour element to cut through the sweet richness. In modern times the ground, dried berries can be used to season rich foods in a similar way.

Legends and Folklore. I have not found any legends or superstitions connected with the barberry tree.

Notes

1. Fröhne D. Pfander H. *A Colour Atlas of Poisonous Plants.* (Wolf Science. 1983). 70.
2. Campbell-Culver M. *The Origin of Plants.* (Headline Book Publishing. 2001). 168.
3. Rackham O. *The History of the Countryside.* (Phoenix Paperback. 1986). 42/3.
4. Hartley D. *Food in England.* (Futura Publications. 1985). 437.
5. Stapley C. (ed), *The Receipt Book of Lady Anne Blencowe.* (Heartsease Books. 2004). 46, 53.
6. Lewer H.W. (ed), *A Book of Simples.* (1700–1750). (London. 1908). 135. (367).

BARBERRY – History of Medicinal Use

Although barberry trees are considered to be native and historically were common in hedgerows and on chalky scrublands, the first mention of the tree for medicine appears to be in the Pharmacopoeia of Paul of Aegina who lived in the seventh century. Medieval surgeons applied the fruits topically on swellings to cool and dry the tissues. Barberry trees were expected to be planted in Elizabethan gardens, as shown in Richard Mabey's edition of Hill's first gardening book. Not entirely for their fruits or medicinal advantages however, as the seeds were to be placed along with those of gooseberry bushes, brambles and haws to grow a thorny and productive hedge.

The barberry was especially recommended as the herb to treat jaundice. Roots of barberry are bright yellow, which brought this herb in agreement with the doctrine of signatures followed at this time that coupled yellow flowered or berried plants with treating the liver and gall bladder.

In *Culpeper's English Physician enlarged* there are recipes for four troches, each containing barberries to treat the digestion. Of the Troches of Barberries he wrote, "They wonderfully cool the heat of the liver, reins, and bladder, breast, and stomach, and stop looseness, cools the heat of fevers"(347).[1] Barberry fruit had been classified as mildly cooling and drying in earlier centuries, however, by this time it had won a place as a cooling and moistening medicine.

Coles begins a long piece on the barberry by explaining the English name of barberry is derived from the Arabic name that Avicenna used for the tree. This was

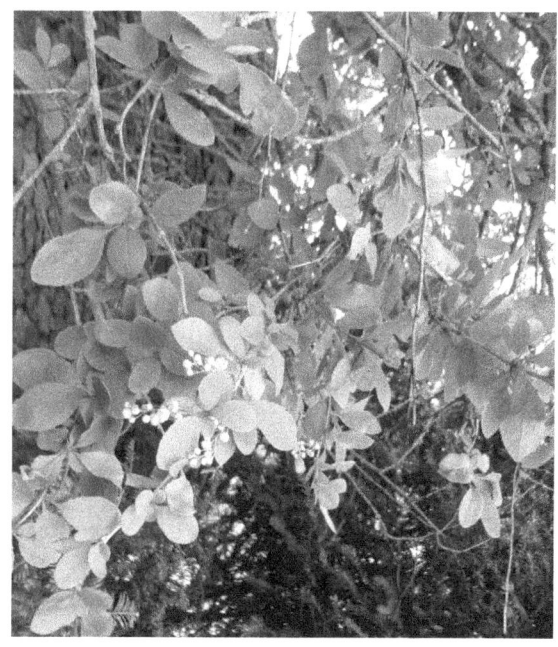

Flowering Barberry. Photo courtesy Lackham Hort. College.

Amyrberis, which referred to the berries. He adds that the barberry can be found across Europe to Austria and then recommends a decoction of the leaves to cool burns and heat from the blood and liver in fevers. While noting the astringency of the fruits, he repeats use of the bark of the roots for jaundice, adding that the green barberry leaf sauce represses sour belching of choler. William Coles specifies it particularly for fevers that have come from "Chollerick and pestilential Vapors" (p.273).[2]

He offers us instructions for giving the tart juice to stimulate appetite. I cannot help thinking that it would be kinder to take it in syrup of violets, which is an alternative. Taken with a little southernwood and sugar it was recommended to kill worms in the body. Coles dissolved the conserved juice of the fruits in water and a little vinegar to make a gargle. He prescribed this to cool inflammations in the mouth and throat. Lastly he refers to the yellow of the branches and roots and relates this to the doctrine of signatures and success in treating jaundice.[2]

In 1694, Pechey repeats these uses in his herbal. By 1722 after a good description of the tree and account of similar uses of the bark, Joseph Miller writes that the only officinal preparation for sale in the apothecary shops is the conserve of the fruit.[3] An Irish herbal a few years later gives the inner bark only for jaundice and the fruits for diarrhoea.[4]

With the profusion of household receipt or recipe books in the eighteenth century there are many recipes for pickling or preserving barberries in sugar, but medicinal recipes also appear. In eighteenth century household collections, there are recipes for preserving the fruits, barberry wine and in one a long and complex recipe which is to be distilled. This was for treating yellow jaundice, colic, obstructions of the liver and spleen, consumption and especially the falling sickness, which we now know as epilepsy. It is clear that the barberry roots, along with agrimony, turmeric, and saffron were aimed at treating the liver, spleen and colic.[5]

At the end of the century, the young surgeon Robert Meyrick quotes both the Egyptian use of the diluted juice of the berries, taken from Alpinus and Ray's recommendation for a decoction in ale of the inner bark as a gentle purge in jaundice. He comments that the acidity of the berries is such that birds refuse to feed on them, a sweet jelly being necessary to enjoy them. He gives us a lotion from the decocted bark to treat itchy skin eruptions.[6]

William Woodville was also writing at this time and was disparaging about the singular efficacy of the berries, writing they were no better than other acidic fruits. He gives this reason as accounting for the Colleges of Physicians both in London and Edinburgh removing the barberry from the Materia medica.[7] However, in 1810 Thornton supports the herb again quoting Alpinus using barberry against the plague, also Pauli in a malignant fever and J. Bauhin for dysentery. He then gives a recipe for barberry jam.[8] Waller in 1822 is also positive in his comments, writing that barberries can be made into comfits, syrup, jelly, and jam which can then be dissolved into drinks. These he recommends for all fevers, especially typhus.[9]

Summary. Use of barberry root bark has been continuous and consistent in treating the liver, spleen, jaundice, and bilious colic, since the sixteenth century. The leaves have been employed for their cooling action when eaten or taken in sauces. The acidic nature of the berries recommended them for cooling fevers, relieving thirst and stimulating appetite. A sugar conserve of the fruit was sold in apothecary shops in the eighteenth century and the juice given with southernwood and sugar to kill intestinal worms.

Although the barberry passed out of favour in mainstream medicine at the end of the nineteenth century, herbalists continued to use the root and berries. In the First World War *Berberis vulgaris* was listed among herbs to be gathered for homoeopathic medicine, while *Berberis aquifolium* is a related species, also recorded for herbalist use. Today this is more familiar to the general public as Oregon grape or Mahonia. In general medicine, the salts of the main alkaloid in the barberry, berberine, have been preferred.[10]

Recipes

Extracted from A Collection of Receipts. 1746. "*A very pleasant* Posset *in a* Fever. Put two Ounces of Preserv'd Barberries into one Quart of Milk; let it boil, and strain it; drink when you are thirsty." p.263.[11]

Notes

1. Culpeper N. Culpeper's Complete Herbal and English Physician enlarged. (1652). (London. 1815 edition). 347.
2. Coles W. The Paradise of Plants. (London. 1657). 272–4.
3. Miller J. Botanicum officinale. Bell. (London. 1722). 84.
4. Scott. M. (ed), *An Irish Herbal.* K'Eogh. (1735). (Aquarian. 1986). 26.
5. Lewer H.W. (ed), *A Book of Simples.* [from 1700–1750]. (Sampson Low, Marston & Co. Ltd. 1908). 113, (318), 135, (367), 192 (526).
6. Meyrick R. The New Family Herbal. (Birmingham. 1790). 27.
7. Woodville W. *Medical Botany.* 3 vols + Supplement. (London. 1790). Supplement. Part 2. 62.
8. Thornton R.J. *A New Family Herbal.* (London. 1810). 360.
9. Waller J. *Waller's New British Domestic Herbal.* Cox & Son. (London. 1822). 23.
10. Todd. R.G. (ed), *Extra Pharmacopoeia Martindale.* 25th edition. (Pharmaceutical Press. 1967). 617.
11. Anon. *A Collection of Receipts.* (Printed for the Executrix of Mary Kettilby. 1746). 263.

BERBERIS VULGARIS – Herbalists' Reference

The Part of the Barberry Tree Used for Medicine – Bark of the root is preferred as it is higher in alkaloids, but the stem bark is the sustainable option. Either would be harvested in late autumn. Leaves are taken in May or June and the green or ripe fruits gathered in August or September.

Dosage and Forms – Tea: 1 teaspoon to a cup of cold water, either left to steep overnight, or brought to the boil and left for ten to fifteen minutes, dosage ½–1 cup three times daily. Tincture 1.5 in 25–45% alcohol. Dose 0.5–0.75ml only.

Constituents – Root and stem bark: isoquinoline alkaloids, the chief being berberine, oxyacanthine, essential oil, resin and tannins.

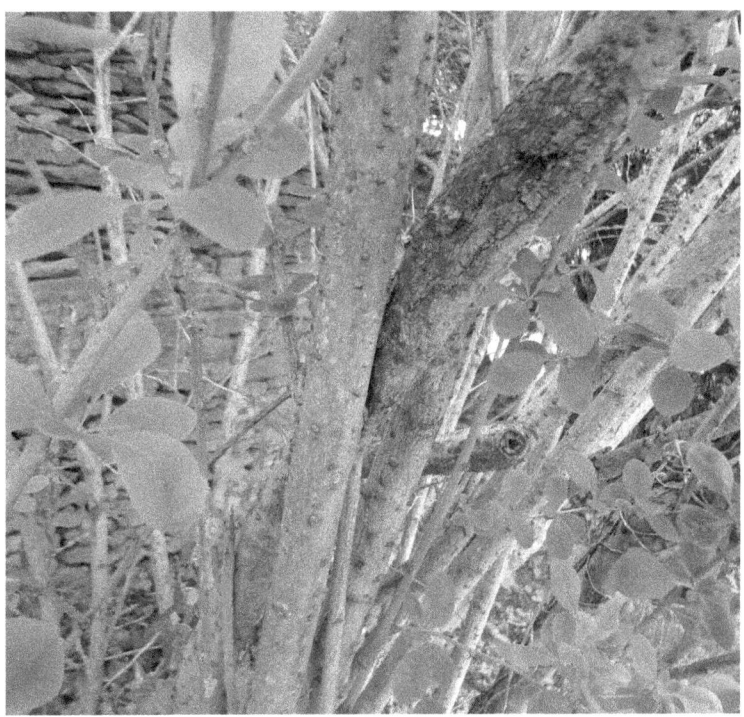

Barberry bark. Photo courtesy Lackham Hort. College.

Leaves: berberine and organic acids. Fruits sugars, gum, pectin, citric, malic and tartaric acid.

Actions and Uses – Since berberine acts strongly against protozoal infection,[1] barberry is used to treat leishmania and giardiasis. It is given in candidiasis and as an anti-microbial. Berberine also kills helicobacter pylori giving it an application in the digestive system in an anti-ulcer role. More than this it is a bitter tonic to the liver and spleen both as a cholagogue and stimulus of splenic contractions. As a digestive tonic it may be applicable in anorexia.

Barberry is anti-emetic and supports the pancreas, also balancing oestrogen levels through action in the liver and large intestine.[2] The range of uses encompasses jaundice, gastritis, gallstones, adjuvant therapy for type two diabetes, metabolic toxicosis, and infectious diarrhoea. Further uses in the urinary system and for discharges make this herb extensive in its range. The astringency and complex action on the smooth muscle of the arteries results in vasodilation.[3] The herb treats varicose veins, haemorrhoids, and heavy periods. In addition small doses stimulate the respiratory system.[4]

Combinations – When treating gall bladder disease barberry combines well with *Chionanthus* and *Leptandra virginica.*[5]

Interactions – Berberine may reinforce the effects of drugs which displace the protein binding action of bilirubin.[6]

Contraindications and Precautions – Caution in acute liver disease, liver cancer intestinal spasm, and unconjugated hyperbilirubinaemia. In large doses, berberine may cause dyspnoea, skin, eye, and gastrointestinal irritation with nausea. Not to be used in pregnancy, when breast feeding or for jaundiced neonates without medical advice.[7]

Notes

1. Buhner S.H. *Herbal Antibiotics* (Storey Books. 1999). 38.
2. Crockett L. *Healing Our Hormones Healing Our Lives.* (John Hunt Publishing O Books. 2009). 170.
3. Barker J. *The Medicinal Flora of Britain and Northwestern Europe.* (Winter Press. 2001). (70).
4. Kelly W.J. (ed. director). *Nursing Herbal Medicine Handbook.* (Springhouse Corporation. 2001). 40.

5. Hoffmann D. *The New Holistic Herbal.* (Element. 1990). 143.
6. Bone K. *A Clinical Guide to Blending Liquid Herbs.* (Churchill Livingstone. 2003). 88.
7. Mills S. & Bone K. *The Essential Guide to Herbal Safety.* (Elsevier Churchill Livingstone. 2005). 256.

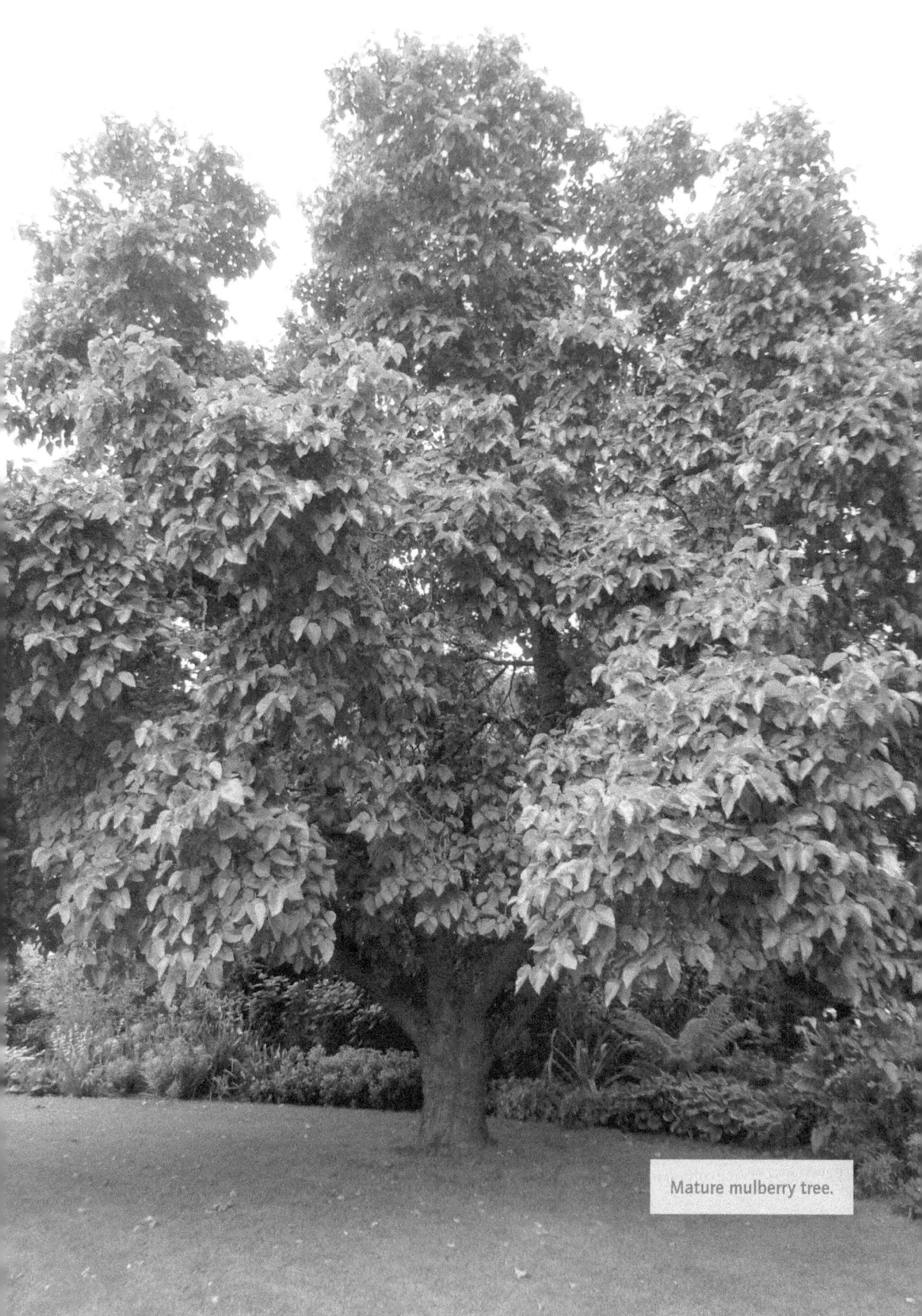

Mature mulberry tree.

Black Mulberry

Morus nigra – Black Mulberry – Moraceae

MULBERRY TREE – *Usefulness* – The soft, rich fruits are delicious as a food. The black mulberry fruit can be larger than that of the white mulberry. The fruits as juice or syrup, leaves and root-bark can be used for medicine. Mulberry wine is made from the fruits. The fruit also gives a good dark red dye. The violet coloured juice was included in turnsole used to colour medieval food, paintings, and manuscripts. The white mulberry leaves are superior as a food for silkworms, but the black mulberry leaves were reported to have been given successfully in Persia.[1] In Greece the black mulberry leaves have also fed silkworms.[2] The dark, sweetly scented wood has been used to make wine casks, it can be turned and used for veneers and marquetry.

Dangers – The tree is frost shy and very late to open its leaves. A young tree should be planted in a sheltered position but requires considerable space in maturity.

Getting to Know the Mulberry Tree – The mulberry was introduced into England by the Romans who enjoyed the fruit. In the medieval period trade guilds had halls where they held meetings and beside these were gardens. One planting of a mulberry in 1364 was recorded in the new garden of the Drapers Hall in. That tree survived for 605 years.[3] Due to the concerted effort of James I to have the black mulberry planted across England to feed silkworms, many seventeenth century houses now in the care of the National Trust are graced with a tree in their gardens. His aim was unfortunately not successful, as silkworms previously fed on white mulberry leaves and cannot cope with those of the black mulberry. In the nineteenth century, one Rev. Townsend on visiting Spain found the white mulberry preferred for silkworms in Valencia but the black mulberry used in Grenada.[4] We may be thankful, however, for the many trees that still survive. They may have a lower branch propped up in their old age but still fruit well. The spread of the crown can be seven metres (twenty feet) across and the height can be up to thirteen metres (forty-two and a half feet). The height of one tree I visited in Dorset could be appreciated only from the top of the adjacent church tower.

Black mulberry trees are easy to distinguish from the white because they have such beautiful perfectly heart shaped, finely toothed leaves, hairy on the underside. The leaves of the white mulberry are longer and narrow, of an oval shape by comparison, although they can be variable. The petiole or stem of the leaf is hairy. The longer catkins are male with rounded female catkins on the same tree. The fruits come ready in late summer and peep out from amongst the dense foliage as if shy to announce their arrival—which may be on your head if you are not careful, since they drop silently when ready. The fruits are rather like a cross between a blackberry and a raspberry and so soft that it has often been the practice to set a cloth on the ground below the tree to catch them, rather than trying to pick from the branches. In winter the deeply fissured bark, which has a typically rugged, gnarled look even on a fairly young tree again, makes it easy to identify.

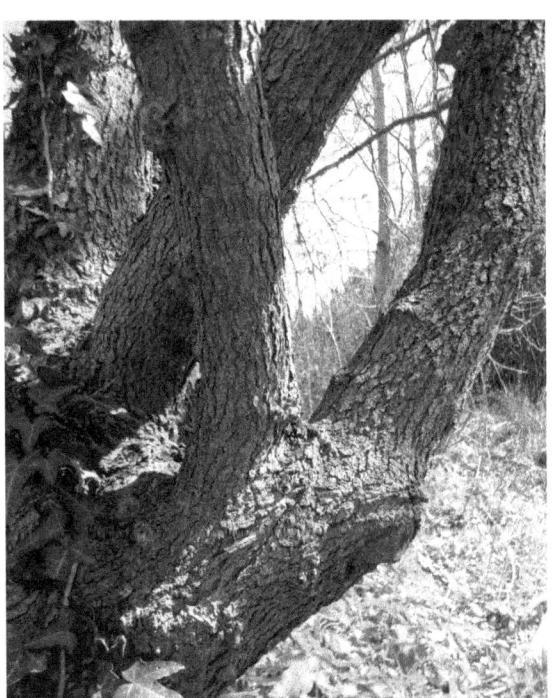
Black mulberry bark.

Inspired by a giant mulberry tree in the large garden of a seventeenth century house where I was designing new herb beds, I planted my own young mulberry tree in 1993 in the hope of fruit some ten years later, since mulberries begin to fruit at around twelve to fifteen years old. True to form it held back from opening its leaves until the second week in May the following spring. This reluctance to acknowledge spring has given it a reputation as the wisest of trees. However, it was not well suited to the chalky ground containing a good deal of flint and some clay at a lower level and did not thrive. The mulberry has roots that tend to be quite brittle and therefore flourishes in rich, light earth. I now have a much smaller garden entirely unsuitable for such a large tree, but thanks to modern developments in horticulture have been able to enjoy growing a potted dwarf mulberry, which was already fruiting on arrival. This means the mulberry is a delight available to all.

The leaves particularly of the white mulberry contain traces of an essential oil that attracts the silkworms, and the twigs and leaves of both have a white sticky sap, which has a rubbery feel and is believed to add a smooth quality to the silk they spin.[5] The leaves make good fodder for much larger animals too. This sap bleeds out when a mulberry is cut in the same way as with the fig and so the tree is only pruned in the dormant season of winter and then simply to remove dead or damaged branches. The somewhat unruly growth of the branches is left intact as the trees fruit on second year growth. The white mulberry is native to China, growing in northern, eastern and western Asia and has had long use in traditional Chinese medicine.[6] Black mulberry is native to southern Asia and is not as hardy.

The black mulberry was grown by the Romans and juice of the fruit was used not only as a mouthwash but applied by ladies as a rouge to redden their cheeks.[7] The fruits were already popular for wine-making in the Anglo-Saxon period and the wood has been used for making casks for red wines. There are many trees with interesting histories. Mulberry trees growing at Syon House, near London include one which is reputed to be the oldest in Britain. William Turner did not mention the mulberry in his account of the botanic garden that he laid out there written in 1548,[8] although some think he might have directed planting the first mulberry there. Kew gardens have mulberry trees which are descended from a mulberry which was planted in Shakespeare's garden in Stratford-upon-Avon in 1609.

Legends and Folklore. The mulberry was dedicated to Minerva, Roman goddess of wisdom, art, and handcrafts, presumably inspired by the late opening of its leaves. From Ovid comes the tragic tale of Pyramus and Thisbe who were to meet at the tomb of Ninus, where a mulberry tree shaded a fountain. Arriving first, Thisbe was frightened by the sight of a lioness feeding nearby, and ran for her life, casting off her long veil as she escaped. Roaring, the lion pounced on it and Pyramus arrived to see the veil in its bloody mouth. Thinking it had eaten his love, he threw himself on his sword in his grief. Thisbe returned to find him dead and also committed suicide, asking the gods to make the white fruits on the tree red in mourning.[9]

There is also a superstition that to protect the house from lightning a mulberry tree should be planted on the north side of the house and a quince on the south.

Notes

1. Miller P. F.R.S. *Gardener's Dictionary.* (London. 1771).
2. Flückiger F.A. & Hanbury D. F.R.S. *A History of Drugs.* (Macmillan & Co. 2nd edition. 1879). 544.
3. Campbell-Culver M. *The Origin of Plants.* (Headline Book Publishing. 2003). 55.
4. Thornton R.J. *A New Family Herbal.* (London. 1810). 756.
5. Lewington A. *Plants for People.* (Eden Project Books. 2003). 80.
6. Bown D. *The RHS Encyclopedia of Herbs.* (Dorling Kindersley. 1996). 313.
7. Stewart S. *Cosmetics & Perfumes in the Roman World.* (Tempus. 2007). 42, 56.
8. Adams J. & Forbes S. (ed), *The Syon Abbey Herbal. A.D. 1517.* (AMCD Publishers Ltd. 2015). 29/30.
9. Moncrieff. A.R. Hope. *Classical Mythology.* (Senate 1994). 169–172.

BLACK MULBERRY – History of Medicinal Use

Archaeological evidence of the pips and seeds of a selection of fruits including the mulberry, confirms mulberry trees (originally from Persia) were being grown and the fruits eaten in second century Southwark, London.[1] Many more excavations from the Roman period have yielded mulberries and the fruits are too soft to have been brought from the Continent, which confirms Roman introduction for this tree. In the first century Celsus writes of mulberries as helpful for encouraging sleep, alongside poppy and lettuce and as a mild laxative. Also, the decoction of the bark with hyssop if the laxative effects were to be extended to discharging worms from the bowel.[2]

Mulberry trees planted by the Romans could have survived for 600 years and supplied fruits for the Anglo-Saxons. It comes as no surprise then to find mulberries (byrig bergena) suggested in morath, an alcoholic drink in this period.[3] In the twelfth century Hildegard recommends a wash made by decocting the leaves, applied vigorously and regularly to cure scabies.[4] A fifteenth century book of cookery recipes gives two recipes for morreye, which one imagines has developed from the earlier morath. True to the period the mulberry juice was spiced, sweetened and mixed with cooked, ground veal, grated bread, and egg yolks.[5] A pottage to be served as a dessert and followed by comfits, fruit, and nuts.

In the Woman's Book of 1540, we find mulberries included with other herbs in a plaster to be laid on a child's stomach to lessen vomiting. Mulberry water is given to a child with milk as a soothing drink after a medicinal bath and other diuretic medicine to ease the child's suffering from a stone interfering with the passage of urine.[6]

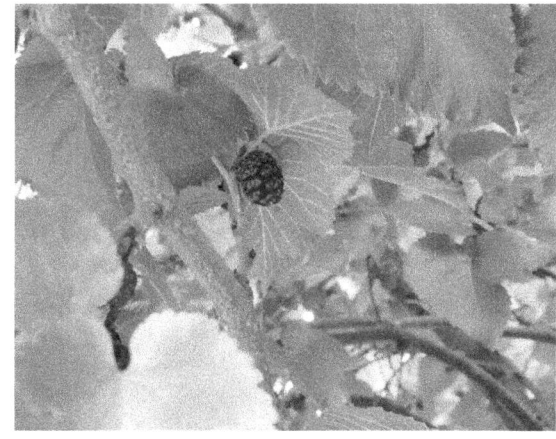

Mulberry fruits.

By the time Culpeper is writing, he makes it clear that the mulberry tree and fruits are commonly seen and tells us that Mercury rules the tree, reflecting the variable medicinal effects of the fruits. While the ripe berries are laxative, the unripe berries are astringent and binding. This duality of results not only applies to the digestive tract but also heavy periods in women. He recommends the bark of the root for expelling broad worms from the digestive system and the juice of the leaves against serpents and aconite poisoning. The leaves beaten with vinegar he applies to burns and a decoction of the bark and leaves for the mouth and toothache. Culpeper repeats earlier recommendations for the juice of the berries or syrup of them for the mouth and throat. He also gives the advice to make a slit in the root bark at harvest time in order to encourage and collect the juice for use with toothache and to purge the belly.[7]

In 1694, Pechey uses honey of mulberries in a complex gargle and says both the syrup and the honey are much used in this way. In 1722, the familiar uses are repeated and the syrup and honey given as officinal preparations in the Pharmacopoeia.[8] Although clearing stoppages has been mentioned before, we find Hill making a more specific comment in writing that the bark of the mulberry root when freshly removed and boiled in water is an "excellent decoction against the jaundice; it opens obstructions of the liver, and works by urine" (p.238). He recommends the syrup of the ripe fruit, one part fruit to two parts sugar, for sore mouths and fevers.[9]

At the end of the eighteenth century, Meyrick in *The Family Herbal* repeats a warning often given before that when mulberries were eaten before a meal they would helpfully ease the food down and through the digestive system, if eaten after a meal, however, they quickly corrupted and were harmful to the stomach. The syrup remains in the Pharmacopoeia of 1791.[10] Thornton writes that the acidity of the mulberries encourages gastric juices and mucus, correcting "putrescency", a powerful cause of thirst. He further writes that the bark of the root is successfully used against worms and tapeworm in particular. He gives the dose as half a drachm of powder.[11]

In America in 1829, the syrup is recorded as being much used to treat angina and aphthae—white patches in the mouth caused by fungal growth.[12]

Summary. Originally from Persia, the mulberry tree was introduced into Britain by the Romans. Pliny, Galen, and Dioscorides give medicinal properties for the parts of the mulberry tree. Over the following centuries the fruits have appeared in several versions of a pottage called murray, which in the original Anglo-Saxon recipe had a medicinal application. The difference in astringency from the unripe fruits to ripe has given rise to the oft-repeated comment that while the unripe fruit is binding, stopping discharges, including diarrhoeas, the ripe fruits are gently laxative. It was not considered advisable, however, to eat the fruit after a meal which was expected to do harm. Eaten before the meal on the other hand, it was helpful to digestion. The juice or syrup of the fruit has had continuous application for inflammation and ulceration in the mouth and throat and curing thirst in fevers. It has also been appreciated as provoking appetite.

The leaves have been credited with action against scabies in the twelfth century and later the decoction was applied to burns for its astringent action. The juice of the leaves was given against serpents and poisoning, particularly poisoning from aconite, for their purging action. The bark of the root has been consistently recommended for use against worms in the digestive tract, specifically tapeworm. At the end of the seventeenth century, it was also recommended for treating jaundice by its action on the liver and as a diuretic. Juice or sap obtained from the root in harvest time was considered good for toothache and use as a purge. Culpeper goes so far as to say to make a hole or slit in the bark to ensure it flows out, hardening in the air.

Recipes

Extracted from A Complete English Dispensatory. 1736. "*Honey of Mulberries.* Take of the Juice of Mulberries, both of the Tree and Shrub, gathered unripe, before Sunrise, and depurated by settling, of each 1 pound and a half, of Honey strain'd and despumated, 2 pounds: let them simmer together, in a gentle Heat, to a due Consistence" (p.406).[13]

Extracted from The Toilet of Flora. 1784. "*A liquid Remedy for decayed Teeth.* Take a pint of the Juice of the Wild Gourd, a quarter of a pound of Mulberry Bark, and Pellitory of Spain, each three ounces; Roch Alum, Sal Gem, and Borax, of each half an ounce. Put these ingredients into a glass vessel, and distill in a sand heat to dryness; take of this liquor and Brandy, each an equal part, and wash the mouth with them warm. This mixture removes all putridity, and cleanses away dead flesh" (p.17) (29).[14]

Notes

1. Alcock J.P. *Food in Roman Britain.* (Tempus. 2001). 66.
2. Spencer W.G. (trans), *Celsus De Medicina* 1 Books 1–1V. (Loeb Classical Library. 1971). 208, 210, 437.
3. Hagen A. *A Handbook of Anglo-Saxon Food.* (Anglo-Saxon Books. 1992). 51, 228.
4. Throop P. (trans), *Hildegard von Bingen's Physica.* (Healing Arts Press. 1998). 113.
5. Austin T. (ed), Two Fifteenth Century Cookery Books. (1888). (Oxford University Press. (Reprint) 1964). 28.
6. Hobby E. (ed), *The Birth of Mankind.* (1560). (Ashgate. 2009). 176, 212.
7. Culpeper N. *Culpeper's Complete Herbal and English Physician enlarged.* (1652). (London. 1815 edition). 123.
8. Miller J. *Botanicum officinale.* Bell. (London. 1722). 229–300.
9. Hill Sir J. *The Family Herbal.* (Bungay edition. Brightly. 1812). 238.
10. Healde T. M.D. F.R.S. *The Pharmacopoeia of the R.C.P. of London.* (1791). 43.
11. Thornton R.J. *A New Family Herbal.* (London. 1810). 761.
12. Togno J. Durand E. (trans) *A Manual of Materia Medica and Pharmacy.* (Philadelphia. 1829). 422.
13. Quincy J. MD. *A Complete Dispensatory.* (10th edition. 1736). 406.
14. Anon. *A Collection of Receipts.* (Printed for the Executrix of Mary Kettilby. 1746). 17.

MORUS NIGRA – Herbalists' Reference

The Parts of the Mulberry Tree Used for Medicine – Fruits, leaves, and bark. The fruits should be allowed to fall from the tree rather than being picked.

Dosage and Forms – 1.7–3.5 g fruit syrup.

Constituents – Fruits: morin, scopoletin, flavonoids. Caffeic acid, tannin, vitamins, and trace minerals.

Actions and Uses – The fruit has some astringency but is also slightly laxative, which makes it suitable as a gentle laxative for children and the elderly. Mulberry can be given when there is diarrhoea and fever as it is also antipyretic and reduces inflammation. As a cooling expectorant, the fruits soothe a sore throat and cough and may prove a suitable alternative to elderberry in this role. The rich syrup may be given both in bronchial infection and inflammation.

The leaves are astringent and vermifuge and in the Balkans have established use in diabetes as they are hypoglycaemic. The syrup can be helpful as a nervine tonic supporting patients with insomnia. The bark is also astringent and anthelmintic.[1]

Contraindications and Precautions – None listed.

Note

1. Barker J. *The Medicinal Flora of Britain and Northwestern Europe.* (Winter Press. 2001). (24).

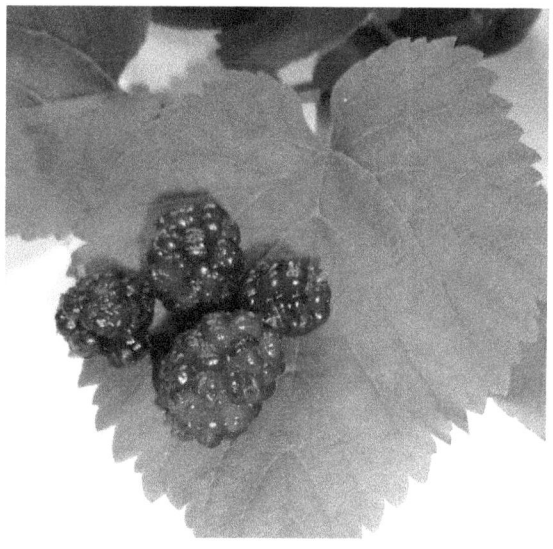

Fruits and leaf.

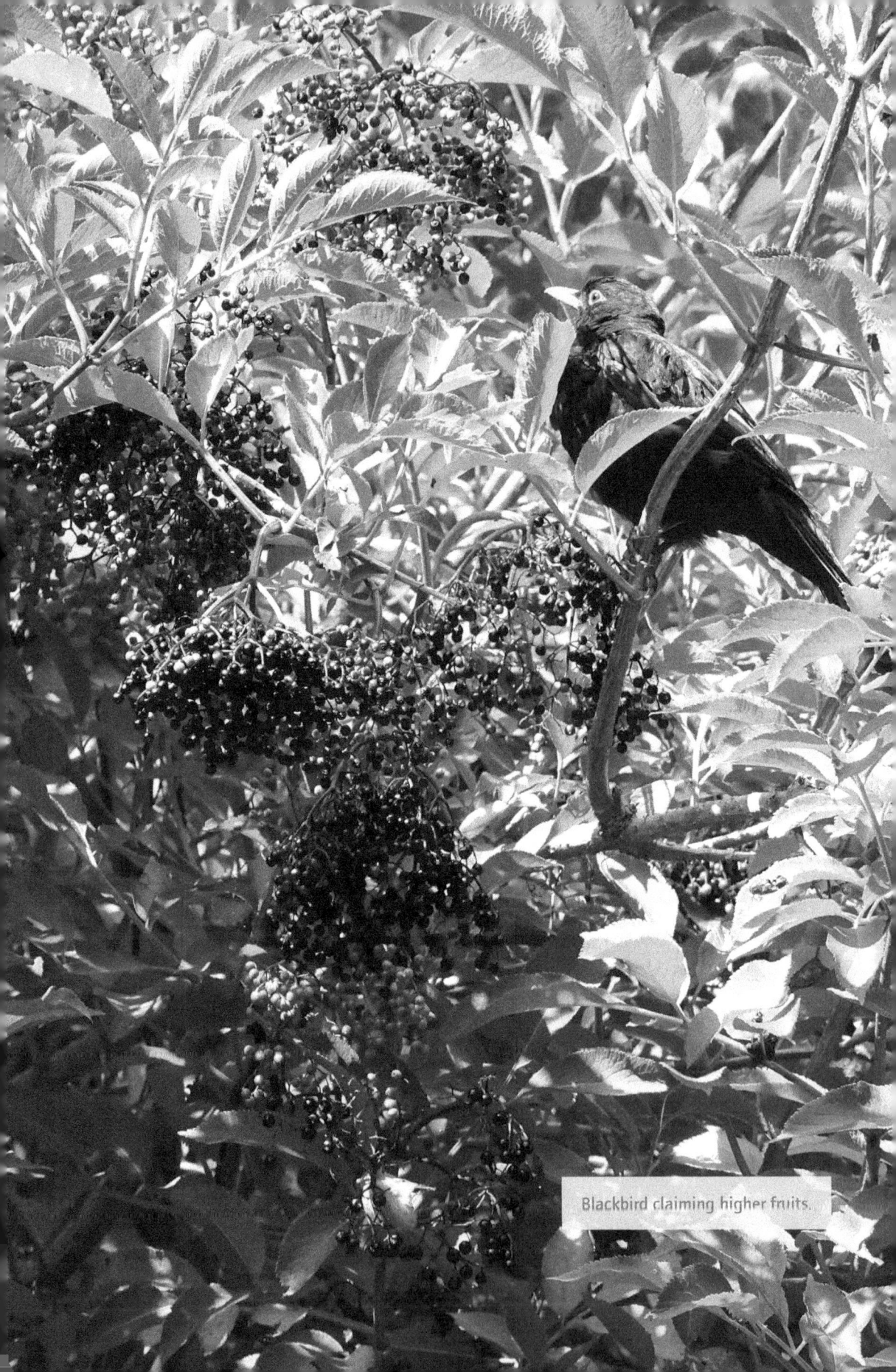
Blackbird claiming higher fruits.

Elderberry

Sambucus nigra – Elderberry – Caprifoliaceae

ELDERBERRY – *Usefulness* – Elderberries are tasty and nutritious as a food. The syrup, juice and tincture from the berries is medicinal. They are used in wines, particularly port and liqueurs and a medicinal wine can be made. The berries provide a dye for wool, silk, cotton and linen giving colours from pink to blue with different mordants. Elder dyes were important in Harris tweed manufacture.[1] The extracted blue colouring is used to indicate alkalis and in their presence gives green, red with acids. Paper and basketry materials can also be dyed pink or blue using the juice with vinegar or salt. The juice gives an attractive long-lasting ink. For uses of other parts of the tree see Elderflower in Spring.

Dangers – Eating a large portion of raw elderberries can give you stomach ache or make you sick. This is due to the resinous substances, which are mainly in the seeds within the berries. Heating destroys the toxic effects so that cooked elderberries are harmless.[2]

Getting to Know the Ider Tree – Field hedges in the countryside commonly contain elder set at intervals. For me, the rich depth of colour and flavour of elderberries epitomises all that is enjoyable, reassuring and satisfying in harvest time as they herald the coming autumn. Over many years I have gathered elderberries with friends and we have sat in the garden for what might be a tedious task of removing the juicy berries from their umbels, if it were not for company. Harvest has always brought people together and this is part of the magic of the elder. The most efficient way of quickly removing the berries is to use a fork, which is another reason for continuing to enjoy the outdoors as elderberry juice sent flying would otherwise readily stain kitchen surfaces.

The umbels of berries should be hanging down a little when they are ready, hopefully with the weight of their juice. If they are not particularly juicy it will help to leave the stripped berries sat in a bowl overnight before including them in a recipe. Each berry contains three seeds. Berries from the purple elder can also be used in cookery. If you do not wish to use them straight away they can either be frozen or dried in a warm oven. Once dried, they look like tiny currants and have been used as a currant substitute in wartime. The berries have yeast on their skin in the same way as grapes so that including them in bread dough can make it rise without further yeast. Elderberry wine was probably made in prehistory using the yeasts on the berries.

Recipes for elderberry wine, port, and ale abound in household books over the centuries. It remains a favourite among home winemakers. I use my mother's excellent recipe for port. This, along with the spiced syrup, has always been available in the winter to treat colds and sore throats, with the added bonus that the port eases rheumatic pain as well. The juice can also be mixed with crab apple juice and honey to make jelly sweets which are tasty and soothing for a sore throat. In the past elderberries have not only been part of the diet of the poor, but they were used as a food colouring by the rich. Sweet pottages were coloured with blends of mulberry, elderberry, bilberry, and blackberry juices, to make the blue dye, turnsole.[3] In medieval royal gardens, the elder was included along with sloe, hawthorn, and rowan in more secluded areas.

As early as Roman times the juice is known to have been used also as a hair colouring, giving a black dye.[4] Culpeper repeats the same use when he directs that the berries be boiled in wine to produce the dye. In an early book on cosmetics (1784), we find the recommendation to rub the eyebrows frequently with ripe elderberries to change them to black. It does not enlighten us as to how you keep the berries after their season is over, but I imagine you simply used the preserved juice to keep the same appearance. If slightly messy, they were perhaps preferable to the alternatives at the time of burnt cork or cloves![5]

Even in the seventeenth century there were already many varieties of elder and William Coles writes that Matthiolus lists eight of them. Miller's *Gardener's Dictionary* (1771) lists the common elder, the cut-leaved *S. laciniata*, which has been called the parsley-leaved elder, and *S. racemosa* or red berried elder. Also *S. Ebulis*, dwarf elder, again bearing berries but not to be used for food, *S. humilis* a dwarf cut-leaved elder and lastly *S. Canadensis*, the American variety, are described as having leaves almost winged. Two hundred years later, *Green's Universal Herbal* omits the cut-leaved elders and adds *S. japonica*, a native elder of Japan. The modern purple, golden, and variegated elders are very attractive and make a fine addition to a large garden border.

Legends and Folklore. In very early times, trees were worshipped and one of those special trees was the elder. Just as the silver birch was linked to the maiden form of the white goddess, so elder was linked to the old crone form, guarding the door to death and the underworld. In Scandinavian myth she was Hyldemoer.[6] Inevitably with Christianity, this pagan goddess, who legend described as teaching the people to spin and weave, was turned into a witch who lived in the elder.

The folklore of this tree is clearly split between good legends that protect the usefulness of the tree in making it protective itself and the portrayal of elder as evil. I have long followed the custom of asking an elder, before gathering or pruning the tree back. It simply feels right and I tell others to do it. My children and grandchildren always liked the idea of this haunted tree, they also enjoyed the mess they could make of themselves helping to prepare berries.

Notes

1. Darwin T. *The Scots Herbal.* (Mercat Press. 1996). 41.
2. Fröhne D. Pfander H. *A Colour Atlas of Poisonous Plants.* (Wolf Science. 1983). 81.
3. McLean T. *Medieval English Gardens.* (Barrie & Jenkins Ltd. 1989). 254.
4. Stewart S. *Cosmetics & Perfumes in the Roman World.* (Tempus. 2007). 45.
5. Anon. *The Toilet of Flora.* (London. 1784). 207.
6. Gifford J. *The Celtic Wisdom of Trees.* (Godsfield Press. 2000). 131.

ELDERBERRY – History of Medicinal Use

Elder is a common tree in most of Britain, the only exception being the northernmost Scottish isles. Archaeological finds leave no doubt it is a native tree and show it has been associated with settlements from very early times. The elder thrives on phosphate-rich soil, which is provided by bones from domestic rubbish heaps and from buried bodies. People are also likely to have encouraged elder close by as a source of food. Finds were so common on Roman sites that it has been presumed the berries were eaten regularly. There is, however, no reason to suppose that use of the berries was for food only. The same applies to elderberries mentioned in the Anglo-Saxon Leechdoms. Ann Hagen reasons that we know fruit wines including elderberry were being made in the Alps in the second millennium BC so why not in Britain.[1] Elderberry wines are commonly accepted as having medicinal use.

Fifteenth century leechbook recipes include treating dropsy and gout. It is specified that the berries must be gathered in Saint Mary's days, between August 15th and September 8th for the second recipe.[2] Culpeper puts the tree under the dominion of Venus and writes at length on all parts of the elder. He uses fresh or dried berries to remove phlegm and choleric humors and recommends the juice of the berries boiled with honey to be used as ear drops to relieve ear-ache. Lastly he decocts the berries in wine for a diuretic drink.[3] William Coles, writing in 1657, repeats that elder is very good in dropsy, the elder being considered hot in the second degree and dry in the third degree. This classification refers to effects produced in the body of the patient. He gives the berries boiled in wine as likely to bring on menstruation.[4]

In 1677, *The Anatomy of the Elder* was published. This is the extraordinary work of Martin Blochwich and gives a wealth of information on the medicinal uses of all parts of the elder tree. For the rob he

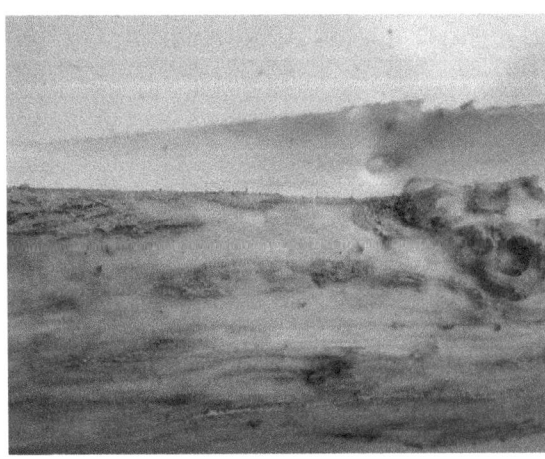

Elder bark peeled away.

instructs to add a little sugar to the pressed and strained juice as it is heated to thicken. He then sets the finished rob together with Spirit of Wine or Spirit of Elder to stand for several days before straining again to provide the tincture. Martin Blochwich continues with instructions for making the spirit of elderberries, the syrup, and more. Finally, there is a recipe for making vomitive oil pressed out of the stones left from the juice extraction. This is not one for the modern medicine cabinet.

His wine recipe instructs us to remove the berries from their stalks and then bruise them in a mortar before placing them in a little barrel and adding must or new wine. The liquors may be boiled together before putting them again into a barrel with must and leaving the yeasts to work. In the second part of the book he gives instruction on treating many disease conditions with one or other of the preparations from the tree. For obstructions of the mesentery and liver, something that occupied much attention at the time, he prescribes a cupful of elderberry wine taken each day for some days or weeks. This was to cut through "thick, tartarous, serous and bilous matter, it cleanseth, evacuateth, and by opening obstructions and purifying the blood, gives the body a more fresh colour" (p.138).[5] This wonderful little book has many other recipes and much advice to give, which we do not have room for here.

In 1694, Pechey quotes the *Anatomy of the Elder* and classes the berries as alexipharmic and sudorific, meaning that they act as an antidote to poisons and induce sweating. He also mentions that spirit drawn from the berries is good in fevers as it provokes sweating, something that the flowers are often given for.[6] A receipt book from the first half of the eighteenth century is not alone in giving a recipe for ebulum. Variations appear in several books. This one requires a heaped bushel of elderberries (fifty-six pounds or over twenty-five kilos) and half a pound (225g) of juniper berries to a hogshead of strong ale (fifty-four gallons or almost 123 litres!). This was clearly for a large household. The berries were first boiled with the ale, hops, and yeast added, and then ginger, nutmegs, mace, and cloves, citron, eringo root, and candied orange peel cut fine, were put into a bag and hung in the liquor for a time before bottling.[7] This sounds like a Christmas punch recipe with a powerful difference and would have been seen as suitable for treating the spleen and dropsy.

Joseph Miller writes that the berries are cordial, which the syrup certainly is, and that they are useful in hysteric disorders, meaning nervous conditions. He notes they are frequently put into gargles for sore mouths and throats. He gives both the berries and the inner bark for dropsies.[8] At this point in 1722 the syrup is still in the Pharmacopoeia. Elderberry wine recipes abound through the centuries following, both in home and published collections, being recommended as a cordial or for dropsy.

In 1822, William Waller writes of the spiced, mulled wine being given to aid perspiration and ease pain. Also rob or jelly to treat fevers. He repeats the laxative and emetic oil from the seeds, which was in the *Anatomy of the Elder*.[9] Thomson notes in 1826 that the berries had previously been much used in fevers, eruptive diseases, rheumatism, and gout but were now scarcely ever ordered.[10]

Mrs. Grieve recommended the inner bark be collected from young trees in the autumn and dried in the sun. It contains a trace of volatile oil, which gives it the distinctive elder smell when first the bark is peeled back to reveal the inner surface.

Summary. The berries have supplied a nutritious food and probably been a source of medicinal wine for more than two thousand years. Certainly from the fifteenth century the efficacy of elderberry juice, whether simply sweetened or fermented, has been recognised for treating dropsy. Gout and rheumatic pain have also been consistently eased by taking elderberry preparations. In the seventeenth century a wealth of knowledge on the elder tree was published in *Anatomy of the Elder*, revealing the interest at that time. The tincture, rob, syrup, spirit, and wine of the berries are all detailed and their actions and uses are given.

It is surprising that many current herbals include use of the flowers only, in spite of the fact that berry preparations such as the syrup, rob, and wine are so popular and well supported through history. They were recommended well into the last century as being analgesic, sudorific, diuretic, etc. They have meanwhile enjoyed continued use in home medicine. See Herbalists' Reference.

Recipes

Extracted from A New Family Herbal. 1810. "Inspissated Juice of Elderberries, commonly called Elder Rob. Take of juice of ripe elder berries, five pounds; double refined sugar, one pound: Evaporate, with a gentle heat, to the consistence of pretty thick honey" (p.324).[11]

Thornton notes the inspissated juice contains the virtues of the elder in a very concentrated state ... making it acidulous, cooling, and laxative.

Extracted from Anatomy of the Elder Tree. 1677. "Elder Berry Wine. Take the Elder Berries cleaned of their stalks, beat them in a stone mortar, or earthen vessel, with a wooden pestle, till all the Kernels be well bruised; with this succulent matter fill the 8, 10, or 12 part of a little barrel, as you will have it of more, or less efficacy, fill up the rest with Must, or new Wine, that they may work together.

Some boyle equal parts of this succulent matter and Must together, till the consumption of a third part of the whole, on a slow fire; then straining it through a thin linnen cloth, they put it (as is said) in a greater quantity into a Barrel, put Must thereon, and so suffer them to work" (p.13).[5]

Notes

1. Hagen A. *Anglo-Saxon Food and Drink.* (Anglo-Saxon Books. 1995). 228.
2. Dawson W. (ed), *A Leechbook of the XVth Century.* (Macmillan & Co. 1934). 95, (251), 141, (385).
3. Culpeper N. *Culpeper's Complete Herbal and English Physician enlarged.* (1652). (London. 1815 edition). 68.
4. Coles W. *The Paradise of Plants.* (London. 1657). 296.
5. Blochwich M. M.D. *Anatomy of the Elder Tree.* (London. 1677). 11–17, 138. 13.
6. Pechey J. *The English Herbal of Physical Plants.* (London. 1694). 72.
7. Smith E. *The Compleat Housewife.* (London. 1739). 222.
8. Miller J. *Botanicum officinale.* Bell. (London. 1722). 388.
9. Waller J. *Waller's New British Domestic Herbal.* Cox & Son. (London. 1822). 128/9.
10. Thomson A.T. M.D. F.L.S. *The London Dispensatory.* (4th edition. London. 1826). 549.
11. Thornton R.J. *A New Family Herbal.* (London. 1810). 324.

SAMBUCUS NIGRA – Herbalists' Reference

The Parts of the Elder Tree Used for Medicine – Berries. (For flowers, leaf, and bark see Elderflower in Spring).

Dosage and Forms – Elderberry juice can be taken with honey. Tincture 1:3 in 25% alcohol. Dose Prophylactic 20ml per week. Acute 10ml twice daily. Tea of dried berries 1–2 teasp per cup. Sweeten with honey. 1–2 cups per day. Elderberry Syrup (spiced or plain) 10ml once or twice a day as needed. Elderberry gel as sweets. Medicinal wine, 1 glass as needed.

Constituents – Sambunigrine, isoquercetrin, sugar, organic acids. Anthocyanins, sambucin, cyanogenic glycosides, Vitamins A, C, and factors of B complex. Tannins.

Actions and Uses – The analgesic and anti-inflammatory qualities of elderberries were made clear in history and are still appreciated. In the past, it was noticed that port adulterated with elderberries could be identified by the good effects it had on the rheumatic and arthritic pain of those who drank it. In the nineteenth century Thomson noted elderberries being given for gout and rheumatism.[1] Elderberries contain B complex vitamins and iron helpful to the nervous system and are included in iron tonics.

The immunomodulatory effects of elder mean the tincture is indicated particularly for those patients who require a tonic in winter for support both against infection and the pain of neuralgia. Elderberry is also given either as a soothing syrup, wine, or tincture for bronchial colds and throat infections. In this role, it is bronchostimulant

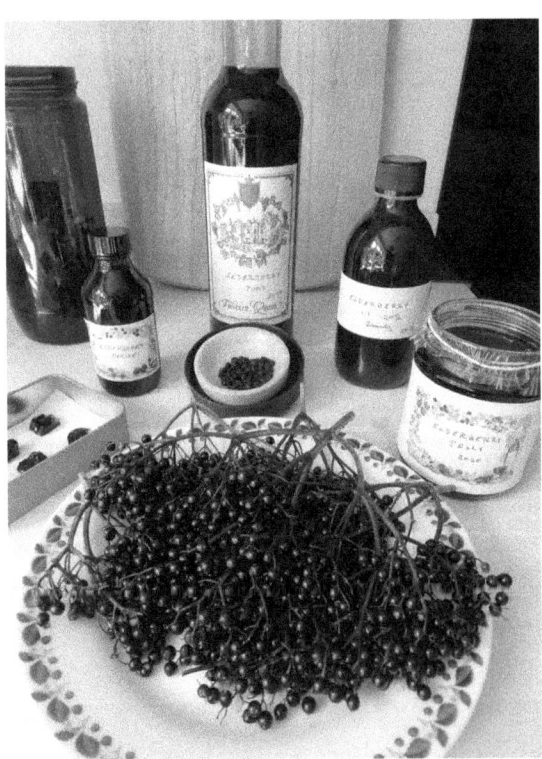
Elderberry gum sweets, jelly, syrup, tincture and wine.

and antipyretic. Sambucus is a valued treatment or prophylactic against influenza. Elderberry extracts have been shown to inhibit certain strains of human influenza virus and decrease inflammatory cytokines.[2]

Taking elderberry regularly can be laxative, but in addition may normalise the bowel action after diarrhoea.[3]

Combinations – With Cinnamomum, Eugenia and Zingiber in the syrup.[4]

Contraindications and Precautions – My experience with patients who have a sensitive bladder suggests elderberry should not be taken by them in any form for more than two weeks without a break. No cautions or contraindications recorded.

Notes

1. Thomson A.T. M.D. F.L.S. *The London Dispensatory*. (London. 4th edition. 1826). 550.
2. Kelly W.J. (ed. director). *Nursing Herbal Medicine Handbook*. (Springhouse Corporation. 2001). 169.
3. Barker J. *The Medicinal Flora of Britain and Northwestern Europe*. (Winter Press. 2001). 375.
4. Stapley C. *Herbcraft Naturally*. (Heartsease Books. 1994). 215.

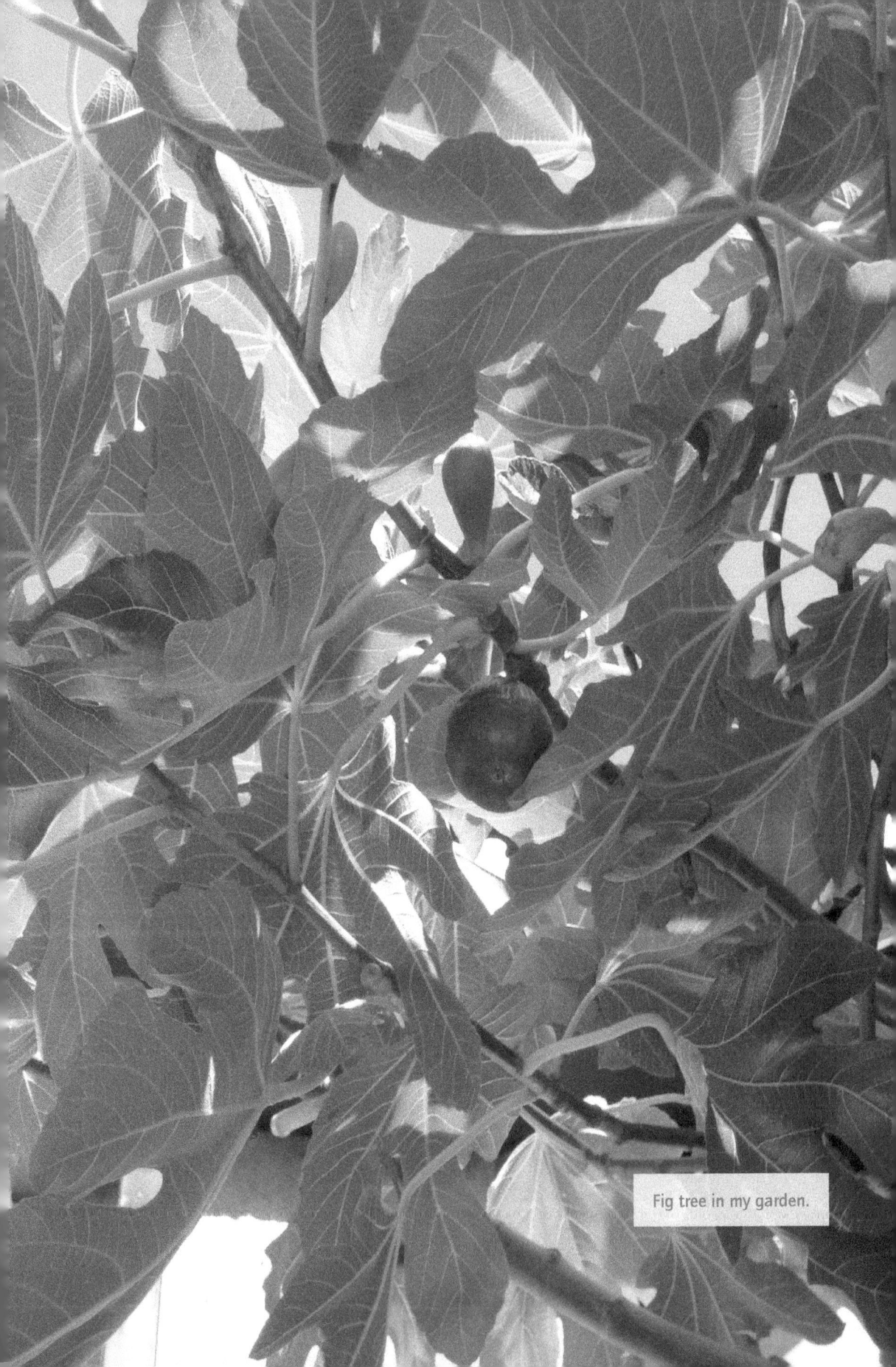
Fig tree in my garden.

Fig

Ficus carica – Fig – Moraceae

FIG – Usefulness – The fruits are nutritious. Syrup of figs is a well-known laxative and the open ripe fruits and leaves have been used as soothing poultices. Ficin in the sap or latex is made up of enzymes that can break down proteins and has been applied to mature meat ready for cooking and eating. It also provides a remedy against roundworms and whipworms. It is used in a similar way to papain for blood group diagnosis.[1] Sap is applied medicinally, directly to remove warts, corns, and verrucas with the surrounding skin protected.

Dangers – The milky sap that oozes from cut leaves and branches is caustic and both that and the leaves may cause allergic irritation in sunlight. Sap is extremely irritant to the eyes. Care should be taken to wear gloves when cutting the tree as fig is phototoxic.[2] The fig should be left until it is quite ripe by which time there is no caustic latex left within the fruit, which now contains 50% sugars as well as vitamins A and C.[3]

Getting to Know the Fig Tree – Herculaneum has to be one of the most impressive archaeological recovery sites in the world. To me it almost overshadowed Pompeii, perhaps in part because there were fewer other visitors to distract me. On the walls of the houses there are amazingly preserved murals in both places. These included platters of food, some showing delicious ripe figs. Looking at them I was reminded that Pliny, who died nearby during the eruption of Vesuvius, praised the figs grown at Herculaneum, and wine made from the fruits. The fruits were also a major crop in Ancient Greece. We find growing the tree is mentioned in the Odyssey and Theophrastus writes of the flexible branches being used to support garlands.

Fig trees may well have been planted in villa gardens in southern England and some historians are convinced of this. However, we have no documented proof. Although the Emperor Julian said that figs could be grown as far north as Paris, the particular wasp that pollinated those fig trees did not exist in Britain.[4] Thanks to the benefit of modern self-fertile cultivars this is no longer a difficulty. On moving into my present home, I found myself the proud owner of the most enormous fig tree I had yet seen.

It had been left to grow in a sheltered, south-west facing garden immediately against the house, to a height of some six metres (twenty feet) tall with branches spreading to reach the upstairs windows of three rooms. From the base, branches had grown out, touched the ground, and rooted. They then arched up and along, rooting again for a distance of some ten feet. I was able to cut these rooted runners and pot them as new young trees.

Fig trees flourish on the Isle of Wight where the climate is largely frost free and they are to be seen in the gardens of Osborne House there. The trees have also grown as wildings in several counties up and down the country. As Richard Mabey has noted in his *Flora Britannica*, this is often alongside rivers. He mentions especially the large trees, fruiting twice a year alongside the River Don. Their germination was due to the raised temperature of the water from nearby steelworks in the past, as it carried the seeds from a sewage outflow to the river banks.[5] Fig trees also grow in tropical rainforest conditions. In South America mantled howler monkeys use the power of the sap in decomposing proteins to cure themselves of worms by eating both the fruits and leaves.[6]

The fruit aside, the tree itself is a pleasure in the garden. The bark of the trunk and branches is remarkably smooth and pleasing to touch, being a soft grey in colour. I love the glossy, large leaves with their distinctive round lobes, perfect for wrapping around fruit. They are easily recognised and often pictured protecting the modesty of Adam and Eve in art. Their beauty has been further celebrated through carvings in wood and stone over the centuries, both in churches and other buildings.

We are accustomed to fruit following flowers, but for the fig this is not so. The flowers are extraordinary, hidden away as if in a secret compartment inside the hollow skin of the future fruit. A wonderful story could be written of the journey of the gall wasp down through the tiny opening surrounded by guards of fleshy scales in the top of the pear shaped fruit. The insect crawls in past the male flowers, which are mainly in the upper part of the receptacle, brushing on their pollen to fertilise the female flowers on their stalks, which never feel the sun directly upon them. It then uses the fruit as a nursery for its young, which are laid inside.

At this point they have the protection of the tough green outer skin of the fruit. The one-celled ovary ripens to a tiny hard nut—the seed of the fruit. With ripening, the fruit itself grows and softens and the acrid, milky sap changes to a sweet fluid. Turning colour, depending on the variety, the fig may become purple, brown, yellow, or remain green. It is now safe to eat. Left unpicked in a hot country the figs will gradually shrivel and dry naturally, possibly to the condition of figs dried on trays in the sun and air.

Legends and Folklore. Figs and fig trees appear a number of times in the Bible, in both the Old and New Testaments. In Genesis, Adam and Eve use fig leaves to cover their nakedness. In the New Testament Jesus condemns the fig tree, which is not bearing fruit to wither away. The meaning of this has, however, been interpreted as a reference to the unfaithful Church, which would die away through heresy. Just like the elder, in more recent centuries the fig tree has been seen both to be protective and the home of a servant of the devil.

To the Romans it was a sacred tree, which had protected the wolf that suckled Romulus and Remus, the founders of Rome. The milky sap from the cut branches was likened to the sperm of the god of war, Mars, their mythical father.

Notes

1. Samuelsson G. *Drugs of Natural Origin.* (Apotekarsocieteten.1999). 366.
2. Avalos J. Maibach H.I. (eds), *Dermatologic Botany.* (CRC Press. 2000). 59.

3. Trease & Evans W.C. *Pharmacognosy.* (W.B. Saunders. 14th edition. 1999). 217.
4. Alcock J.P. *Food in Roman Britain.* (Tempus. 2001). 67.
5. Mabey R. *Flora Britannica* (concise edition). (Chatto & Windus. 1998). 148.
6. Engel C. *Wild Health.* (Houghton Mifflin Co. 1979). 133/4.

FIG – History of Medicinal Use

Originally from south west Asia, the fig appears on Egyptian wall paintings and the fruits were used in recipes to treat the heart and lungs.[1] The tree has been common in the Mediterranean area for many centuries. Dioscorides wrote of the medicinal use of the milky sap and the juice of the leaves in addition to the fruits.[2] The Roman army of occupation in Britain also enjoyed eating figs in the second century. We know this from the seeds, which remained to be discovered

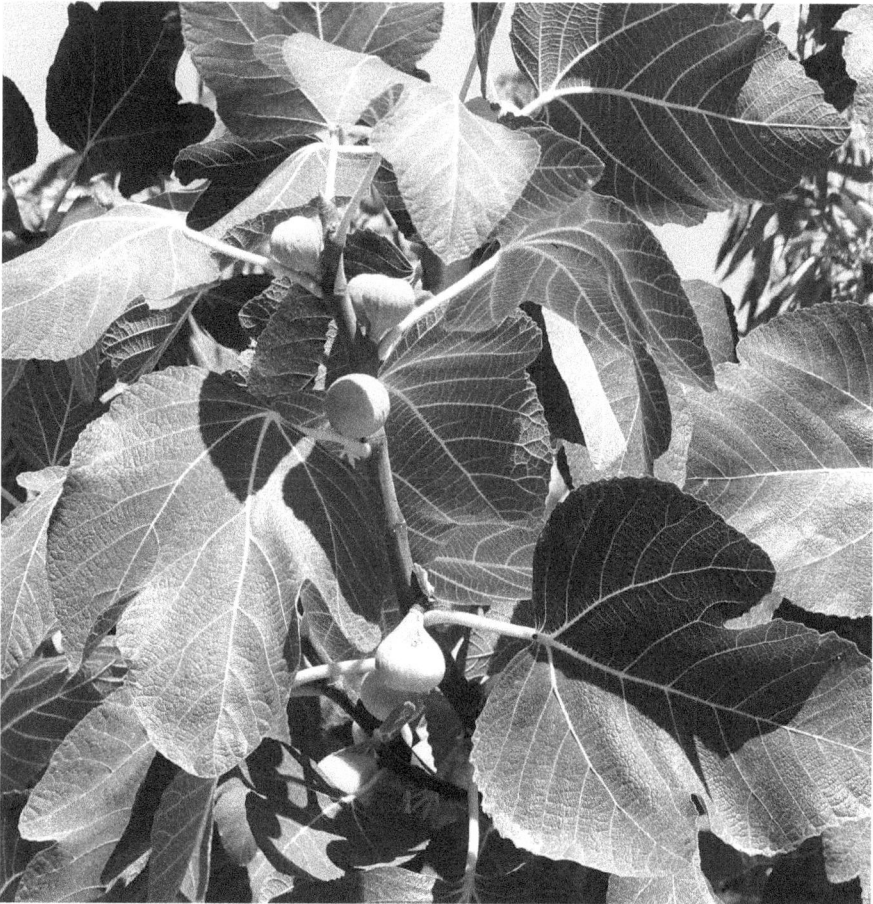

Figs on tree in Chios.

by archaeologists digging in a Roman latrine at Bearsden on the Antonine Wall.[3] Archaeology from other British sites has also revealed figs in the diet of this period and these may have been eaten for their laxative properties.

The fruits would certainly have been familiar to Christian pilgrims, not only because they appear numerous times in the Bible. They are included on Charlemagne's list of plants and trees for the ideal monastery in the ninth century. It is then not surprising that Sussex claims the oldest tradition for introduction after the Roman period either by an Abbot of Sompting, or possibly Thomas Becket at West Tarring.[4] Aelfric includes them in his vocabulary of daily life for students at Winchester around 995 A.D.[5]

The written reference, which is often quoted as the earliest, to a fig tree in Britain appears to relate to another Archbishop of Canterbury, Reginald Pole in 1525. He brought trees from Italy to Lambeth Palace, one of which grew to be huge, at some fifty feet. However, in Fluckiger and Hanbury's *History of Drugs* published in 1879, there is mention from an earlier history by Matthew Paris that in 1257 the weather was so bad that a number of fruits, including the fig, failed to ripen. The average price of imported figs between 1264 A.D. and 1398 was about 1¾ d per lb, one penny cheaper than raisins and currants.[6]

We find figs being recommended in medicinal use in Britain in the fourteenth century. They are included in recipes for the chest to ease breathing and for nausea. A combination of fig with honey, elecampane, and anise appears, which in another form makes useful cough sweets. Figs are also given alongside liquorice in a complex remedy. One manuscript quotes health advice from Galen, recommending eating figs and raisins especially in the month of March.[7]

By the seventeenth century when Culpeper is writing of the fig, he regards growing the trees as so common in England that he does not bother to describe its form. He writes that the fruits prosper well enough for medicine, but cannot recommend them to eat. Culpeper puts the tree under the dominion of Jupiter. He adds that the decoction of the leaves may be useful as a wash for sore heads and leprosy.[8] This might cover a wider range of skin conditions than the disease we understand it to be.

Culpeper and Coles agree on a long list of further problems, from chilblains to warts and toothache to be treated with ointments, decoctions, syrups of figs, the ashes, or the juice. While Culpeper writes only of trees grown at home, Coles describes the way in which the manured tree grows in Italy and Spain, where the fruit was laid out to dry in the sun before being exported. He wrote of growth here—"the fruit though many times it appear before the leaves; yet seldom commeth to perfection, unless it be planted under a hot Wall" (p.140).[9] He tells us the shape of the leaf—with five divisions, rather like the fingers of a hand are a sign it may be used to treat joint pains. Coles writes, "Figs bruised and applyed with Barly Meal, and the powder of *Fennygreek* seed do mollify the hard tumours and Kernells under the Throat and Ears, and elsewhere by Signature;" He also notes "Figs stamped with fair Rue, and the kernels of Nuts, withstand Poyson and corruption of the Air"(p.140).[9] It is likely this idea has come from the famed antidote of Mithridate against poisons and venoms.

The eighteenth century sees figs appearing in published recipes for consumption of the lungs, gout, and rheumatism, surfeit water to treat indigestion and rickets.[10] Fig trees had become popular in walled gardens of the wealthy by this time and we see them listed alongside apricots and medlars. We even find fig leaves included in a recipe in the *Toilet of Flora* 1784, along with walnut shells, oak galls, ivy berries, cypress-nuts, mulberry, and other leaves for dyeing the hair black and preventing falling hair.[11]

In the nineteenth century, imported figs were certainly popular with 163,763 hundredweight, being imported in 1876 at a cost of £318,717. There was still mention of applying them to swellings and to using their laxative properties in *Confectio Sennae*.[6]

Summary. Originally from south-west Asia figs were enjoyed and used in medicine by the first century A.D. Aelfric includes figs in his Latin grammar based on daily life around 995 A.D. but the first written evidence of trees in Britain comes from 1525. In addition to medieval use for treating coughs, constipation, and bruising, they were recommended for easing passage of kidney stones and gravel. Their milky sap meanwhile has always been used as a caustic to remove warts. Fig trees were common by the seventeenth century and Culpeper and Coles used them in a range of preparations including syrup, ointments, decoctions of the leaves, the ashes, and the juice. These treated many conditions from chilblains to consumption and rickets. Laxative use has remained dominant.

Recipes

Extracted from A Leechbook of the XVth Century. (140). "Bruises or Wens, to heal them. Take good figs and bray them right small till the kernels be also broken, and then stamp as much of boar's grease and half so much of the yolks of eggs, and lay thereof a plaster to the sore. And t'will break it and then heal it" (p.59).[12]

Extracted from A Collection of Recipes. 1746. "*A Posset*-Drink *for a* Cough. Take one Handful of Hyssop, four Sprigs of Minth, (Mint) as much Savoury and Angelica, one Handful of ston'd Raisins, and twelve Figs; infuse all these in three Pints of clear Posset-drink; add, when strain'd, one Ounce of Syrup of Maiden-hair, as much Syrup of Violets: Drink often" (p.162).[10]

Notes

1. Manniche L. 1989. *An Ancient Egyptian Herbal.* (British Museum Press. 1989). 103.
2. Gunther R.T. (ed), *Dioscorides Greek Herbal.* (Hafner. 1968). 90.
3. Alcock J.P. *Food in Roman Britain.* (Tempus. 2001). 29, 67, 155.
4. Campbell-Culver M. *The Origin of Plants.* (Headline Book Publishing. 2001). 24.
5. Harvey J. *Mediaeval Gardens.* (Batsford. 1981). 4.
6. Flückiger & Hanbury. *A History of Drugs.* 2nd edition. (Macmillan & Co. 1879). 542/3. 544.
7. Henslow G. Rev. Prof. M.A. *Medical Works of the Fourteenth Century.* (Burt Franklin. New York. 1972). Ms. A. 43, 47, 63. Ms. D. 140.
8. Culpeper N. *Culpeper's Complete Herbal and English Physician enlarged.* (1652). (London. 1815 edition). 76.
9. Coles W. *The Paradise of Plants.* (London. 1657). 139.

10. Anon. *A Collection of Receipts.* (Printed for the Executrix of Mary Kettilby. 1746). 102, 138, 149, 254. 162.
11. Anon. *The Toilet of Flora.* (London. 1784). 11.
12. Dawson W. (ed), *A Leechbook of the XVth Century.* (Macmillan & Co. 1934). 59. (140).

FICUS CARICA – Herbalists' Reference

The Parts of the Fig Tree Used for Medicine – Fruits, leaves, and sap.

Dosage and Forms – Syrup of figs. See also topical applications.

Constituents – The sap oozes readily from cut leaves and contains proteolytic enzymes, lipase, protease, and amylase. The fruits contain organic acids, alkaloids, apigenin glycosides, approx. 50% sugars, vit B_6 other vitamins, and minerals.

Actions and Uses – The well-known laxative properties of fig seeds have made the fruits a favourite in treating constipation. Dried or fresh figs may be eaten in this role or the syrup used. Dried figs can also be mashed with a little honey and used as a slightly laxative carrier for powdered herbs. This is especially helpful when the patient cannot afford tinctures, or alcohol is unsuitable for them and the taste of the dried, powdered herb in a tea would be unpleasant. Such "sweets"

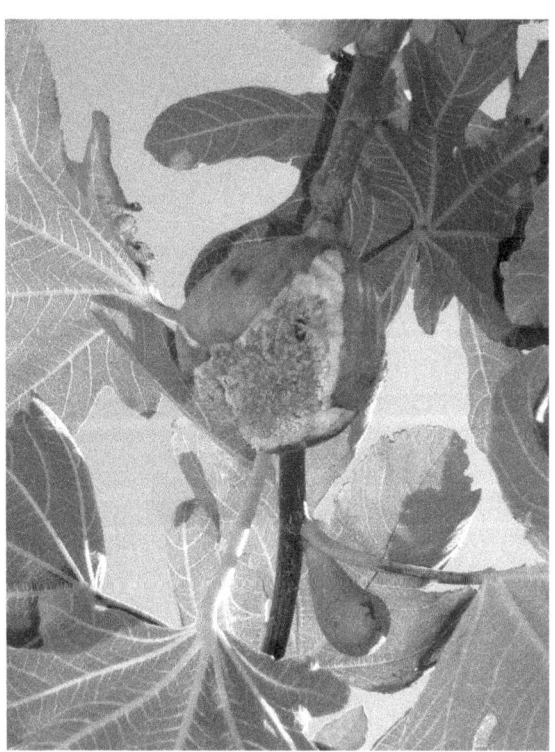

Ripe fig split open.

may be welcomed for children or more particularly the elderly, and they are effective so long as the powder is evenly distributed. The demulcent and expectorant actions of the syrup also extend use to easing inflammation of the trachea, bronchial infections, coughs, and asthma. For these uses, a little thyme can be added to the syrup.

In aiding cleansing of the system, being catabolic, digestive, and diuretic, figs have a role in addressing the problems of boils, carbuncles, acne, and abscesses. They are additionally vermifuge and candidicide. Fig has been used in the past to deodorise and possibly ease malignant cancers.[1]

Topical Application – Roasted figs may be cut in half and the soft pulp used to poultice boils.² A test should be made on an area of skin which is not inflamed to check for allergic response before this is tried. The leaves may also irritate the skin.

The milky sap is applied with very different effect directly to warts, corns, and verrucae. The surrounding skin should be protected as when using other caustic herbs in this situation.

Contraindications and Precautions – Furanocoumarins and bergapten make the leaves and sap a skin irritant in sunlight, also a potential skin allergen. Sap must be kept away from the eyes.

Notes

1. Duke J.A. *Handbook of Medicinal Herbs* (CRC Press LLC. 2ⁿᵈ edition. 2002). 300/1.
2. Grieve M. *A Modern Herbal.* (1ˢᵗ pub. 1934 Jonathan Cape. Saavas. 1984). 312.

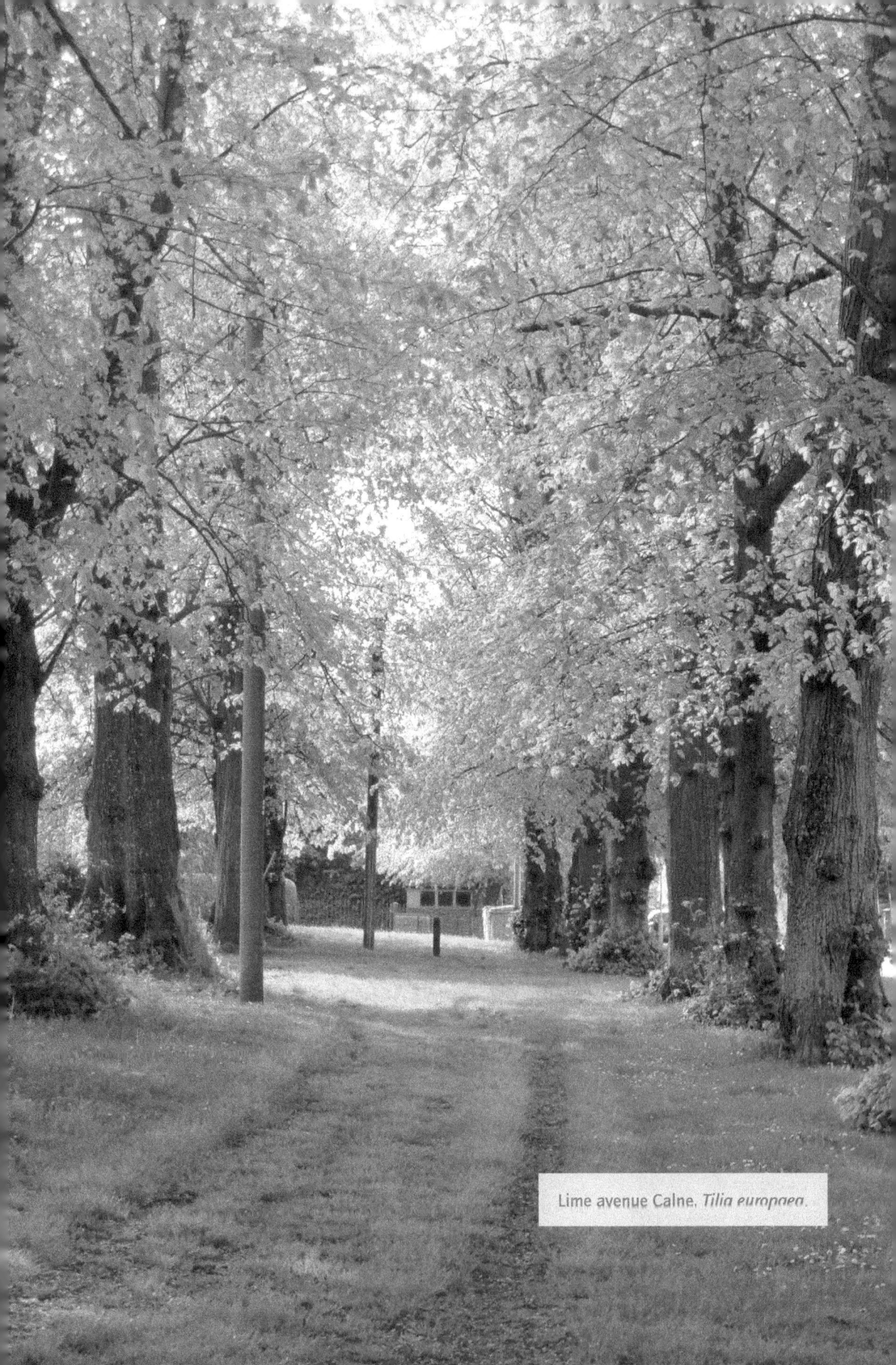
Lime avenue Calne. *Tilia europaea*.

Limeflower

Tilia europaea, T. cordata. T. platyphyllos – Linden – Limeflower – Tiliaceae

LIMEFLOWER – Usefulness – The lime has been called a tree of a thousand uses. The flowers and bracts have valuable medicinal properties and all parts of the tree have been used in medicine. Linden-flower tea is enjoyed as a refreshing and soothing drink. Brandy has been distilled from the flowers. The leaves provide animal fodder. The young leaves and small fruits are edible. The flowers have cosmetic use. Baskets are made of lime bast from the inner bark. The bark can be beaten and steamed to produce fibres for cloth and paper. Twisted into strong threads, ropes, and cords it has been used in fishing nets for bowstrings and wrapping tool handles for thousands of years.[1] The wood is suitable for elaborate decorative carvings found in cathedrals and stately homes, as well as for turning and making various items. For centuries it has supplied boxes, bread boards, and sounding boards for pianos.

Dangers – The flowers become narcotic if left to dry on the tree.[2] Lime trees are notorious for the honeydew, which drips from their leaves in summer and is very difficult to remove from cars that have been parked beneath.

Getting to Know the Limeflower Tree – *Tilia europaea* is the most familiar of the limes as it is planted alongside roads and in parkland. It is in fact a hybrid of *T. cordata* and *T. platyphyllos*, both of which are native to parts of Britain. The *europaea* is easily recognised by the young growth around the base of the trunk, which forms what is termed a bole. For identification of those lime trees without a bole you need to examine the leaves or, in winter, the bark.

T. platyphyllos or large-leaved lime has large leaves green on both sides, with hairs on the upper surface. The bark is rougher and grey compared to that of *cordata*. *T. cordata* also known as small-leaved lime has smaller heart-shaped leaves, which are smooth on the upper surface; the bark of young trees is comparatively smooth, darkening and cracking with age. The small-leaved lime tends to be the smaller tree at up to twenty-five or thirty metres (eighty-two to ninety-eight feet) and limited to certain areas, where you may find it has been pollarded over a long period. It tends to reproduce by means of suckers. The small-leaved lime and the *T. europaea* both harbour aphids, which are responsible for the sticky honeydew that drips down to cover anything left beneath. Before, or even after the honeydew adds sweetness, the soft leaves can be eaten in sandwiches. They are too soft for salad leaves. Try adding lemon juice and spicy herbs to give them a lift.

There are both male and female limes. The wood of the female is whiter and the bark thinner and more flexible, so it was preferred in the past for making containers.[3] Female trees bear hermaphrodite flowers, which are pollinated by bees eager for limeflower nectar. The bees also drink honeydew made by the aphids. Lime-flower honey is a great favourite. Lime-flower wine is almost mead with a very honeyed flavour.

The flowers have a further application in cosmetics, being included in moisturising creams and lotions for their hydrating mucilage and anti-inflammatory properties.[4] In the nineteenth century, a French chemist tried to make a chocolate substitute from the fruits and flowers ground together.[5] Within each of the fruits clustered in a bunch, which are also charmingly known as "hen's apples", is a little black seed. There may be three seeds but usually only one ripens. The pressed seeds give good quality oil but the quantity required makes this an unlikely home activity. They have also been used in medicine, taken or applied powdered to stop bleeding. The fruits can supply a yellow dye.

Lime wood, or perhaps the inner bark, was cut into thin sheets in the Roman period to be folded for the inner sides to take writing. Comparable written tablets found on the Roman wall in Britain, however, were of birch or alder due to the absence of lime in that area.[6] Considerable use of lime bast over the centuries meant lime trees were pollarded, which extends their lives possibly to 1,000 years.

The scent of lime blossom is soothing and the tea calming, helping to lower blood pressure. It seems animals are aware of this effect too. A friend has noticed that when her horse is upset or anxious it goes to stand beneath a lime tree, breathing in the scent. This offers the possibility that horses first led people to find the calming influence of lime flowers and use them medicinally. Flowers and bracts can be used in medicine from all three trees. These should have been harvested soon after the flowers open and dried carefully, as with too much heat (over twenty-seven degrees) they readily spoil.[7]

In Goodyer's translation of *Dioscorides Book 1*, boxes of lime wood are recommended for keeping delicate dried flowers and over a thousand years later lime was still used for making apothecary boxes. When I first attempted to learn woodcarving, I was given lime wood as the easiest wood for a beginner to work. An expert can produce wonderful carvings, I recall seeing the carvers at work during the restoration of Uppark after a serious fire some years ago. In the medieval period lime was often chosen for carving statues of the Virgin Mary, giving it the common name of *Lignum sacrum* or sacred wood. Lime wood was used to panel rooms when panelled walls were fashionable. It is light in colour and smooth, which is most attractive, the wood is also sufficiently light in weight to be chosen for making musical instruments.

Once burned, the wood produces a fine charcoal used for smoking foodstuffs, by artists for sketching and formerly for making gunpowder.

Legends and Folklore. The lime was once dedicated to the Germanic goddess of love and fertility, Freya. Lime flowers were strewn before newly wedded couples to wish them

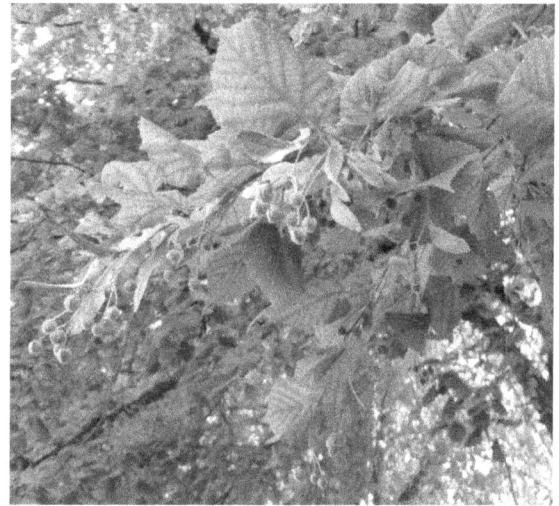

Hen's apples on lime.

handsome children. In some places a wooden floor was constructed over the lowest branches of a large lime tree so that the musicians could sit there and play for dancing at the wedding reception.[8]

Notes

1. Spindler K. *The Man in the Ice.* (Weidenfeld & Nicolson. 1994). 233.
2. Burlando B. et al. *Herbal Principles in Cosmetics.* (CRC Press. 2010). 233.
3. Hort A. (trans), *Theophrastus. Enquiry Into Plants.* Books 1–5. (Loeb Classical Library. 1999). III x 3–4. 225.
4. Hampton A. *Natural Organic Hair and Skin Care.* (Organica Press. 1987). 150.
5. Mabey R. *Flora Britannica* (concise edition). (Chatto & Windus. 1998). 128.
6. Bowman A.K. *Life and Letters on the Roman Frontier.* (The British Museum Press. 2003). 80.
7. Mills S. *Out of this Earth.* (Viking. Penguin. 1991). 405.
8. DeCleene M. & Lejeune M.C. *Compendium of Symbolic and Ritual Plants in Europe.* (Man and Culture Publishers, Ghent. Belgium. 2003). 384.

LIME FLOWER – History of Medicinal Use

Pollen, wood, and charcoal of Tilia species has been found at numerous sites from the Mesolithic and Neolithic ages onwards. Careful examination of the pollen has revealed both *Tilia cordata* and *T. platyphyllos*, together with their hybrid progeny *T. vulgaris* in prehistory.[1] Such an association with human settlements is not surprising as the leaves make good fodder for animals, and the bark also offers bast fibres for use in ropes, threads, and baskets. The hollowed out tree trunks have been found used to line wells from the Neolithic period.[2]

The body of the man found preserved in the ice of the Alps, who lived during the Bronze Age, had a bark container with him that had been sewn together with lime bast and his bowstring was also made from lime.[3] Our earliest reference to Tilia for medicine comes from Pliny who compares the actions of the leaves to those of the olive. Hildegard of Bingen suggested covering the eyes and face with the leaves at night, presumably as a compress to clear the eyes.[4] In Gerard's Herbal, we find the first mention of the flowers and water distilled from them to treat headache, apoplexy, dizziness, and epilepsy.[5]

This use of the flowers continues, while at the end of the century Pechey adds use of a mucilage of the bark for treating burns and wounds, the leaves to reduce swelling of the feet, and the small fruits to stop bleeding. In spite of these details, twenty-five or so years later Miller records that parts of the tree other than the flowers are seldom used. Another application for these has been found in treating palpitations of the heart. The flowers are

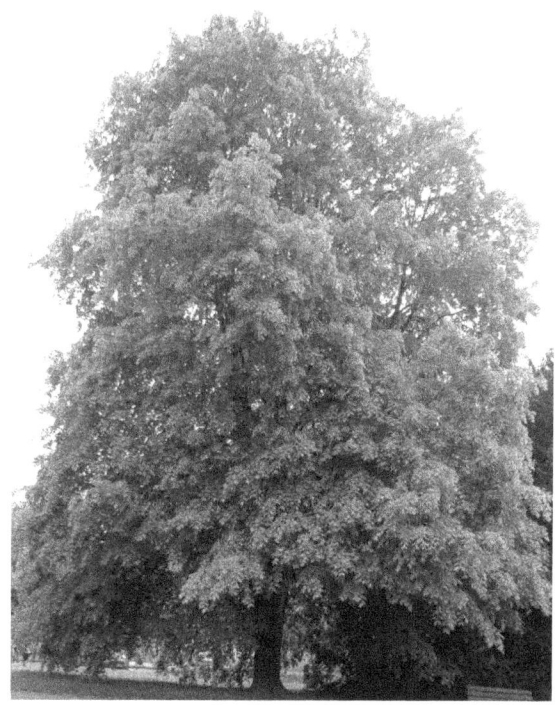

Tilia platyphyllos.

by then included in two complex waters, *Aqua Paeon. Comp* and the *Spirit Lavandulae*.[6] It might have seemed that the use of lime flowers was increasing and yet in 1751 Hill records that the use of the distilled water "is now disregarded" (p.429) and the flowers only included in old recipes.[7]

In 1778, Gilbert White notes in his *Journal* news of the use of lime flowers to treat coughs and fevers in the south of France. Impressed by the story of how avenues of limes were plundered for their flowers in France, Gilbert White tried making the tea and found it very pleasant with a taste resembling liquorice.[8] Forty years later, Waller takes up the thread of French use, writing that lime flowers are much used on the Continent and that in addition to prescribing them for nervous disorders, French physicians value them for calming fevers following surgery or violent injuries. The tea was recommended to be taken with the addition of a small amount of sliced liquorice. Interestingly, the distilled water has continued in use in France. Waller also gives us a repeat of the much earlier use of the inner bark macerated in water to apply to burns, fomentation of the leaves to ease painful tumours, and a cure for distressing constipation. This was achieved by sitting over steam from the leaves, which apparently produced instant relief. He ends by suggesting that juice tapped from close to the roots of the lime was worth a trial as a cure for epilepsy.[9]

Brook gives lime flower for asthma, comments on the mucilaginous nature of all parts of the tree, and supports use of the inner bark not only for burns, but for treating gouty and rheumatic joints.[10] In the twentieth century, during the First World War lime flowers are described as in use in herbal medicine and homoeopathy in England and as a popular bed-time drink in Belgium.[11] Mrs. Grieve gives the leaves and shoots for poultices and fomentations and flowers for a tea.[12]

Summary. Use has been made of various parts of the lime tree from early times. Chewing the leaves or preparing them as a decoction dates back 2,000 years to Pliny. Gerard adds use of the flowers and water distilled from them. Appreciation of the lime flowers and distilled waters containing them has long been stronger on the Continent than in Britain, where it has been inconsistent over time. We also find mucilage from the inner bark of the tree applied to burns and wounds, and later to painful rheumatic joints. The flowers have been valued for treating headaches and conditions associated with the nervous system such as vertigo and epilepsy. Apoplexy and palpitations of the heart also involve the circulation, and lime flowers were included in prescriptions for treating these conditions.

Recipe

Extracted from Brook's Herbal Complete. 1872. "INFUSION OF LIME FLOWERS. Take of lime flowers four drachms; liquorice root four drachms; Boiling water three pints. Infuse for a quarter of an hour. This is a pleasant and wholesome drink for asthmatic people, and must be taken warm" p.170.[10]

Notes

1. Godwin Sir H. *History of the British Flora.* (Cambridge University Press. (2nd edition). 1975). 160/161.
2. Adams M. *The Wisdom of Trees.* (Head of Zeus Ltd. 2014). 140.
3. Spindler K. *The Man in the Ice.* (Weidenfeld & Nicolson. 1994). 233.
4. Throop P. (trans), *Hildegard von Bingen's Physica.* (Healing Arts Press. 1998). 122.
5. Johnson T. (ed), *The Herbal.* John Gerard. (1633 edition). (Dover Publications, New York. 1975). 1482.
6. Miller J. *Botanicum officinale.* Bell. (London. 1722). 438.
7. Hil J. M.D. *A History of the Materia Medica.* (London. 1751). 429.
8. White G. Rev. M.A. The *Natural History and Antiquities of Selborne.* (1778). (Swan Sonnenschein & Co. 1911). 359.
9. Waller J. *Waller's New British Domestic Herbal.* Cox & Son. (London. 1822). 223/4.
10. Brook R. *Brook's Family Herbal.* (revised edition. J.A. Brook, Richardson & Co. London. 1876). 170.
11. Teetgen A.B. *Profitable Herb-Growing and Collecting.* (London. 1916). 179.
12. Grieve. M. *A Modern Herbal.* (1st published 1934 Jonathan Cape. Saavas. 1984). 486.

Tilia Europaea, syn. T. Vulgaris, T. Cordata, T. Platyphyllos – Herbalists' Reference

The Parts of the Lime Flower Tree Used for Medicine – Flowers with bracts are used dried. These are gathered in midsummer as soon as the flowers open. *Tilia cordata* flowers slightly later than *T. platyphyllos*.

Dosage and Forms – The tea is made with 1–2 teaspoons dried herb per cup. Infuse for 5–10 minutes. 1–2ml of Tincture: 1:5 in 45% alcohol three times daily. Tincture 1:2, Dose 15–30ml per week.

Constituents – Volatile oil includes citral, eugenol, and limonene. All species have low tannins and varying mucilage polysaccharides, flavonoids, amino, and phenolic acids. Tilia has more than 150 to 1 ratio of potassium to sodium when taken as a decoction.

Actions and Uses – The diaphoretic action may result from the presence of quercetin, p-coumaric acid and kaempferol.[1] Lime flower is additionally a stimulant for the immune system.

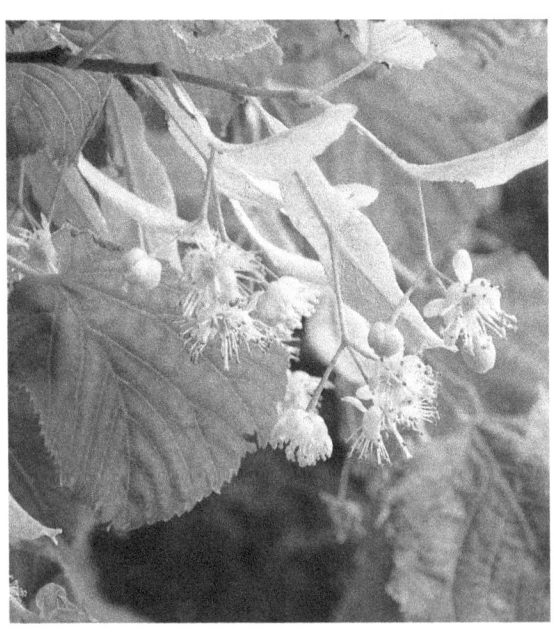

Lime flowers and bracts.

Lime flower is particularly regarded as a herb for the wellbeing and support of the circulatory system, this is often in the area of reducing blood pressure, when the additional tonic nervine action makes it especially effective. The smooth syrupy consistency of a good tincture adding a slight sweetness to the mix gives a calming message in itself to the patient taking the medicine. The flavonoids are also helpful to the health of the blood vessels and the vasodilatory effects are valued in peripheral circulatory problems. Soothing and calming, the antispasmodic effect can be appreciated where there is nervous angina.

Lime flower has been credited with action to dissolve hard deposits and is viewed as helpful in breaking down fats in the bloodstream and reducing cholesterol. With anticoagulant action in the blood it is recommended for coronary deficiency and it is regarded as a specific spasmolytic and neurocardiac herb.[2] The high potassium ratio and the presence of terpineol in the herb may produce the diuretic effect. Lime flower tea is popular as a mild sedative preparing the patient for sleep. It also aids digestion. Tilia may be used to treat migraine, arteriosclerosis, angina from anxiety, dysmenorrhoea, agitated depression, and insomnia.

Specific Indication – In nervous tension associated with arteriosclerosis and high blood pressure.[3]

Combinations – With Crataegus for the heart. With Sambucus, Salvia and Matricaria for colds, it can be prepared using the dried herbs as an inhalation. With feverish conditions there is the option of a hand-bath of Tilia with Achillea and Matricaria, which together help to reduce the temperature and ease symptoms.

Topical applications – Lime flower tea may be used as a soothing wash for burns and damaged, irritated skin.

Contraindications and Precautions – Moderate doses only should be observed with cardiac patients. Although the polyphenol content is associated with lowering iron absorption from eating bread, at 52% this is still lower than the action of black tea.[4]

Notes

1. Kelly W.J. (ed. director). *Nursing Herbal Medicine Handbook*. (Springhouse Corporation. 2001). 271.
2. Holmes P. *The Energetics of Western Herbs*. Vol. 1&2. (Snow Press. Boulder. Revised 3rd edition. 1989). Vol. 1. 175–7.
3. *British Herbal Pharmacopoeia*. (British Herbal Medicine Association. 1983). 214.
4. Bone K. *A Clinical Guide to Blending Liquid Herbs*. (Churchill Livingstone. 2003). 318.

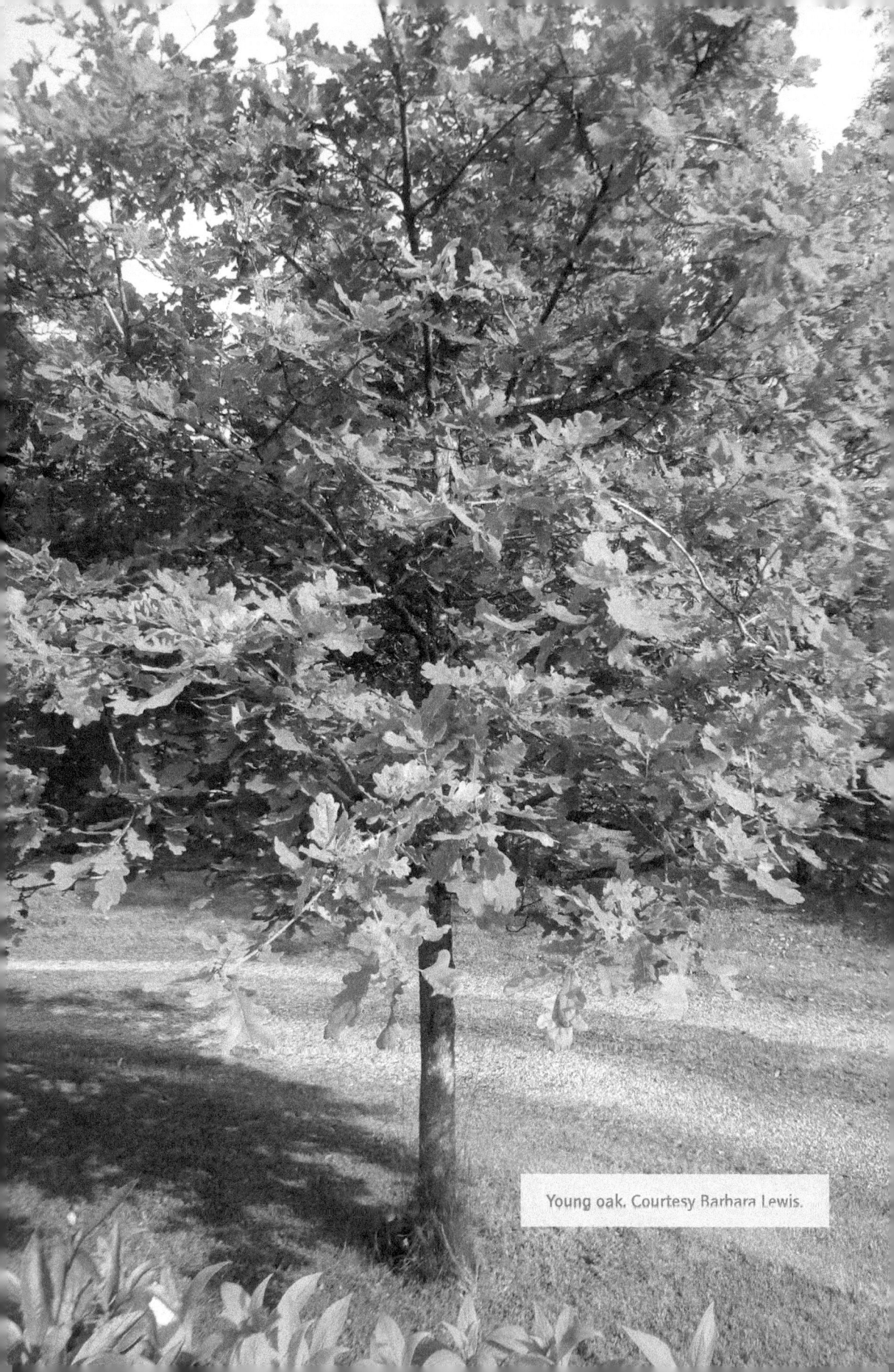

Young oak. Courtesy Barbara Lewis.

Oak

Quercus robur – Oak – Fagaceae

OAK – Usefulness – The inner bark, leaves, and fruits are used in herbal medicine. The oak supports more insects and fungi than any other tree. Acorns provide food for wildlife and some domestic animals in small amounts. They have also provided a famine food for people when prepared properly. Acorns can be roasted and ground as a coffee substitute. Wine can be made from the leaves and ale from young oak bark. The oak tree has been a major source of wood for ship and house building in the past. More recently, oak has been valued for turning, carving, and making quality furniture. All parts of the tree can provide dye for fabrics and threads. The bark can be used to tan leather. The gall that grows on the oak has been a major source of ink, particularly galls imported from Aleppo.

Dangers – Overgrazing by cattle on acorns can make them ill.

Getting to Know the Oak Tree – There is perhaps no tree as famous in England. It has been used many times to signify strength of purpose and the identity of the nation. For twenty years I lived in a 400-year-old thatched cottage with a frame made of oak. The strength and solidity of the beams was soundly reassuring in an age when newly built houses have become flimsy and will be fleeting by comparison.

Oak trees are not generally considered to be suitable for planting in gardens for over time they can grow to a height of thirty-six metres (118 feet), while the spread of the fully mature tree may be almost as much. They tend to be planted in public places to celebrate special occasions. In the past they were also planted to mark parish boundaries, since they live for up to 2,000 years. I was then delighted to find that a friend with a large garden had planted four acorns twelve years before and now has three beautiful young oak trees. Where once there were two oaks beside the curving drive up to her house, the space available has lately dictated that only one should remain there. It is pictured above. The two native oaks in Britain are the pedunculate *Quercus robur*, which can thrive in heavy clay soils and the sessile *Q. Petraea* with leaves that are less deeply lobed and have a wide, rounded appearance at the tips. The sessile oak has long stalks to the leaves and no auricles. The oak tree I am referring to here has leaves on short stalks with two auricles at the base.

Almost everyone is familiar with acorns, which are borne by all oak species. On *Q. Robur* they have long stems, unlike the clusters of acorns on the sessile oaks that are without them. However, there are many hybrids between the two species to confuse us. Acorns aside, the attractive catkins in spring may pass unnoticed. A single tree may bear both male and female flowers and is pollinated by the wind. Once pollination has occurred, the male catkins die off. The female flower sits above the leaf in the picture below while the long male catkins hang down.

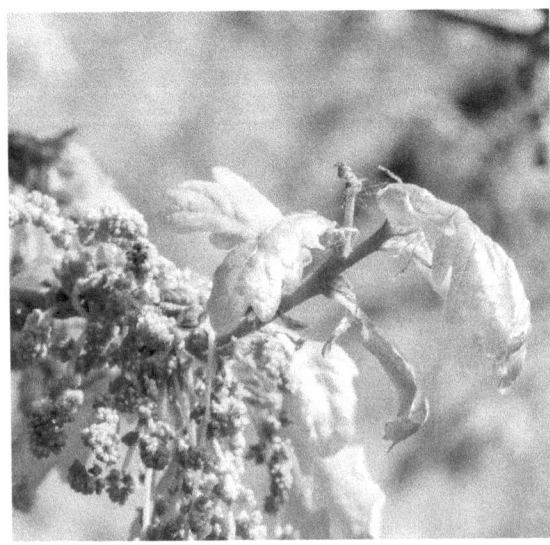

Flowering Oak. Photo David Papworth.

The flowers may appear before the leaves or at the same time as the first flush of leaves.

The oak is host to a myriad of wildlife, one beautiful insect that feeds on the oak is the purple hairstreak butterfly. It is not unusual for an insect infestation on a grand scale to eat the early leaves and the trees then produce new leaves in summer. These are sometimes referred to as Lammas leaves. In fact, part of the secret of the longevity of the oak is its capacity for re-growing after set-backs. New growth from a damaged trunk, even when a fire has left the tree burnt, can produce a coppice tree. Oak trees also hang onto their leaves late in the year, many species being evergreen.

Living as I do, close to the Savernake Forest I cannot help but admire the famous Big Belly oak every time I pass by, as it stands close to the main road. It has an iron band around the hollow trunk and is truly ancient, yet still produces fresh leaves each year. Further into the forest is the Cathedral oak with an even wider girth, judged to be over 1,000 years old. In old age, pedunculate oaks can have dead branches left reaching out at angles high up in the canopy making them look like the antlers of a stag. There are many descriptive names attached to old oaks up and down the country, which testify to the affection in which they are held.

I have long known large oaks that have supplied me with leaves at midsummer. There is a tradition, which no doubt came about through experience initially, that oak leaves are best gathered for wine-making during the week of the twenty first of June. I only know that wine made with the leaves at that time is very good and so I continue to follow the instruction.

We were reminded of the links with the oak as symbol of the Celtic supreme deity Esus and the former worship of oaks in the late 1990s when on the Norfolk coast the discovery and subsequent removal of Seahenge took place. A circle of fifty-five wooden posts surrounded a huge inverted oak tree, which had been set into a peat bed now covered by sea at high tide. The site had clearly been sacred and after the initial excavation in 1998 concern that it would soon be lost to the sea led to the removal of the oak.[1] A full size replica was reconstructed for Channel Four. I was tutoring historical workshops at Flag Fen at that time and went to see the large oak that had been transported to the Field Centre there. I found the sight of the tree hung in the air wrapped by strong chains as if a captive, while being sprayed with water to preserve it, unexpectedly hard to bear.

Legends and Folklore. The oak tree is not only identified as a special tree in England, but has been regarded so across Europe. It is more often struck by lightning than any other tree and so it is not surprising that the oak was seen as the tree belonging to Thor, god of thunder and the Celtic thunder god Taranis.[2] The gods Zeus and Jupiter were also associated with the oak, which was revered by the Greeks, Romans,

Anglo-Saxons, Germans, and Norsemen, as well as the Celts. Pliny wrote that the Celts would not perform any ritual act without oak leaves. The name "Druids" is derived from the Welsh derw meaning an oak tree.[3]

Notes

1. Pryor F. *Seahenge*. (Harper Collins. 2001). 245–262.
2. Gifford J. *The Celtic Wisdom of Trees*. (Godsfield Press. 2000). 67.
3. Miles A. *The British Oak*. (Constable & Robinson Ltd. 2013). 81.

OAK – History of Medicinal Use

The relationship between man and the oak began in prehistory due to the suitability of the timber for constructing houses, boats, and trackways, as well as the smaller essential shields, tubs, and so on. Archaeology confirms use from the Neolithic period onwards. Pliny writes in the first century that the most potent medicinal part of the acorn is the peel and the skin just beneath. There is considerable detail in his classification of various gall nuts and ways of preparing them whether underripe or fully ripened.[1] We find them used in every situation where the effects of the tannins could be of service in tightening and protecting tissues, healing, and acting to reduce discharges.

Much of what Pliny wrote about the oak can be found in *Dioscorides*, writing in the same century. In his herbal he gives the information under Dyer's Oak, *Quercus aegilops*.[2] In the Anglo-Saxon Leechbooks mentions of oak are in contrast to classical sources, using the leaves or twigs of the oak rather than the gall nuts. Again, the astringency supports the uses. The medieval surgeon Lanfranche classifies galls under cicatrizers and includes them with arsenic, alum, sulphur, and vinegar in a corrosive to treat gangrene. Another surgeon Henri de Mondeville sets the Quercus—large and small (robur) oaks under repercussives. He prefers the galls from the large oak but says the small oak sometimes bears them. They are cooling and drying.[3] It seems inevitable that we find parts of the oak used in recipes for restraining uncontrolled bleeding in the *Woman's Book* of 1540. This time it is the acorn cups that are mixed with haemostatic herbs in baths.[4]

In the enlarged edition of Gerard's Herbal, it recommends women with a prolapsed womb to sit over a very hot decoction of oak to

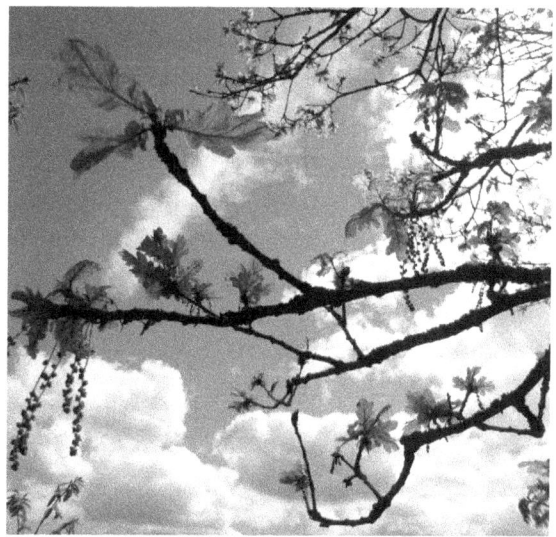

Male catkins in spring.

produce a reversal and cure.[5] It is difficult to imagine this working without a good deal of assistance. So far, the emphasis has been on halting bleeding and tightening tissues, but the astringent oak had more to offer. Culpeper adds the distilled water of oak buds as an anti-inflammatory when used inwardly or outwardly, which also acts to cool the heat of fevers.[6] At the same period, (1653), Coles gives the powder of acorns drunk in wine for stitch and pain in the side, especially if mixed with bay-berries.[7] This treatment appears to have been successful if any conclusion can be drawn from a similar recipe surviving the next century. In 1746, a collection of contributed recipes was published and we find another recipe for stitch. This time the powdered acorn is mixed with an equal quantity of powdered angelica seed and a glass of black cherry water is taken afterwards.[8]

Summary. There is plentiful evidence of the use of native oak by prehistoric man. All parts of the tree are easily recognisable and feature in the archeobotanical record. Our first recorded use of the oak for medicine comes, not surprisingly, from Pliny. There is a clear pattern, which is repeated throughout history of using the binding and drying properties of the tannins in the oak for treating multiple problems. Dysentery and fluxes, which are discharges of various kinds, which can include bleeding, are obvious candidates for this. Various preparations of the acorns, bark, leaves, or gall nuts were used in roles such as tightening and healing inflamed tissues, particularly the gums, relieving toothache and restraining prolapses or miscarriage.

Applied externally the oak has dried and treated superficial abscesses, burns, snake bites, and malignancy. Medieval surgeons used oak galls with corrosive arsenic, alum, and vinegar to clean gangrenous wounds. From the nineteenth century onwards, use concentrates on the bark rather than other parts of the tree. Although only prescribed today in small doses, modern use supports the historical picture and can be found in the Herbalists' Reference.

Recipes

Extracted from Thornton's Family Herbal. 1810. "Rx 1. Take of oak bark, in pieces—ounce ½, boiling water … a pint … Let it remain for four hours, then strain; add to this Alum in powder … a drachm:

To be used as a lotion cold to limbs after the gout, and also to scrophulous glands."

"Rx 2. Take of galls, in powder … drachms 2, Hog's lard … ounce ½: Make into an ointment, to be applied by means of lint to the external piles, or even pressed somewhat up the fundament every night. This has done wonders in the piles, taking at the same time the following" (p.769).[9] There follows a mix containing quassia, aromatic confection and ginger to take internally twice daily.

Notes

1. Jones W.H.S. (trans), *Pliny Natural History* VI Books XXIV–XXVII. (Loeb Classical Library. 1989). Xxiv iii. 7–10.
2. Gunther R.T. (ed), *Dioscorides Greek Herbal*. (Hafner. 1968). 77.
3. Rosenman Leonard D. MD. *A Medieval Surgical Pharmacopoeia and Formulary*. 1170–1325. (San Francisco. 1999). 76, 78.
4. Hobby E. (ed), *The Birth of Mankind*. (1560). (Ashgate. 2009). 129.
5. Johnson T. (ed), *The Herbal*. John Gerard. (1633 edition). (Dover Publications, New York. 1975). 1339.
6. Culpeper N. *Culpeper's Complete Herbal and English Physician enlarged*. (1652). (London. 1815 edition). 128.
7. Coles W. *The Paradise of Plants*. (London. 1657). 375.
8. Anon. *A Collection of Receipts*. (Printed for the Executrix of Mary Kettilby. 1746). 162.
9. Thornton R.J. *A New Family Herbal*. (London. 1810). 769.

Quercus robur, Q. Petraea – Herbalists' Reference

The Parts of the Oak Tree Used for Medicine – Inner bark from young thin branches should be gathered in spring. Leaves are harvested in June for drying. Gather fruits in September.

Dosage and Forms – Acorn tincture 1:5 in 45% alcohol. Dose is 15–30 drops three times daily.

Constituents – Condensed tannins, saponins, quillaic acid is the main sapogenin, resin.

Actions and Uses – The astringency of oak from the tannin content has seen it recommended and approved by the German Commission E for treating acute diarrhoea, given internally in small doses. Local treatment of genital and anal inflammation, as well as that of the mouth and pharynx in a mouthwash or gargle has also been approved.[1] Oak is rarely given internally however as the taste is objectionable. In topical applications, oak not only helps to stop bleeding and discharges, but promotes repair of damaged tissue through the action of the tannins. It may be used for chilblains, sweaty feet, weeping eczema or eczema close to leg ulcers, burns, leucorrhoea, vaginitis, urethritis, prolapse and haemorrhoids.

Combinations – May be given with ginger before meals.[2]

Topical Applications – Tincture for external application is diluted one part to twenty of boiled water. Powdered inner bark or acorns can be applied to ulcers and wounds. Also used in an ointment or lotion.

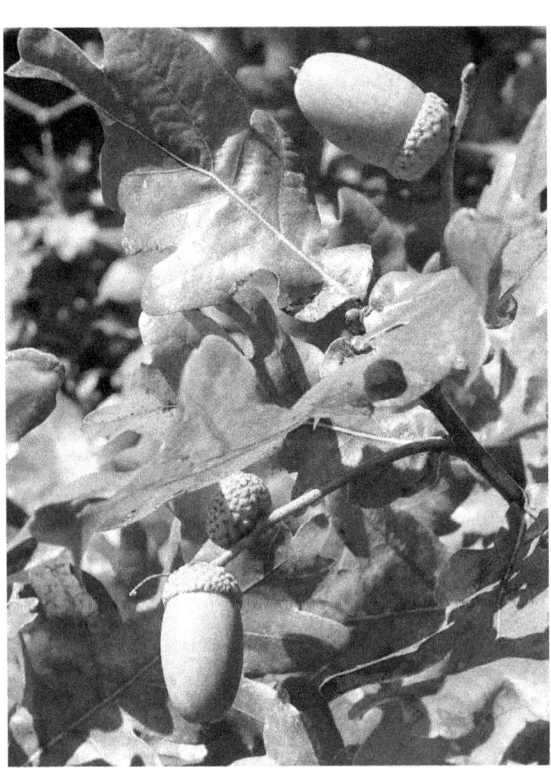
Acorns on the oak.

Make a decoction for use as a compress, or in a Sitz bath for acute perianal inflammation. Add a small handful of chopped bark to one litre of water. Cool before use. This can also be applied to ease inflammatory skin conditions. Oak compresses should never be covered with waterproof material. They should only be applied loosely in order for the fluid to evaporate.[3]

Contraindications and Precautions – Do not mix oak extracts with those containing alkaloids as these are precipitated by the tannins.[4] Absorption of alkaline drugs may be inhibited after internal use. Avoid continuous use. Not to be added to a full body bath or applied over a large damaged area.[1]

Notes

1. Blumenthal et al. *Herbal Medicine. Expanded Commission E monographs.* (Integrative Medicine Commission. 2000). 278.
2. Hoffmann D. *The New Holistic Herbal.* (Element. 1990). 219.
3. Weiss R.F. M.D. *Herbal Medicine.* (Thieme. 2nd edition revised and expanded. 2000).295.
4. Mills S. & Bone K. *Principles & Practice of Phytotherapy.* (Churchill Livingstone. 2000). 34/5.

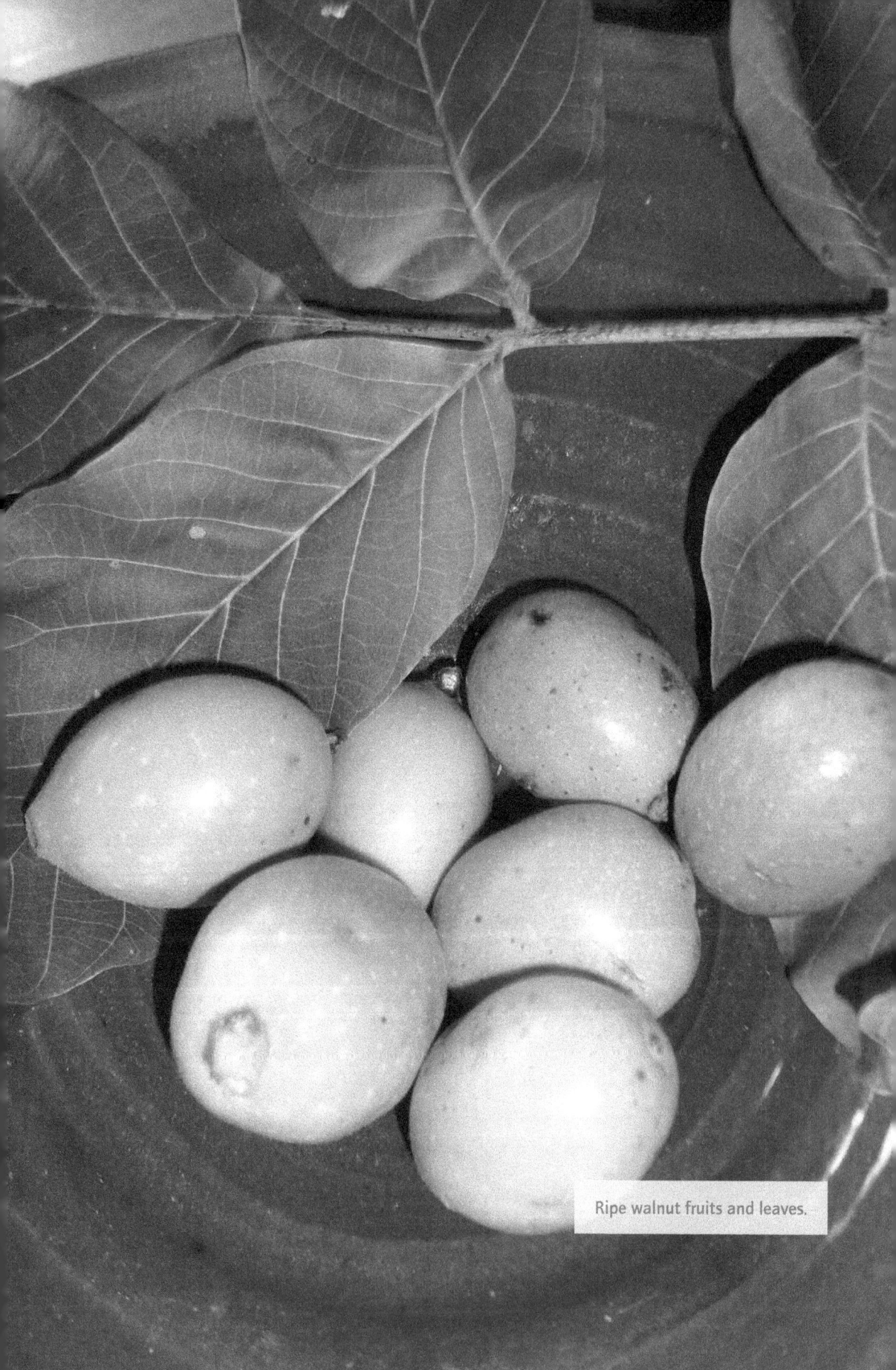

Ripe walnut fruits and leaves.

Walnut

Juglans regia – Juglandaceae

WALNUT – Usefulness – The unripe fruits can be pickled. The ripe seeds or nuts are rich in vitamins and minerals, and considered a tonic and aphrodisiac food. The leaves provide medicine and insect repellent. Oil from the nuts is flavoursome for salads, has medicinal applications, and is used to polish wood, but does not keep well. The husks of the fruits provide a fast dye, which does not require a mordant. The leaves and bark provide hair, wool, and wood dyes.[1]

Dangers – Juglones from the leaves and roots react with the soil to produce chemicals that inhibit growth of other plants nearby. Internal medication from the leaves should be limited to short term use under the guidance of a herbal practitioner.[2] Gathering up husks from the walnuts will powerfully stain your hands.

Getting to Know the Walnut Tree – Originating in Asia, walnut trees are now naturalised in Southeast Europe and have been planted in Britain for over 1,000 years. My wish to grow a walnut tree in my garden was granted recently, I think by squirrels, who kindly planted six walnuts for me that sprouted as young trees. Rooks and crows also like walnuts and bury them as food stores. Unable to believe my eyes, I carefully removed the first seedling from the pot in which it had been buried, to check identification. The open nutshell attached between stem and root left me in no doubt. Re-planted in more suitable compost it was none the worse for the short exposure.

Fully grown, however, even one tree would be far too large for a modest garden as they can reach twenty-five to thirty metres (eighty to 100 feet) tall, with a wide spread of leafy branches. A long-lived tree, the walnut matures slowly and it will be twenty years before these young trees will bear fruit. Grafted trees can be bought and will crop sooner. Walnuts will flourish best in rich, loamy soil, rather than clay. Some are self-fertile, others better with cross-pollination. The drooping male catkins seen in late April and early May form on buds from the previous year, while the smaller female flowers are produced on new shoots. The leaves are dark and leathery to touch when mature and are borne in groups of five to nine elliptical leaflets, smooth around their edges, making them quite distinctive. The bruised or crushed leaf will give out an aroma, which is repellent to insects.[3]

The bark of walnut is brownish and quite smooth when the trees are young, becoming rougher and grey with age. The trees were grown for their timber more than for the nuts in earlier centuries, the wood providing elegant furniture, wainscots, the wheels, and bodies of coaches and gunstocks. Cabinet makers also used it for inlay work and walnut is suitable for carving and turning. By 1824, Green states that walnut is now out of fashion in favour of mahogany in England, although still in favour on the Continent.

My windfall of trees required me to find them homes before they were too large for pots, as the clay soil here would not suit them. A friend has planted them on her land in Devon. I was sad to see them go as walnuts can add flavour and nutrition to so many dishes, both savoury and sweet. They can be sprinkled on everything from salads to breakfast cereal, included in stuffings and ketchup, or blended into cheese. They are also tasty in sweet biscuits, cakes, toffee, other confections, ice cream, and desserts. It is fortunate that I have always known someone with a tree, for in addition to finding the nuts delicious in healthy snacks and other foods, there is an earlier harvest of the green, swelled, but as yet unripe fruits, which are gathered from the trees in June or early July. These are tasty when pickled and have been enjoyed for centuries. A recipe from 1609 specifies the walnuts should be about the size of a large cobnut and they are seethed initially to remove tannins, so that the first water must be thrown away—or for me as a dyer—better still, saved to be used as dye liquor.[4]

They are cooked again in fresh water, before adding vinegar and honey. This has been a successful recipe, made during my stillroom workshops at the Weald and Downland Living Museum. Pickled walnuts remain popular today. Sir Hugh Plat in 1609 may have been inspired by earlier recipes from the Continent where walnuts were being candied. Green walnuts were pricked as above, steeped in water and then boiled with a generous amount of honey, adding spices.[5]

Anyone with a walnut tree is always glad of someone willing to come and clear away the many husks left, usually on a lawn as the ripe fruit falls. These give a beautiful range of brown shades, which are fast. On silk, however, I sometimes prefer the results from that first strong water taken during pickling. It seems from the reference in a book of cosmetic recipes from the eighteenth century, the green shells of walnuts were preferred for dyeing hair also. These were amongst a list of possible herbal dyes, to be boiled in rain-water, wine, or vinegar and herbs known for treating headaches and problems with eyes, ears, etc, such as lemon balm, betony, and clove gilliflowers added for a holistic recipe.[6]

Legends and Folklore. It seems odd and unhappy for the tree that it was regarded as necessary in the past to beat the nuts off the tree with sticks and it was again beaten on Christmas Day in order to be fruitful. Coles and others refer to young boys enjoying the task. Keeping a walnut in your pocket for good luck was something practised by my father-in-law years ago. We kept the walnut as a memento after he died.

The Greeks and Romans dedicated the tree to Zeus/Jupiter, and so walnuts are occasionally referred to as Jupiter's nuts and connected with fertility. Roman writers refer to walnuts being scattered at weddings.

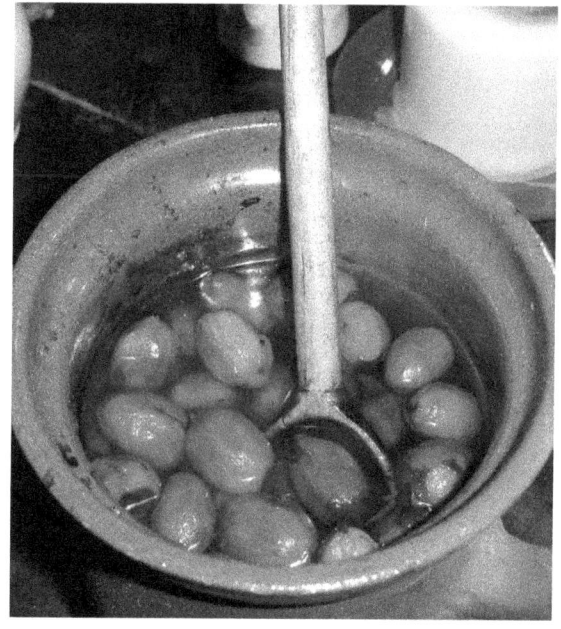
Pickling unripe walnuts. Photo courtesy Weald and Downland Living Museum.

This is interpreted as symbolising brides leaving the sphere of Diana's influence for that of Hymen, goddess of marriage.[7]

Notes

1. Green T. *Universal Herbal or Botanical Dictionary*. 2 vols, (Caxton, London. 2nd edition. 1824.) Vol. 1. 766.
2. Barker J. *The Medicinal Flora of Britain and Northwestern Europe*. (Winter Press. 2001). 12.
3. Chiej R. *The Macdonald Encyclopedia of Medicinal Plants*. (Macdonald Publishing. London. 1984). 163.
4. Plat Sir H. *Delights for Ladies*. (1609). (Crosby Lockwood. 1948). 40.
5. Warde W. & Anglosse R. (trans), *The Secretes of Maister Alexis of Piemont*. (Atenar. 2000). 89.
6. Anon. *The Toilet of Flora*. (London. 1784). 11.
7. Baker R St. Barbe. *Trees A Book of the Seasons*. (Lindsay Drummond Ltd. 1948). 16.

WALNUT – History of Medicinal Use

The walnut was supposed to have been introduced to Italy by Vitellius and appears quickly to have become valued both for its nuts and wood. The Romans are thought to have introduced the trees in turn to Britain, although substantiating written record for their presence here in the early years of the first millennium is missing. Walnut trees were on the list for the ideal monastery garden drawn up by Charlemagne between 816 and 836 A.D. and Aelfric's partnering the Latin and colloquial terms for walnuts in 995 A.D. supports them being established

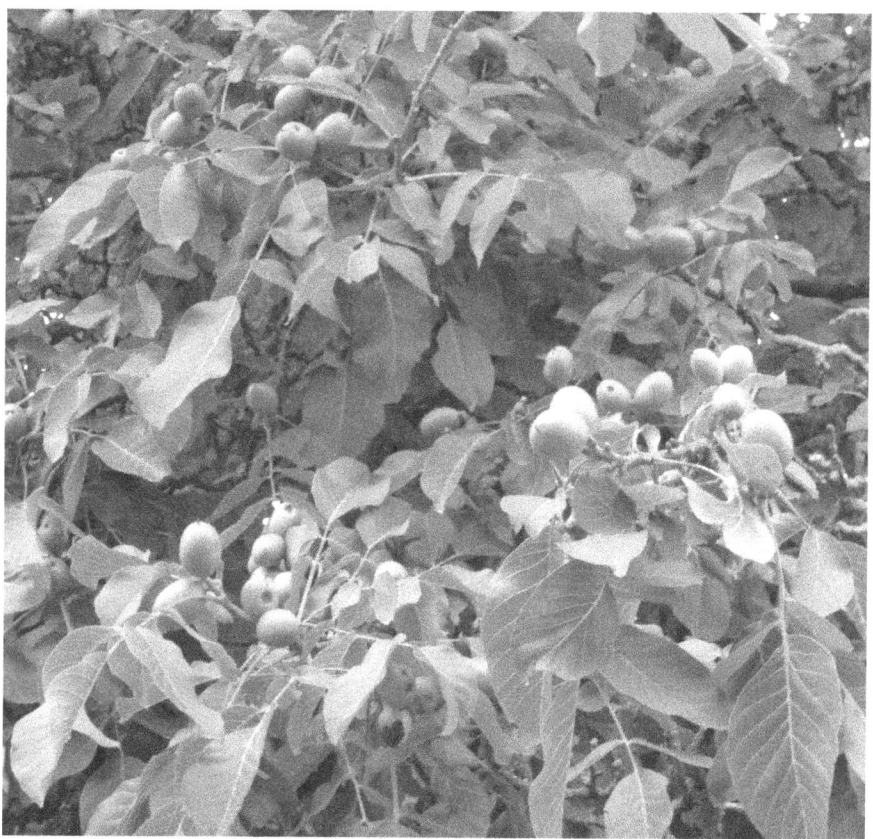

Fruits on the tree near Bayleaf House. Photo courtesy Weald and Downland Living Museum.

here. A possible reference to the walnut in the Earl of Lincoln's garden in Holborn dates to 1295.[1]

That the leaves contain poisonous substances is commented on by Pliny, who also regarded the dried nuts as oily and injurious to the stomach. Nevertheless, he recommended them for removing phlegm and easing colic.[2] The use of walnuts against tapeworms began in this era and has remained with walnuts ever since. Several of his other remedies have not lasted the test of time. Dioscorides joins Pliny in prescribing walnuts as antidotes to poisons, also the burnt husk beaten in oil and wine to be applied to the head as a stimulant to hair growth in alopecia.[3]

Hildegard of Bingen included young walnut leaves or the bark in a worming drink. She regarded walnut oil as fattening and likely to congest the lungs with mucus.[4] By 1443, aromatic water was being distilled from walnut leaves gathered on midsummer day or into the following night. This precious water was taken to cure madness.[5]

In the following century, walnuts given with figs and rue were eaten against the plague. There were more hair care recipes in this *Book of Secrets*, but this time the hair stimulant involved the addition of the ashes of several animals. The hair dye was made only with the walnut leaves.[6] Gerard writes that the walnut tree is by then common in orchards. A milk resembling that from the almond is being made, which he says is cooling and pleasing to the sick body.[7]

Coles comments on the nut having a close resemblance to the form of the brain, which according to the doctrine of signatures suggested this to be supportive of the head. He tells us that salt from the husks or walnut bark was applied to head wounds. He gives the authority of the famous School of Medicine in Salerno, Italy, for the belief that walnuts were effective against poisons. He suggests using old walnut kernels to heal gangrene and carbuncles, applying them together with rue and figs, reasoning they were previously applied to old ulcers.[8] Pechey writes in his herbal of tapping the sap but says it is not as pleasant as that of birch.[9] There is no mention of this practice after that date. However, I have been told by a Lithuanian tree surgeon that this is still done in his home country.

In 1722, Joseph Miller, head of the Chelsea Physic garden, is still recommending the green nuts as cordial and alexipharmic, that is of particular use against "malignant Distempers, and the Plague it self"(p.147). He records that they are one of the main ingredients in the widely regarded and expensive treacle water or Theriac, made in Venice and London with great ceremony and sold by Apothecaries to the rich. He also writes of the bark as strongly emetic and oil expressed from the ripe nuts as a good medicine for the stone and gravel in the kidneys.[10]

In 1790, Woodville supports use of the unripe fruit for killing worms, pointing out the wealth of earlier recommendations. He compares the nut to the almond and writes that the oil, which does not congeal in cold temperatures, may be substituted for almond oil in medicine.[11] The 1791 Pharmacopoeia includes a watery extract from the unripe fruit, given in cinnamon water in drop doses to bring away worms in children. A purgative was to be added on the third or fifth day to ensure complete removal.[12] In the early nineteenth century, Waller quotes the German seventeenth century professor of surgery, Etmuller, saying that perforations made in the roots in February "yield a copious juice" (p.354), which was recommended for chronic toothache and pain from the urinary stone and gravel. He does not say however that he has witnessed the practice in Britain.[13]

Summary. It seems the Romans both introduced cultivation of the tree in Britain and, through the works of Pliny and Dioscorides, the use of parts of the walnut tree in medicine. The power of the fruit rinds and oil to eliminate tapeworms has been a consistent reference over the centuries. Antibacterial qualities are evident from the general regard of walnut to be eaten as an antidote to infectious diseases, to the extent that walnut was an ingredient in the famed panacea Theriac.

Old kernels were also applied to gangrene, carbuncles, and external ulcers. Mrs. Grieve writes in the twentieth century of the quills of bark available commercially for providing a decoction used to heal indolent ulcers. The leaves could also provide a decoction for the same.[14] Recipes for stimulating hair growth, conditioning and dyeing hair are frequent. Aromatic water was distilled from the unripe fruits in June from the fifteenth century onwards. The brain-like shape of walnut kernels was seen as an indication for using them to treat the head. They were accordingly administered for mental illness and with the addition of rue and figs to prevent plague. Both oil and milk extracted from walnuts were compared favourably to those made from almonds and used in medicine. Almond oil in particular has been recommended for easing passage of urinary stones.

Recipe

Extracted from Anon. 1746. "*For the* Cholick. Take the thin Peel that comes off the Kernels of a ripe Wallnut, dry'd, and beat to Powder; the thin Yellow Peel of Orange powder'd; of each a like Quantity: Mix it in a Cup of hot Ale, and drink it up. A small Spoonful of the Powders, mix'd, is a Dose" (p.162).[15]

Notes

1. Harvey J. *Mediaeval Gardens.* (Batsford. 1981). 32, 84.
2. Jones W.H.S. (trans), *Pliny Natural History* VI Books XX–XXIII. (Loeb Classical Library. 1989). XXIII. LXXV. 513.
3. Gunther R.T. (ed), *Dioscorides Greek Herbal.* (Hafner. 1968). 87. 88.
4. Throop P. (trans), *Hildegard von Bingen's Physica.* (Healing Arts Press. 1998). 108/9.
5. Dawson W. (ed), *A Leechbook of the XVth Century.* (Macmillan & Co. 1934). 319. (1043).
6. Warde W. & Anglosse R. (trans), *The Secretes of Maister Alexis of Piemont.* (Atenar. 2000). 93.
7. Johnson T. (ed), *The Herbal.* John Gerard. (1633 edition). (Dover Publications, New York. 1975). 1440.
8. Coles W. *The Paradise of Plants.* (London. 1657). 3.
9. Pechey J. *The English Herbal of Physical Plants.* (London. 1694). 190.
10. Miller J. *Botanicum officinale.* Bell. (London. 1722). 246.
11. Woodville W. *Medical Botany.* 3 vols + Supplement. (London. 1790). Vol. 2. 348/9.

12. Healde T. M.D. F.R.S. *The Pharmacopoeia of the R.C.P. of London.* (1791). 37.
13. Waller J. *Waller's New British Domestic Herbal.* Cox & Son. (London. 1822). 353.
14. Grieve. M. *A Modern Herbal.* (1st published 1934 Jonathan Cape. Saavas. 1984). 843.
15. Anon. *A Collection of Receipts.* (Printed for the Executrix of Mary Kettilby. 1746). 162.

JUGLANS REGIA – Herbalists' Reference

The Parts of the Walnut Tree Used for Medicine – Leaf, gathered May-July, green fruit peel, oil.

Dosage and Forms – The leaves can be administered as an infusion or syrup. Decoction of the dried leaf 2–3g per 100ml cold water, bring to the boil and simmer for 15 minutes, to be used in a hand or foot bath or for compresses. Walnut leaf is approved by the German Commission E for external use.

Constituents – Leaf—Ellagitannins, juglone, flavonoids, organic acids, volatile oil.

Fruits – Organic acids, carbohydrate, fat, vitamins, hydrojuglone, minerals, eugenol.

Actions and Uses – Leaf—This is a bitter astringent, which is also laxative and expectorant. The decoction may be taken for constipation and chronic coughs. Use of the leaf may help to dissolve urinary stones but walnut should only be taken in the short term.[1] It may also be hypoglycaemic, and as a taenifuge is given to destroy tapeworm.[2] Green peel of the fruit has been used for diarrhoea and anaemia. The leaves are both bactericidal and insect repellent. Juglone in the leaves has been shown to have antifungal and antiviral properties.[3] Washes are used externally for herpes, eruptive skin complaints, and hair loss.

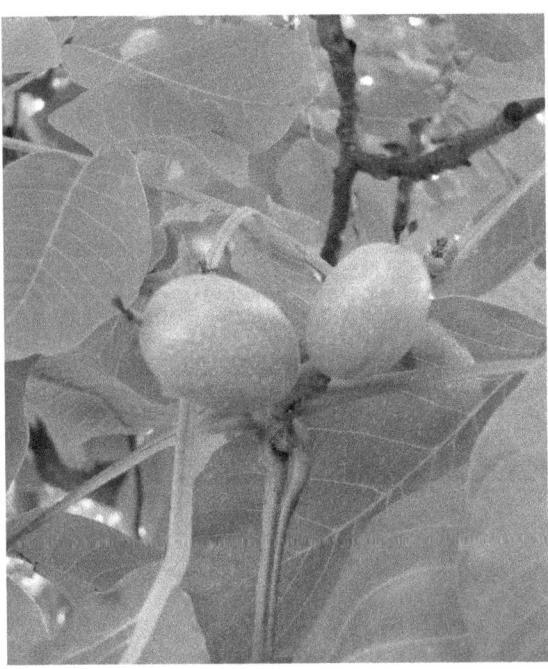

Close up of walnut fruits. Photo Courtesy Weald and Downland Living Museum.

Topical Applications – The oil is helpful for dry skin conditions. The leaves may be applied in compresses, on dressings, or as a decocted wash for eczema, herpes and eruptive skin conditions, excessive perspiration of hands and feet, chilblains, and varicose ulcers.

Combinations – Walnut leaf and *Viola tricolor* are suggested together in equal parts applied for skin complaints.[3]

Contraindications and Precautions – Walnut is incompatible with many other herbal remedies, also with antacids. Not for long term internal use.[4]

Notes

1. Bown D. *The RHS Encyclopedia of Herbs.* (Dorling Kindersley. 1996). 298.
2. Barker J. *The Medicinal Flora of Britain and Northwestern Europe.* (Winter Press. 2001). (12).
3. Blumenthal et al. *Herbal Medicine. Expanded Commission E monographs.* (Integrative Medicine Commission. 2000). 401.
4. Barker J. *The Medicinal Flora of Britain and Northwestern Europe.* (Winter Press. 2001). (12).

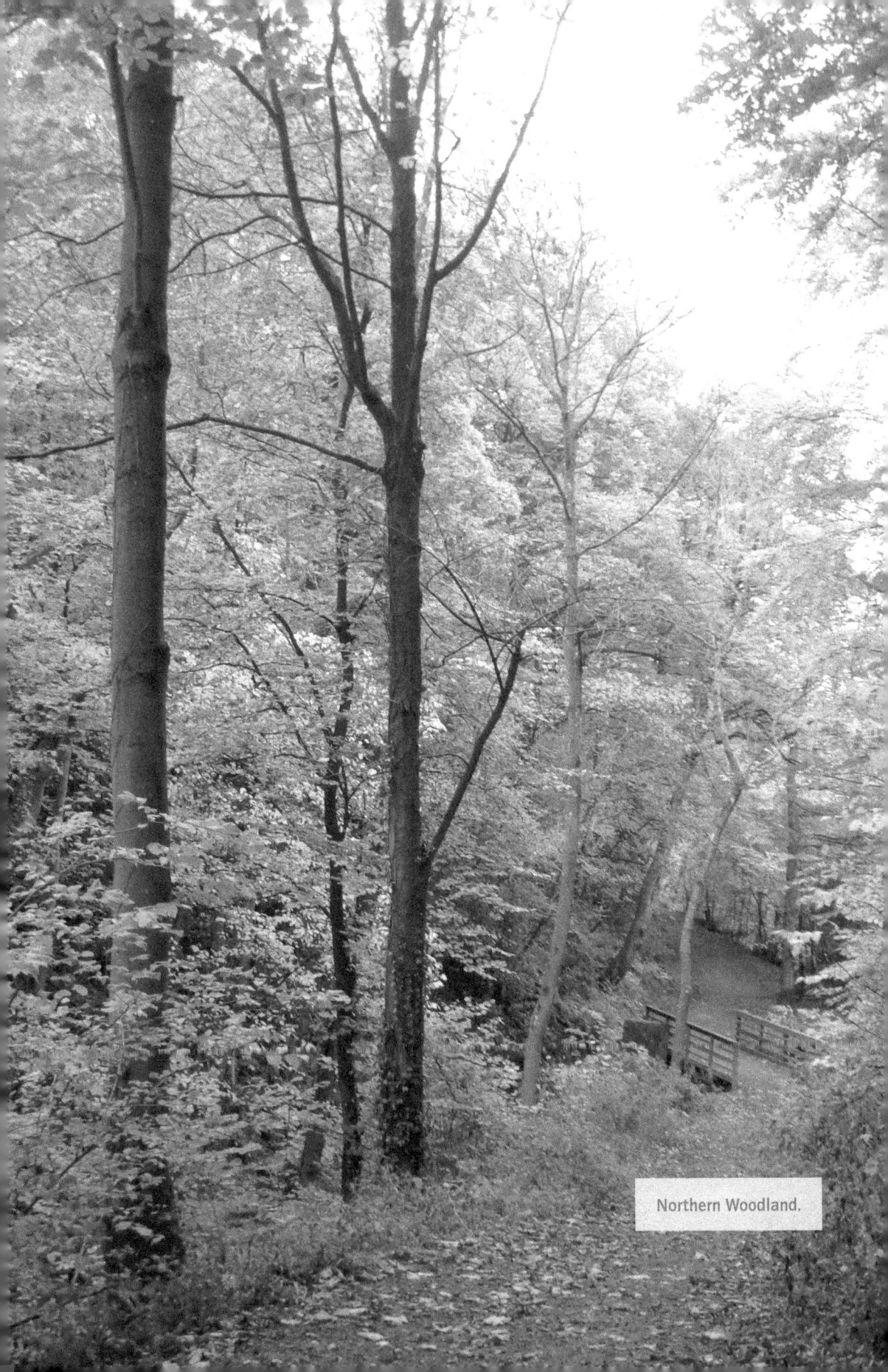
Northern Woodland.

AUTUMN

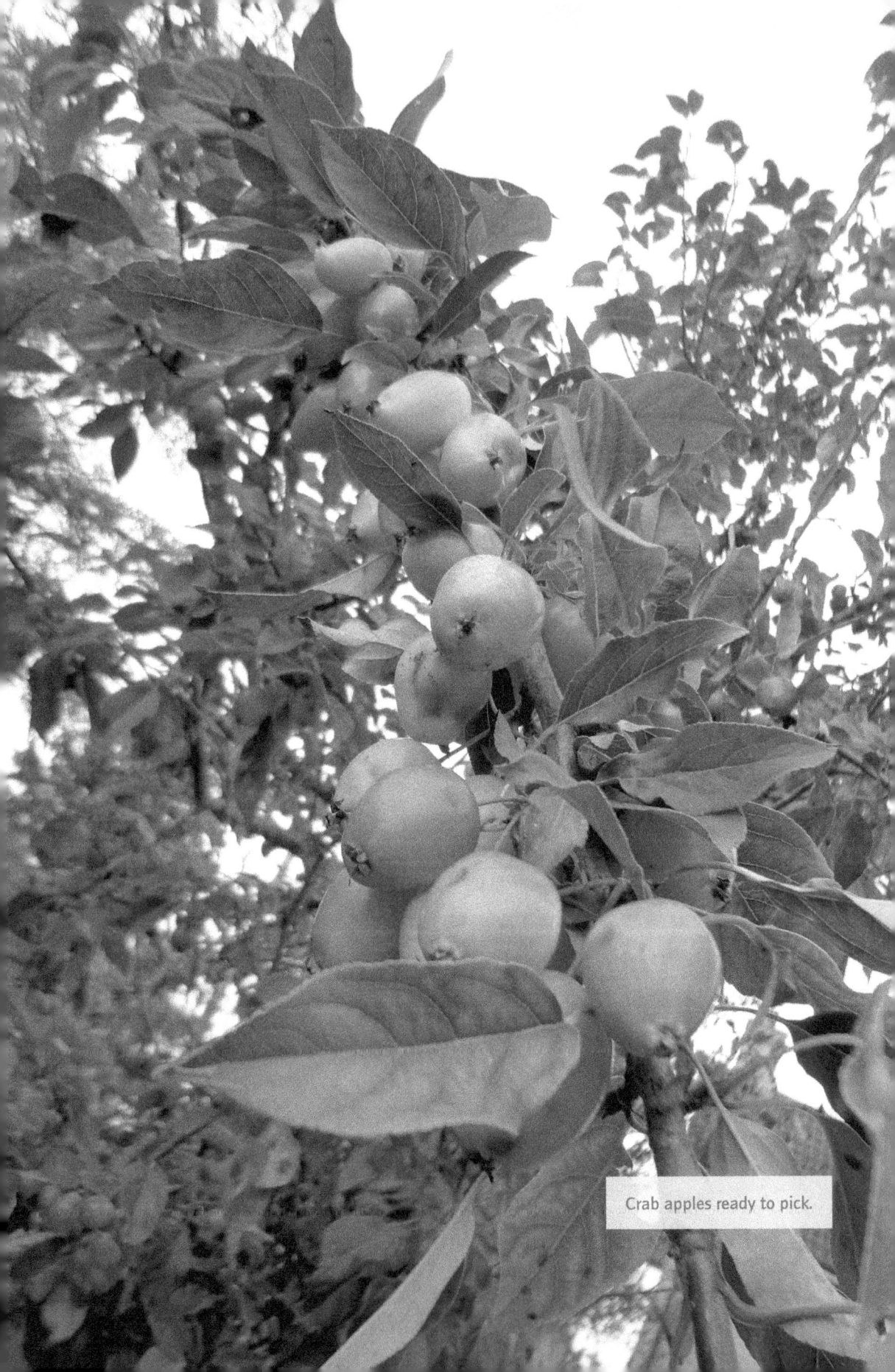

Crab apples ready to pick.

Crab Apple

Malus Sylvestris – Crab Apple – Rosaceae

CRAB APPLE – *Usefulness* – The fruit juice provides sour vinegar, known as verjuice for preserving. The whole, unpeeled fruits offer pectin-rich liquor valued over the centuries for setting jellies and jams. The fruits are used to make cider and wine. The bark gives a yellow dye. The leaves and flowers may also be used for dyeing. The wood can be turned. It has been used in wood engraving and a wide range of objects, from tools to musical instruments have been made from crab apple.

Dangers – The seeds of apples contain amygdalin in common with other members of the *Rosaceae* family. A few seeds do no harm but eating a cupful has proved fatal.[1]

Getting to Know the Crab Apple Tree – The crab apple grows wild across much of Europe, reaching a height of about ten metres and living sometimes for as long as a century. Distinguishing a truly wild crab apple tree from one that has grown from the pip of a discarded apple can be difficult as such "wildings" tend to revert. There are in fact two sub-species, the native *Malus sylvestris*, the fruit of which is more yellow when ripe and quite long, and the *Malus mitis*, which has a rounder, larger fruit. Generally apples less than five centimetres (two inches) across are considered crab apples.

The form of the tree also varies, being different in woodland where it is encouraged to be slender, reaching for light, to a tree in a hedgerow, which can spread its branches and still receive light from all sides. The grey-brown bark cracks as it grows upwards, to leave narrow, raised plates that can peel off. There may be spines on the twigs and branches, amounting to thorns, announcing its membership of the rose family. You may not recognise it as an apple tree until the white or pinkish blossom appears, or you see the yellowish green fruits with a blush of red colour where the sun catches them in autumn.

In prehistory, crab apples were gathered for food and boiling them would have given a thickener for honey syrups. While preparing for an autumn Celtic workshop almost thirty years ago, I decided to blend crab apple juice with elderberry juice and honey to make a thick extract which would keep well. On tipping the pan to pour it I realised this was considerably thicker than I had expected as the mix fell into shiny round drops maintaining their shape. I had in fact made jelly sweets. The idea that the early Celts could have made such delicious sweets in this way was a novel one and a useful lesson in not taking it for granted that such delights were not open to our ancestors.

The cultivated apple may well have been brought by the Romans, if crabs had not been taken into cultivation before. Saxons and Celts planted orchards but the crab apples often remained in the wild, their usefulness appearing only in lists compiled by the monks. One such, written at St. Albans in 1382, sets the crab with sloe amongst wild fruit trees.[2]

The medieval simile "as sour as a crab" refers to the taste of these small apples, which had an uncomplimentary nickname of "choke apples". Despite their sour taste, crab apples have been part of our diet as well as being used in medicine for many centuries. In Medieval cookery they are partnered with spices such as nutmeg, cloves, and cumin and this too gives a perceived medicinal effect on the stomach. Still, wild food guides abound with recipes containing them, for the fruits can be usefully partnered with any hedgerow berries, guaranteeing a set jelly or jam. They are not limited to jellies and syrup. We find other suggestions given in Thomas Tusser's *Five Hundred Points of Good Husbandry*. His instructions to the farmer in the month of October are to pound the crab apples for making verjuice and cider.[3] Almost 500 years later both the vinegar-like verjuice and cider are still made and the best cider may be said to come from a blend of cultivated apples and wild crab apples.

Tastes vary in different counties, in Gloucester the astringency of the Hagloe-crab was popular in the 1950s and 60s.[4] The wine, declared by Green in 1824 to be little inferior to Rhenish wine—with the proper addition of sugar, still appears in books of country recipes.

The tree is so pretty that often smaller cultivars are commonly grown in gardens and the fruits vary in their size, shape, and taste. Some crab apples are really sour and others a good deal sweeter. Meanwhile, the wild crab apple has a history of being used as a stock for grafting less hardy apples onto. In Millers *Gardener's Dictionary* of 1771, there is the instruction to obtain the seeds of the crab apple when the fruits are pressed for verjuice and sow these in light earth, covering them with only half an inch of soil in November or December if the weather is reasonably dry. The advice to wait until early spring if the winter is already proving wet is to protect them from turning mouldy. Crab apple is used in nurseries as a dwarfing rootstock for new varieties of eating and cooking apples, taking advantage of its hardy, frost-resistant nature.

In recent years while collaborating with a project designed to bring experience of nature into the hospice environment, I was given two tiny saplings. These had grown from crab apple seeds sown by patients and I have gladly nurtured them as they are growing into trees. I look forward to gathering my own crab apples in the not too distant future, where previously I have depended upon the kindness of friends to give me a portion of their harvest.

Legends and Folklore. Something which may be more likely as the climate changes and plants and trees receive confused signals is that one branch may blossom while fruits remain on the tree. This was once thought to predict the death of a member of the household. Presenting the last apple each year to the Apple Tree Man contained in the oldest tree of the orchard has been a custom carried out to sustain fertility and clearly is a superstition of great antiquity.[5] Young girls setting crab apples in the loft in the shape of the initials of possible husbands is recorded for the west of England. At the old Michaelmas Day, which falls in October, the best preserved initials name the husband to be.[6]

Notes

1. Fröhne D. Pfander H. *A Colour Atlas of Poisonous Plants.* (Wolf Science. 1983). 190.
2. Harvey J. *Mediaeval Gardens.* (Batsford. 1981). 122.
3. Tusser T. *Five Hundred Points of Good Husbandry.* (Original 1573). (Oxford University Press. 1984). 40,
4. Aylett M. *Encyclopaedia of Home-Made Wines.* (Odhams Press Ltd. London.1957). 67.
5. Phillips R. *Wild Food.* (Pan Books. 1983). 131.
6. Vickery R. *Oxford Dictionary of Plant-Lore.* (Oxford University Press. 1997). 93.

CRAB APPLE – History of Medicinal Use

After the extensive excavations of the Lake Dwellings in Switzerland at Wangen, Zug, Marin, and Moringen, it was concluded that wild crab apples had considerable importance in Bronze Age food.[1] In Britain, no stores of crab apples have been found at the comparable site of the Glastonbury Lake Village. However, the use of apple pips to impress decorative patterns into pottery elsewhere has been taken to support the assumption that the fruits were gathered in quantity, at least for food. As with other herb foods, it would seem to be inevitable that when the apples were eaten, their medicinal properties and possibilities would in time become clear. The comment of Dioscorides that wild (crab) apples bind the bowel, and if using them for this action they must not be fully ripe, gives them a place in medicine in the first century A.D.[2] Pliny also gives wild apples against loose bowels, and agrees, writing they must be used unripe.[3]

Coming forward into the period of written history in Britain, we find the first mention of the tree in medicine is for crab apple bark harvested from the lower east side of the tree. This is mixed with other tree barks, ash, willow, and oak in an Anglo-Saxon salve for headache and diseases of the limbs.[4]

In the later medieval period crab apples are considered good to cleanse the stomach. Crab apples were commonly stuffed with spices in medicinal recipes; the spices, which are also herbs and part of the treatment, and the apple acting both as a medicinal herb and

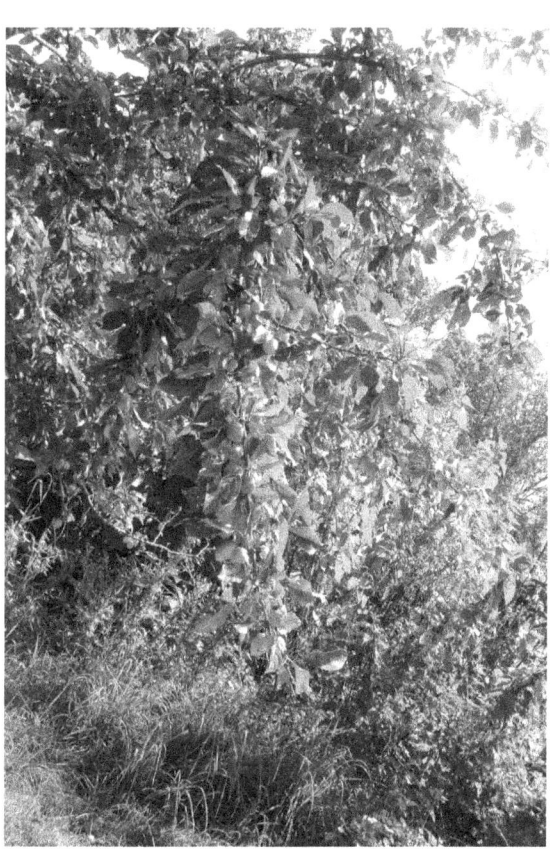

Mature Crab apple tree.

a carrier for others. Heating the stomach was considered to aid the digestion. Sour crab apples were, it must be remembered, considered as binding not only to the bowels, but also when pregnancy was concerned, to the uterus. It was therefore natural to warn pregnant mothers near their time not to eat them.

We also find crab apples valued for their juice used with outward applications, in cooling compresses. In the mid seventeenth century Coles agrees, writing that the juice of crabs known as verjuice, when applied on wet cloths draws out heat from burns and aids healing. Also, "A *rotten Apple* applyed to *Eyes* that are *blood shotten* or *enflamed* with heat, or that are *black* and *blew* by any stroake or fall, all day or all night, helpeth them quickly"(p.259). He continues about the distilled water of good, sound apples to expel melancholy and produce mirth and that of rotten ones to cool heat and inflammation of sores.[5]

In 1722, Miller recorded that while it was valued for external treatments verjuice was rarely given internally, being restricted to gargles for ulcers in the throat and mouth. At the end of the century Meyrick suggests that "few things are better adapted" (p.124) for this purpose, adding strains and bruises to the list of indications for applying the juice.[6]

In the nineteenth century, Green states that the ripe fruit is laxative and "excellent in the dysentery; boiled or roasted, it fortifies a weak stomach; and they are equally efficacious in putrid or malignant fevers, with juice of lemons or currants" (p.432).[7]

Summary. While eating crab apples in prehistory led to the development of sweeter cultivated varieties for food, it also meant that the astringent, cleansing, and healing properties of the crab apple were discovered. At first it was taken internally in Roman medicine to bind loose bowels. Anglo-Saxon medicine contributed a complex recipe using the bark of the tree together with other barks in a salve. The cleansing of the stomach comes to the fore in the medieval period, giving the fruits a place in treating fevers.

Although the notion of eating the apples or taking their juice internally does not altogether vanish, emphasis changes to the outward application of the juice to remove heat from inflamed, infected, burnt, or scalded skin in the seventeenth century. Use as a gargle for an ulcerated mouth or throat is also supported. In the nineteenth century the earlier comments that the juice had proved useful in dysentery, the cooked apple fortified a weak stomach, and was equally effective in malignant fevers, is repeated by Green. In the twentieth century, Mrs. Grieve endorses use for diarrhoea and writes the bark may be decocted for treating bilious fevers.[8] For the modern use see Herbalists' Reference.

Recipe

Extracted from The Paradise of Plants. 1657. "And if they be roasted and eaten with the Juice of Liquorice and Sugar, morning and evening, two houres before meat, they wonderfully helpe those that are troubled with the Cough, or any paine in their Breast" (p.258).[5]

Notes

1. Keller Dr. F. (trans), Lee E. *The Lake Dwellings of Switzerland &c.* (Longmans Green & Co. 1878). Vol. 1. 44, 66, 522.
2. Gunther R.T. (ed), *Dioscorides Greek Herbal.* (Hafner. 1968). 84.
3. Jones W.H.S. (trans), *Pliny Natural History* VI Books XX–XXIII. (Loeb Classical Library. 1989).XXIII LIV. LV. 483.
4. Pollington S. *Leechcraft.* (Anglo Saxon Books. 2000). 195. *Lacnunga* 31.
5. Coles W. *The Paradise of Plants.* (London. 1657). 257.
6. Meyrick W. *The New Family Herbal.* (Birmingham. 1790). 124.
7. Green T. *Universal Herbal or Botanical Dictionary.* 2 vols, (Caxton, London. 2nd edition). (1824). Vol. 2. 432.
8. Grieve M. *A Modern Herbal.* (1st published 1934 Jonathan Cape. Saavas. 1984). 47.

MALUS SYLVESTRIS – Herbalist's Reference

The Parts of Crab Apple Used for Medicine – These are the leaves, fruit, and fruit peel. Also, the fruit juice.

Dosage and Forms – The powdered dried fruit. Infusion: 1–2 teaspoons of dried leaf per cup, given twice daily. The powdered peel may be included with lemon balm in tea. 2 teaspoons per cup. One cup to be taken at night. Pulped fruit is scalded with very hot, not boiling water to be taken for diarrhoea. Dose ½ cup three times daily, sweetened with honey.

Constituents – Crab apple fruit contains pectin, malic, and citric acids, quercetin, sugars, and fruit enzymes.

Actions and Uses – The fruit pulp is antacid and nutritive in the stomach and it appears from a report from Normandy where sweet cider was popular that this was protective against kidney and bladder stones.[1] Either the powdered dried pulp or the juice may be used to reduce

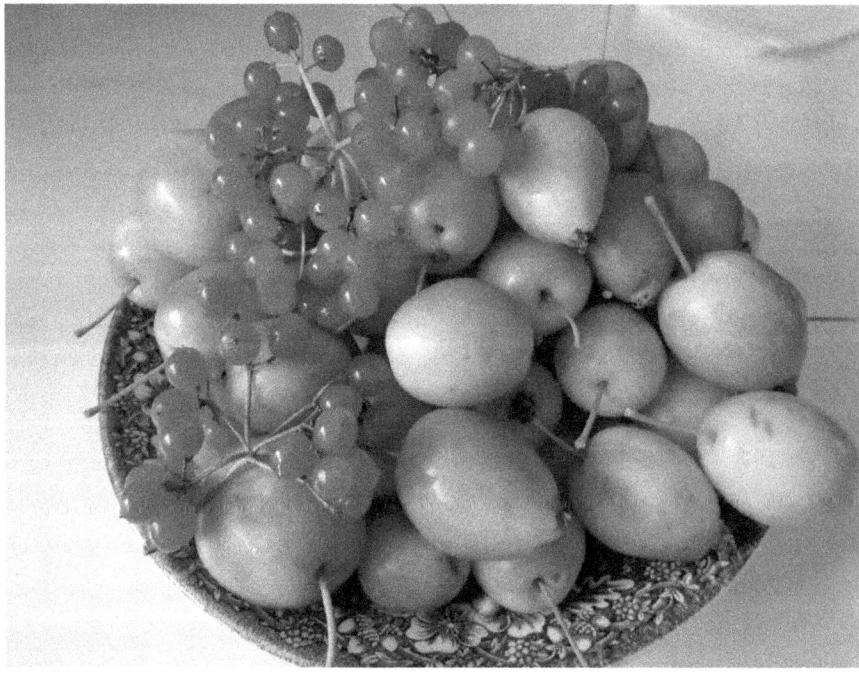

Crab apples with guelder fruits.

symptoms in gastro-enteritis and other stomach inflammations. Apple juice was donated in 2019 by a Somerset apple orchard for a trial with children in the gastro-entrology ward of a hospital in the south west to give relief and restful sleep. Apple leaves and peel assist in removing uric acid from the system, which makes them helpful for treating gout in a mixed tea.[2]

Topical Applications – Pulp of the apple can be applied to reduce inflammation. Historically the juice has also been applied as a compress for burns, scalds, and inflamed skin.

Contraindications and Precautions – None known when eaten or taken in reasonable amounts.

Notes

1. Grieve M. *A Modern Herbal.* (1st pub. 1934 Jonathan Cape. Saavas. 1984). 46.
2. Barker J. *The Medicinal Flora of Britain and Northwestern Europe.* (Winter Press. 2001). (134).

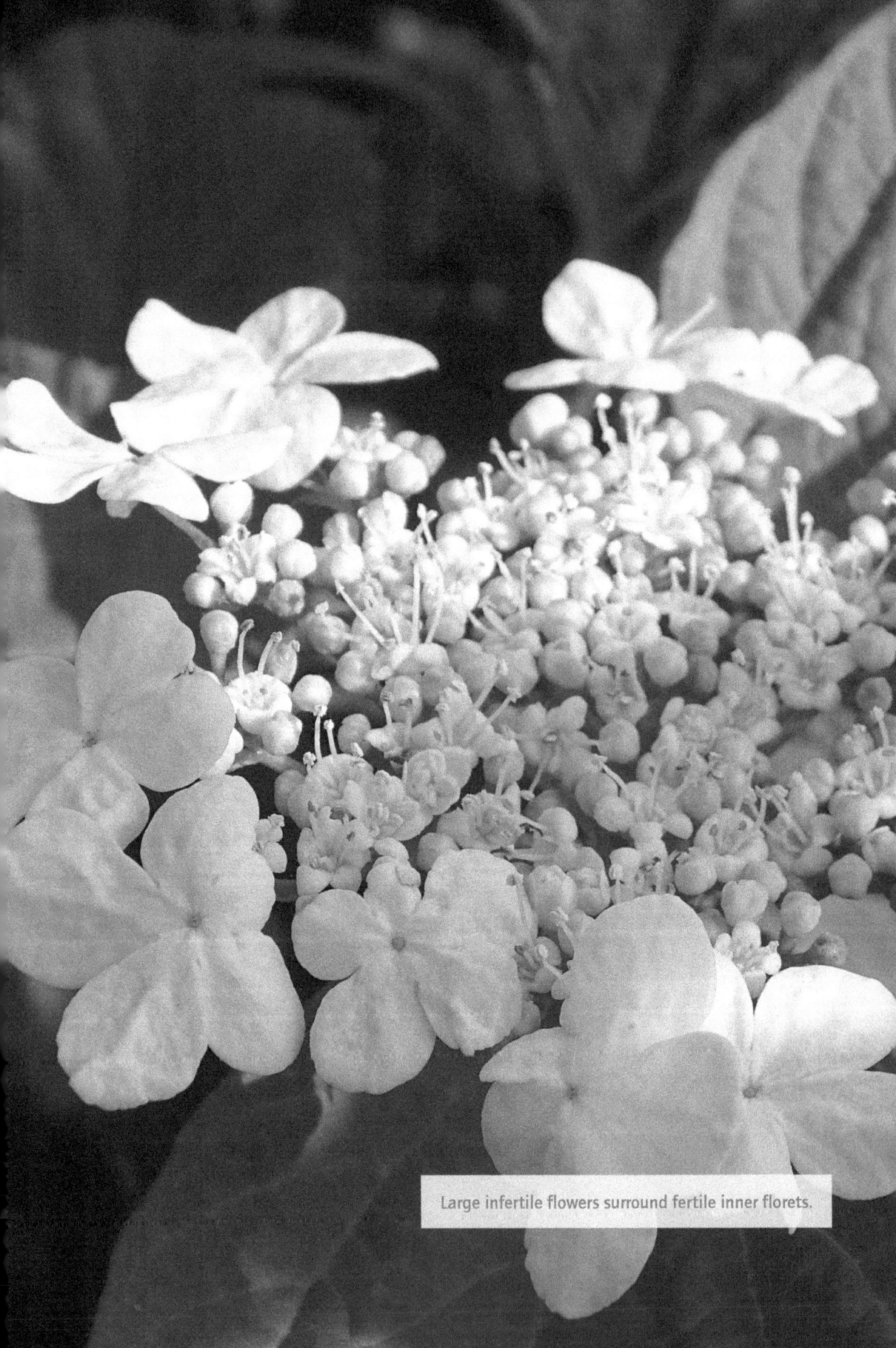

Large infertile flowers surround fertile inner florets.

Cramp Bark

Viburnum Opulus. Guelder Rose – Cramp Bark – Caprifoliaceae

GUELDER ROSE – Usefulness – It is commonly grown as a decorative hedging and in shrubberies. The bark is used in herbal medicine. The berries make a tangy preserve. They can also be distilled to make spirits. The wood was used for making skewers. Dried berries can be used to make ink.

Dangers – If eaten raw the berries cause mild stomach upset.

Getting to Know the Guelder Tree – Despite being so familiar from modern plantings of low maintenance shrubs on roundabouts, around public and commercial buildings, and alongside pathways, guelder berries are rarely gathered today. Their uses seem to be virtually unknown. They are very attractive in appearance certainly, but should anyone try the raw berries, they would find them to be extremely tart to the tongue. The brilliant white flowers open in late spring as I am busily harvesting elderflowers, which belong to the same family.

They are exceptional in having two distinct groups of florets in the same flower head. There is a central core of small flowers rather like those of the elder, which offer nectar to visiting insects and will, when pollinated, produce the berries. The scent is emitted by these inner flowers to draw in the bees. Around this compact inner group is a circle of larger apparent flowers, which on close inspection are actually made up of rather flat bare petals giving the whole head a distinct resemblance to those of the hydrangea. These are not fertile. The two together give a "broiderie anglaise" effect as the outer flowers stand out on stalks around the dense, fertile centre.

The tooth-edged leaves are rather elegant with three distinct lobes, a little like the maple leaf but not as broad. In autumn they turn from the fresh green of summer to yellow/gold or burnt umber, but are often still green when the berries turn bright red. Given a good position in moist soil the tree can grow to four metres (thirteen feet), but is slower than the elder to reach this same height. As a native tree, it grows in marshy areas and damp hedgerows, the other name of marsh elder was recorded by Miller in the mid eighteenth century, referring both to the habitat and likeness of the inner flowers to those of the common elder. The bark, which is harvested in spring, is grey and fairly smooth with a reddish inner layer. This is the strongly scented part of the tree which is used in herbal medicine to relax the muscles, not only of the skeleton, but those of the blood vessels and around the organs. It is one of the most useful herbs as it treats many conditions in different systems of the body where spasm is a problem. There have been acute situations as well as those with chronic pain when as a herbalist I have been extremely grateful to have such a dependable herb to bring fast relief to my patient.

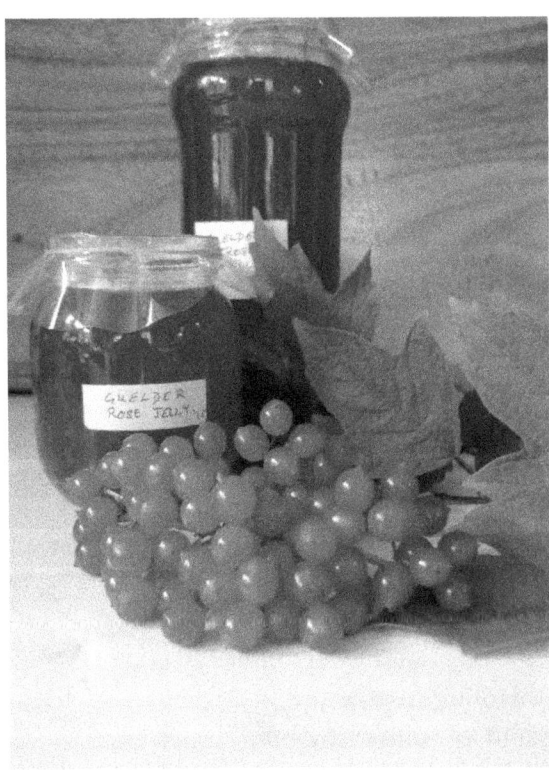

Guelder fruit jelly.

The trees grow in Scandinavia, Russian Asia and across Europe. In 1300 it appears as guelder rose in a list composed by Crescenzi and by early in the sixteenth century it was painted by Bourdichon as guelder rose.[1] The name guelder rose, comes from that of a Dutch province, Gueldersland where the wild tree was first brought into cultivation.[2] The closely related native wayfaring tree *Viburnum lantana* is more common in the wild and may be mistaken for guelder since it also produces berries, however the leaves and flowers are very different. The flowers are all of the same size. The wayfaring tree also has antispasmodic action but tends to be used much less and only for uterine cramps.

When sowing seeds from the guelder berries, these should be sown out of doors for the frost to stimulate germination. I have taken cuttings each time I have moved house, conveniently these can be taken at almost any point in the year and are easy to establish as new trees. Jelly from the vibrant berries, which are rich in vitamin C, is tart and a wonderful colour.

The berries can also be gathered and dried for making ink.[3] Phillips records how in Siberia the berries were fermented with flour before being distilled to make a spirit. See Herbalists' Reference for modern use.

Legends and Folklore. I have been unable to find legends or folklore associated with cramp bark.

Notes

1. Harvey J. *Mediaeval Gardens.* (Batsford. 1981). 164.
2. Phillips R. *Wild Food.* (Pan Books. 1983). 120.
3. Grieve M. *A Modern Herbal.* (1st published 1934 Jonathan Cape. Saavas. 1984). 382.

CRAMP BARK – History of Medicinal Use

Wood from a late Bronze Age trackway on Shapwick Heath close to Glastonbury and seeds from the Glastonbury Lake Village are evidence for an awareness of possible uses of *Viburnum opulus* from very early times.[1] A native tree, it has a close relative, *Viburnum prunifolium* with the common name of the Wayfaring tree and both are well known in the countryside. However, the Marsh Elder as it was first called is not represented in the old herbals. The Wayfaring tree which was also used to treat cramp appears in Pechey's Herbal of 1694. He simply gives *Viburnum* for the Latin name but the description of the berries as first green, then red, and lastly black, leaves no doubt that the title of Wayfaring Tree is correct. He gives astringent medicinal use for the leaves and berries, but does not mention the guelder rose, *Viburnum Opulus*.[2]

The long silence about a herb we find so useful today is surprising. It is not until 1771 that Miller includes *Viburnum opulus* as a variety of Marsh Elder in his *Gardener's Dictionary*. He remarks that it grows naturally close to rivers and in marshy areas of England and is not often kept in gardens. He tells us that at this point it is also known among nurserymen as Guelder Rose to emphasise the difference between this tree and the *Viburnum opulus* with globular flowers.[3] Apparently it gained this name through being first brought into cultivation in a Dutch province called Gueldersland.[4] It is a very attractive bush both when flowering with dazzling white flowers around the creamier centre blooms, and when it bears the bright red berries, and the leaves turn red in autumn.

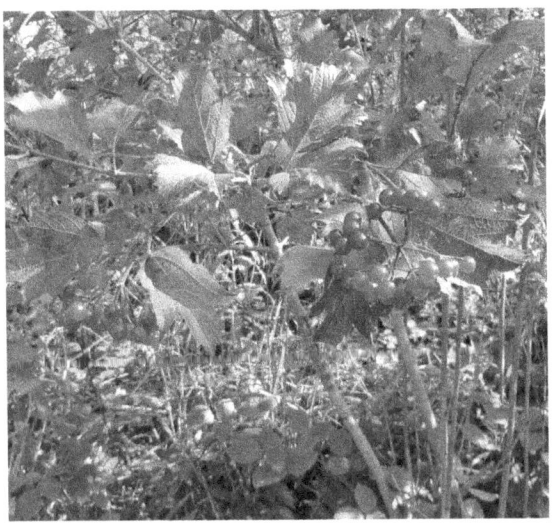

Cramp bark with fruits.

It seems we need to look to America for the origin of herbalists' current use of this herb. Mrs. Grieve points out that the English *Viburnum opulus*, also known as black haw is almost identical to the American black haw, *Viburnum prunifolium* an official drug in the American Pharmacopoeia.[5]

As with much of the herbal knowledge in America, where both varieties grew, use originated in Native American knowledge. Viburnum opulus was also referred to as the high-bush cranberry or Pembina, a corruption by fur traders of the Cree name 'nipiminan' meaning summer berry of a tree growing by the water. Eating the sharp berries is commented on in early reports from 1749 and 1760. In 1868, *V. opulus* was included in a list of Canadian medicinal plants.[6] Although the Menominee and Chippewa treated stomach and menstrual cramps with a tea of a Viburnum, it is not entirely clear whether this refers to the *V. opulus* or *V. prunifolium*.[7]

Amongst the settlers cramp bark, this time definitely meaning Viburnum opulus, had clearly been appreciated, as the Shaker Communities list it as very effective in relaxing cramps and spasms in asthma, pregnancy, and convulsions. A poultice of the fruit was also recommended to be applied to the throat to relieve irritation. 1850 appears to be the first date for cramp bark to be sold as a medicinal herb by the Shakers in Union Village Ohio. Medicines were also made from cramp bark at New Lebanon, Mount Lebanon, Watervliet, and Harvard in the years following up until 1885.[8]

In the Materia Medica of the Physio-medicalists, we find *Viburnum opulus* beside *Viburnum prunifolium*. *V. opulus* is referred to there as cramp bark and *V. prunifolium* as Black haw, which is recommended for treating after pains following birth, prolapsed uterus, enlarged uterus, and passive menorrhagia.

In the entry for *V. opulus* it is described as "an admirable relaxing and stimulating, antispasmodic nervine." It is clearly mostly prescribed during pregnancy at this time, whether for cramping limbs, or to ease pain and prevent miscarriage. A list of possible herb combinations is suggested to give the best result. However, the accompanying recipe is for treating sciatica.[9]

Although the textbook of the Physio-medicalists was not reprinted by the National Association of Medical Herbalists until 1932, it appears contacts between the two had already established use of cramp bark in Britain. In the 1905 *National Botanic Pharmacopoeia* we find the bark of the root of *Viburnum opulus* given thorough recommendation. The list of applications for its effects has grown to include all nervous complaints and debility. We have in the details not only sickness, dizziness, and fainting but fits, lockjaw, rheumatism, and heart disease.[10]

In 1916, Ada Teetgen cataloguing plants to be collected for herbalists, homoeopaths, and mainstream medicine during the First World War writes that the wayfaring tree is commonly seen in the countryside, and that both this tree and the Guelder rose are valued in medicine for the constituent substance viburnin contained in their barks.[11]

Summary. Although a native tree, which has probably been used for food from the Bronze Age onwards in Britain, medicinal use here for cramp bark is not recorded in early herbals. Only the closely related Wayfaring Tree is mentioned in Pechey's Herbal of 1694. In North America, however, the First Nations regarded the "nipiminan", a Cree name that also refers to the bush growing by water, as medicinal. Shaker settlers sold cramp bark for relaxing cramps and spasms due to conditions ranging from asthma to convulsions from 1850 onwards. It was included in a list of Canadian medicines in 1868 and entered the United States Pharmacopoeia in 1894 and had a place in the *Materia Medica of the Physio-Medicalists* in 1897. By 1905, British herbalists are using cramp bark and we find it listed in the *Botanic Pharmacopoeia* for that year. The therapeutic range has widened from spasms mentioned above to include lockjaw, neuralgic pain at the heart, and rheumatism. For modern use see Herbalists' Reference.

Notes

1. Godwin Sir H. *History of the British Flora.* (Cambridge University Press. 2nd edition. 1975). 337.
2. Pechey J. *The English Herbal of Physical Plants.* (London. 1694). 191.
3. Miller P. F.R.S. *Gardener's Dictionary.* (London. 1771).
4. Phillips R. *Wild Food.* (Pan Books, 1983). 120.
5. Grieve M. *A Modern Herbal.* (1st published 1934 Jonathan Cape. Saavas. 1984). 382.
6. Erichson-Brown C. *Medicinal and other uses of North American Plants.* (Dover Publications. 1979). 148.
7. Harris M. *Botanica of North America.* (Harper Resource. 2003). 70.
8. Miller A.B. *Shaker Herbs.* A History and a Compendium. (Potter. 1976). 162.

9. Lyle T.J. A.M.M.D. 1897. *Physio-medical Therapeutics, Materia Medica and Pharmacy.* Ohio. 389. herbaltherapeutics.net/media/library/Physio-Medical-Therapeutics.pdf accessed 24/2/2020.
10. Scurrah J.W. F.N.A.M.H. *The National Botanic Pharmacopoeia.* (Bradford. 1905). 26.
11. Teetgen A.B. *Profitable Herb-Growing and Collecting.* (London. 1916). 170/71.

VIBURNUM OPULUS – Herbalists' Reference

The Parts of the Guelder Rose or Cramp Bark Used for Medicine – Dried bark that has been collected in spring.

Dosage and Forms – 2–4g. 1–2 teaspoon per cup for decoction, not recommended due to the taste. 1:1 in 25% alcohol 2–4ml three times daily. 1:5 in 45% 5–10ml three times daily. The powdered dried bark can be added to fig with a little honey or added date for a medicinal conserve to be eaten as sweets three times a day.

Constituents – Tannins,- catechin and epicatechin (unlike Viburnum prunifolium). Viburnin, scopoletin and hydroquinones, arbutin, trace minerals. Salicosides, resin, tannins.

Actions and Uses – Guelder rose is mainly used for its sedative and spasmolytic properties in relaxing both nerves and muscles. Since it acts on the visceral muscle as well as the skeletal muscle, it has applications not only in spasmodic muscular cramp and muscular rheumatism but also in several body systems. Action on the blood vessels helps to reduce high blood pressure and the antispasmodic action can be helpful in intermittent claudication.

In the lungs, relaxation is useful in asthma and bronchitis. In the genito-urinary system *Viburnum opulus* is given for menopausal flooding, painful menstruation, threatened miscarriage, and is useful in any uterine dysfunction. It is particularly helpful for difficulty in swallowing and colic in the gut or gall bladder. Since it addresses both nerves and muscles it may be indicated for treating a neurogenic bladder and bed wetting.

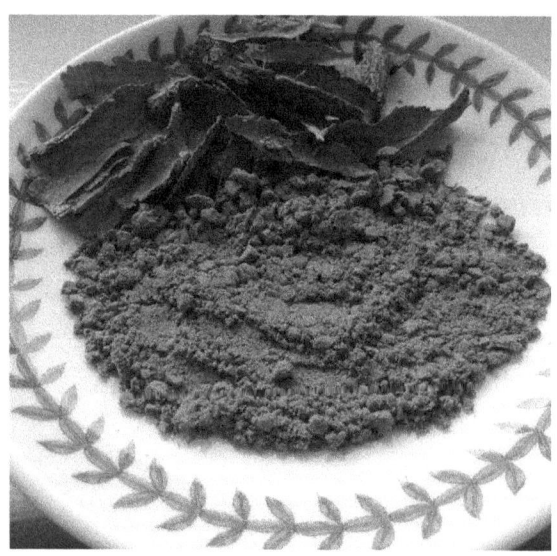
Dried bark.

Specific Indications – Cramp in skeletal muscle and the genito-urinary system.[1]

Combinations – It may be combined with Zanthoxylum to treat cramp, particularly in Raynaud's disease. Many combinations have been given, experience has suggested Crataegus, Tilia, and Achillea. Taken with *Althaea* tea in spasm of the cardiac sphincter muscle of the stomach it has given swift relief. With Boswellia it has proved beneficial after severe muscular injury.

Interactions – None known.

Contraindications and Precautions – None given.

Note

1. *British Herbal Pharmacopoeia*. (British Herbal Medicine Association. 1983). 230.

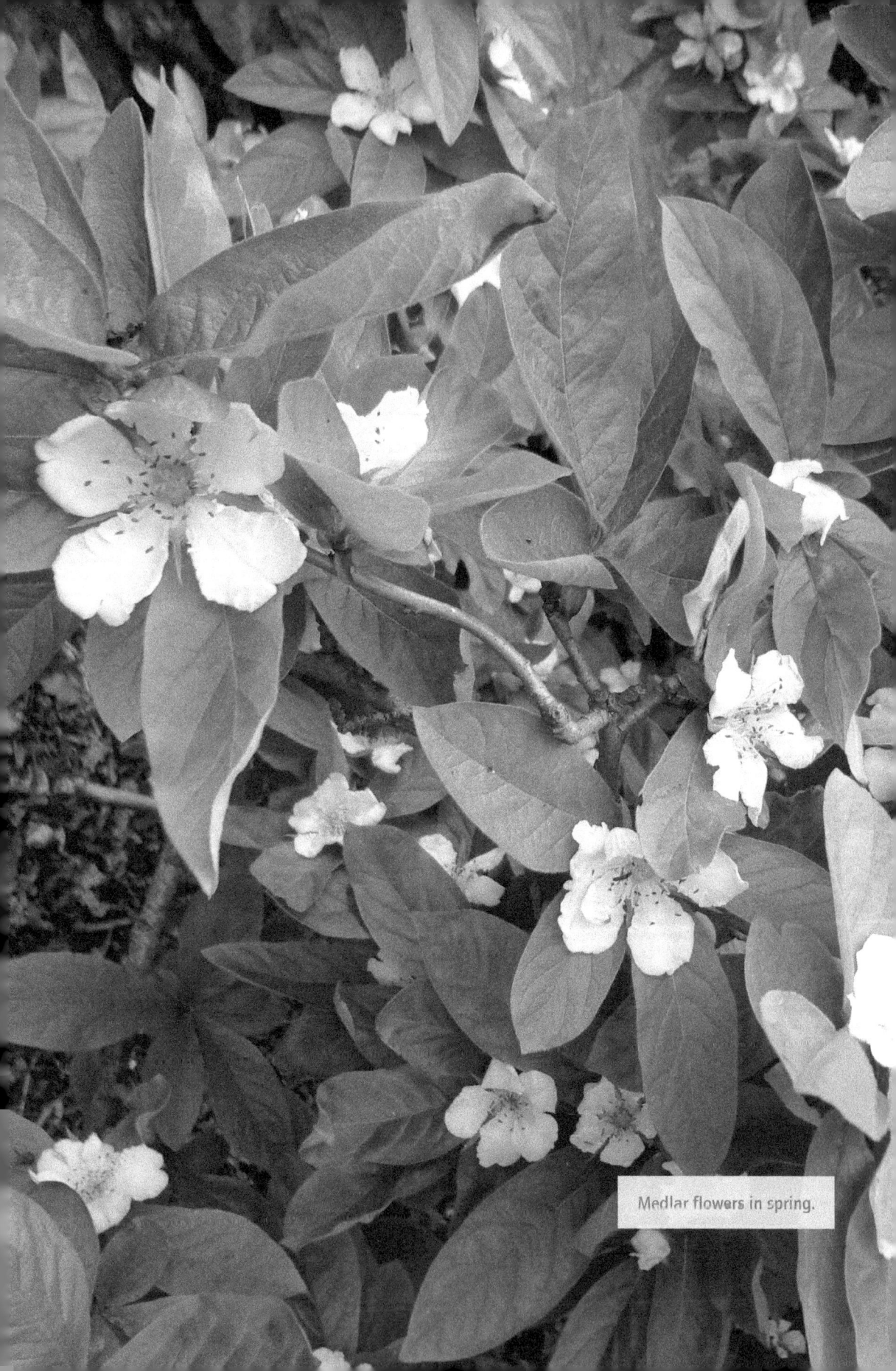
Medlar flowers in spring.

Medlar

Mespilus germanica – Medlar – Rosaceae

MEDLAR – Usefulness – The fruit makes a tasty jelly that has medicinal properties. A delicious wine can also be made from medlar fruits. This small tree has been grown for the ornamental value of the stunning white blossom in spring.

Dangers – None known.

Getting to Know the Medlar Tree – The medlar can grow to be nine metres (twenty-nine and a half feet) tall with a wide spread of branches, but they can equally well be pruned back to be no higher than three metres (ten feet) and kept more controlled. In my experience of growing the tree, it produces many fruits within a few years of planting and with care the canopy tends to become attractively rounded overall. The abundant blossoms in May resemble small perfect white roses, having a faint apple scent and are set amongst the clusters of long, lanceolate leaves. These are thicker than those of the quince and a soft green above yet almost grey on the underside, as this is covered in silky hairs. Stroking a leaf is rather like stroking the ear of a rabbit, a comforting sensation.

It is hard to associate the elegance of blossom and leaf with the crazy haphazard growth of the branches as the tree ages. In autumn they are hung with a generous crop of small fruits, which, it has to be said, are less than attractive. The flower receptacle and calyx below remain and grow to enclose the true fruit, which makes their form both fascinating and in many eyes amusing. The crown shape left by the petals around the upper hollow space within has attracted the uncomplimentary name of Open-arse. We find this name used both in Chaucer and in many herbals.

In his translation of the health instruction from the hospital and medical school at Salerno, the *'Regimen Sanitatis Salerni'*, Sir John Harington gives us "Eate *Medlers*, if you have a loosenesse gotten,…. They have one name more fit to be forgotten"(p.43).[1]

The fruits have been eaten in Britain since the Roman occupation and recognised for their special digestive properties. When stewed in wine and sweetened with honey, they have been a medicine to be enjoyed and were one of the ideal fruits in monastery orchards. Medlars have featured in the past as fruits to be especially recommended in pregnancy, earlier rather than later, as they were thought to help against nausea and cravings for unusual foods. Late in pregnancy their astringency was suspected of delaying labour.

Although the medlars can be picked and eaten straight from the tree in southern Europe where the trees originate, in our climate, despite one form of the tree having naturalised here,[2] they require a long preparation. Picked late in October, hopefully before the squirrels can harvest them, they can be laid on newspaper, kept in shade and left to "blet". Other methods are to pack them in moist bran which shortens the time taken to ripen, or to cover them with straw. When first picked they are still rock hard and must soften to be ready for making jelly, cooking with apples or other fruits or making wine.

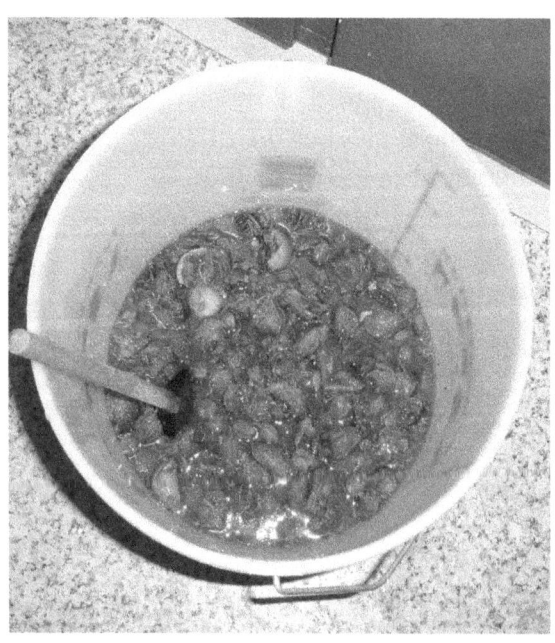
Making medlar wine.

Cut open they reveal inside five seeds often referred to as nutlets. The flesh of the fruit by this time is quite brownish and mushy. The jelly and wine I have always found well worth the effort of making, but once you have processed any amount of the fruits you can understand how apples became more popular for everyday cookery. The flavour is more intense than apple, as if it has been roasted. Medlars make an excellent dessert wine which involves less work than the jelly and proves quite as satisfying. The bletted fruit can also be spiced by sticking them with cloves before keeping them for two months in a preserving jar covered with sugar and topped up with brandy. If you just have a few fruits they will also be good baked as you would an apple or quince with a little butter, sugar, and spices.

In a sixteenth century book of secrets we find a method of using medlar fruits to refresh and remove the hint of mouldiness in wine made of other fruits. The bletted, opened fruits are hung beneath the bung of the wine vessel for a month to achieve this.[3]

Gerard recommended that medlar trees should be grafted onto hawthorn to make them have larger fruit, while Evelyn, writing in the seventeenth century wrote that the medlar and crab apple were more closely related. All three trees are part of the *Rosaceae* family. In 1697, the nurseryman Telford grew both English standard medlars and the Dutch, the English was slightly more expensive as it was believed to be the better variety. The Dutch medlar is listed as the variety generally cultivated in English gardens by 1769.[4] Medlar trees can be seen in many National Trust gardens, there is an excellent specimen at Brockhampton Manor, Worcestershire.

Legends and Folklore. In the past medlar trees have been seen as protective against witches. Culpeper gives the amusing idea that because the tree is ruled by Saturn and old man Saturn disapproved of women having longings and fancies that the fruit would restrain these. At some time along the way a related belief grew that this needed their husbands to plant the tree in their garden. In order to avoid this playful outcome, I made sure that I planted my own.

Notes

1. Harington Sir J. The School of Salernum. *Regimen Sanitatis Salerni.* (Ente Provinciale per Il Turismo. Salerno. Rome. 1957). 43.
2. Grigson G. *The Englishman's Flora.* (The Folio Society. 1987). 171.
3. Warde W. & Anglosse R. (trans), *The Secretes of Maister Alexis of Piemont.* (Atenar. 2000). 86.
4. Harvey J. *Early Gardening Catalogues.* (Phillimore & Co. 1972). 37.

MEDLAR TREE – History of Medicinal Use

The medlar grows naturally in south-east Europe and south-west Asia and we find Dioscorides referring to a medlar tree the size of an apple tree in Italy. There the fruits can be eaten straight from the tree but in that state would be quite astringent.[1] Pliny repeats the use for checking loose bowels and writes that they are beneficial to the stomach.[2]

Medlars appear to have been grown by the Romans during their occupation of Britain as seeds have been found at Silchester.[3] Medlar trees may have subsequently died out but evidence of the fruits in the Anglo-Saxon leechdoms suggests otherwise. Leechbook recipes include medlars with other fruits, such as apples and pears, when they were cooked in vinegar or sharp wine for astringency.[4] The astringent quality was exploited by medieval surgeons in topical applications as well as with internal use. Being styptic, cooling, and drying, the fruits were applied to reduce inflammation and swelling, reducing fluid engorgement.[5]

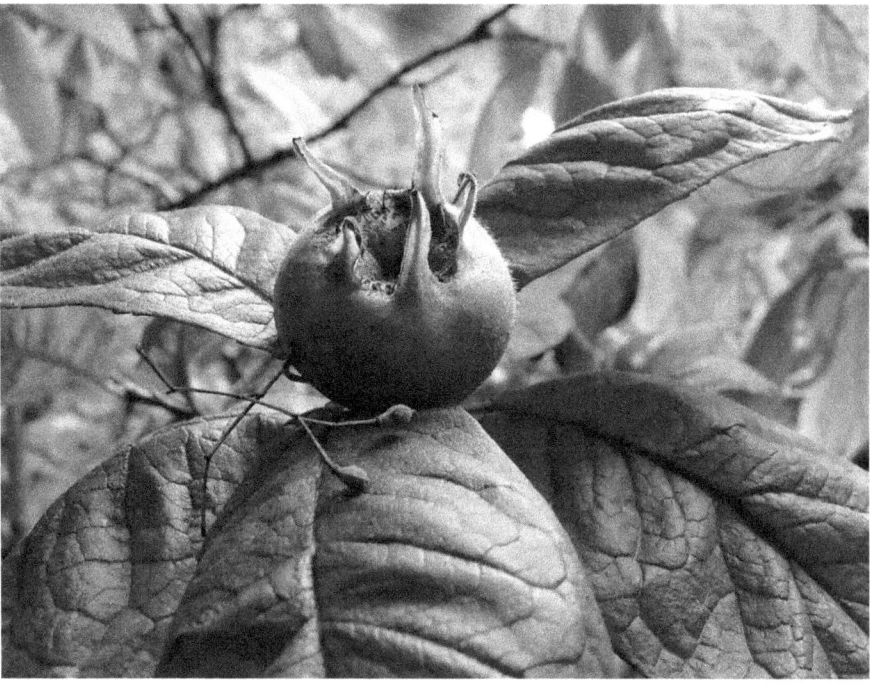

Fruit ready to be picked.

Hildegard of Bingen regarded medlars as heating rather than cooling and saw all the strength of the tree as going into the fruit, which meant she had little regard for the properties of the leaves but suggested the bark in medicine.[6] Abbey gardens were certainly expected to grow medlars, although it seems more likely that this was for food than for using them in the infirmary. The medlar does appear in the librarian Thomas Betson's list of plants at Syon Abbey, which seems to be copied from that of John Bray, but it does not find a place in the remedies listed.[7] It has to be remembered, however, that Syon Abbey had a mother house in Sweden and many of the remedies differ from those generally used in Britain at the time. Alexander Neckham put medlars with cherries and plums—all to be eaten when ripe to the point of being rotten.

Chaucer lists them as homely trees including medlars as native in Britain and they were valued not only for the fruit but for the beauty of their blossom in the fourteenth and fifteenth centuries.[8] In the sixteenth century, *The Woman's Book* includes a recipe containing medlars with other tart fruits in a bath to restrain menorrhagia.[9] Culpeper describes another similar kind of medlar growing in England that bears thorns and has smaller, less pleasant fruit. He classifies the tree as belonging to Saturn and recommends the retentive and restraining qualities of the fruits for stopping bleeding, miscarriage, and excess humours. He recommends the leaves as well as the fruit for astringency in a decoction as a gargle or mouthwash. He adds parsley root to an earlier recipe for urinary stones.[10]

At the same period William Coles repeats much of the above, adding to the poultice of dried medlars which Culpeper gives, the recipe given below. Besides all these recipes and supporting the power of the leaves to speed healing of wounds, Coles thoroughly recommends eating medlars to pregnant mothers. This was not only to stop them miscarrying, but to halt their longings for unusual foods. He does not appear to be aware of a warning in The Woman's Book on eating them too close to the birth.[11] In 1694, Pechey recommends medlars against vomiting and diarrhoea.[12] Use of the fruits and the seeds for breaking urinary stones is echoed in the eighteenth century in an Irish herbal.[13]

Summary. Medlar trees appear to have been brought to England by the Romans and the knowledge of these cooling, drying fruits in medicine dates back to that time. They are mentioned in the Anglo-Saxon Leechbooks and were used by medieval surgeons in poultices for reducing swelling and inflammation. The fruits were also put into medicinal baths and feature in obstetric medicine to restrain bleeding and miscarriage. Culpeper recommends the leaves as well as the fruits for their astringency in healing wounds and as a mouthwash or gargle. Coles has an elaborate poultice recipe and directs pregnant women to eat them for their better health and to stop longings for unusual foods.

Although these uses continue into the eighteenth century, in the nineteenth Brook records that there are so many more powerful remedies to hand, the medlar is going out of use.[14] However, medlars still find a place in the Herbalists' Reference for today.

Recipe

Extracted from The Paradise of Plants. 1657. For vomiting, to fortify the digestion and preserve the humours from putrefaction: a "Pultis, or Plaster be made with dryed Medlars, beaten and mixed with the juyce of Red Roses, whereunto a few Cloves and Nutmegs, may be added, and a little red Corall also, and applyed to the stomach, it will work more effectually" (p.82).[11]

Notes

1. Gunther R.T. (ed), *Dioscorides Greek Herbal.* (Hafner. 1968). 85.
2. Jones W.H.S. (trans), *Pliny Natural History* VI Books XX-XXIII. (Loeb Classical Library. 1989). LXXIII. 509.
3. Alcock J.P. *Food in Roman Britain.* (Tempus. 2001). 66.
4. Hagen A. *A Handbook of Anglo-Saxon Food.* (Anglo-Saxon Books. 1992). 59.
5. Rosenman Leonard D. MD. *A Medieval Surgical Pharmacopoeia and Formulary.* 1170–1325. (San Francisco. 1999). 85, 26.
6. Throop P. (trans), *Hildegard von Bingen's Physica.* (Healing Arts Press. 1998). 115.
7. Adams J. & Forbes S. (ed), *The Syon Abbey Herbal. A.D. 1517.* (AMCD Publishers Ltd. 2015). 155.
8. McLean T. *Medieval English Gardens.* (Barrie & Jenkins. 1989). 236.
9. Hobby E. (ed), *The Birth of Mankind.* (1560). (Ashgat. 2009). 129.

10. Culpeper N. *Culpeper's Complete Herbal and English Physician enlarged.* (1652). (London. 1815 edition). 115.
11. Coles W. *The Paradise of Plants.* (London. 1657). 81.
12. Pechey J. *The English Herbal of Physical Plants.* (London. 1694). 126.
13. Scott M. (ed), *An Irish Herbal.* K'Eogh. (1735). (Aquarian. 1986). 100.
14. Brook R. *Brook's Family Herbal.* (J.A. Brook, Richardson & Co. London. Revised edition. 1876). 152.

MESPILUS GERMANICA – Herbalists' Reference

The Parts of Medlar Used for Medicine – Leaves gathered in May, fruits and seeds in October.

Dosage and Forms – Medlar jelly and wine as needed. A standard infusion of the leaves 25g (1oz) leaves to 600ml (1 pint) boiling water, can be left to stand for 10 minutes before using it as a wash.

Constituents – Tannins in leaves and fruits, citric and malic acid, peptic substances, sugars, and vitamins in the fruit.

Actions and Uses – The pulp of the fruit has an astringent effect from the tannins with an osmotic action, bringing more water into the bowel, so that while reducing diarrhoea it does not then cause constipation. It may be useful in normalising bowel action after dysentery[1] or in chronic conditions, such as irritable bowl syndrome (IBS) or in cancer of the bowel, while the patient awaits or undertakes orthodox treatment. The leaves are astringent for healing wounds. As with several other native tree barks, medlar has been tried as a possible substitute for quinine. The results were uncertain for treating fevers. As the history of this fruit has related, the pulverised seeds or nutlets have been prescribed repeatedly in the past for breaking urinary stones.

Contraindications and Precautions – Use as a lithontripic to remove small stones from the body should only be undertaken under medical supervision.[2]

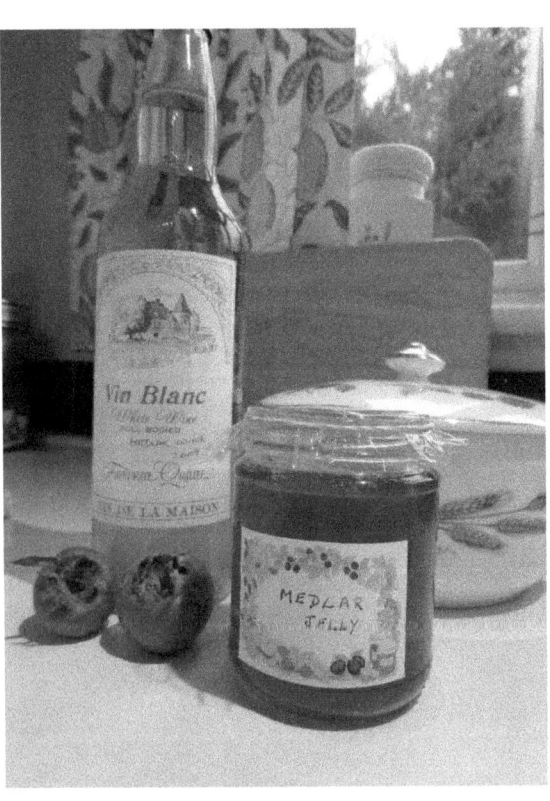

Medlar wine and jelly.

Notes

1. Barker J. 2001. *The Medicinal Flora of Britain and Northwestern Europe.* Winter Press. (136).
2. Chiej R. *The Macdonald Encyclopedia of Medicinal Plants.* (Macdonald Publishing. London. 1984). 196.

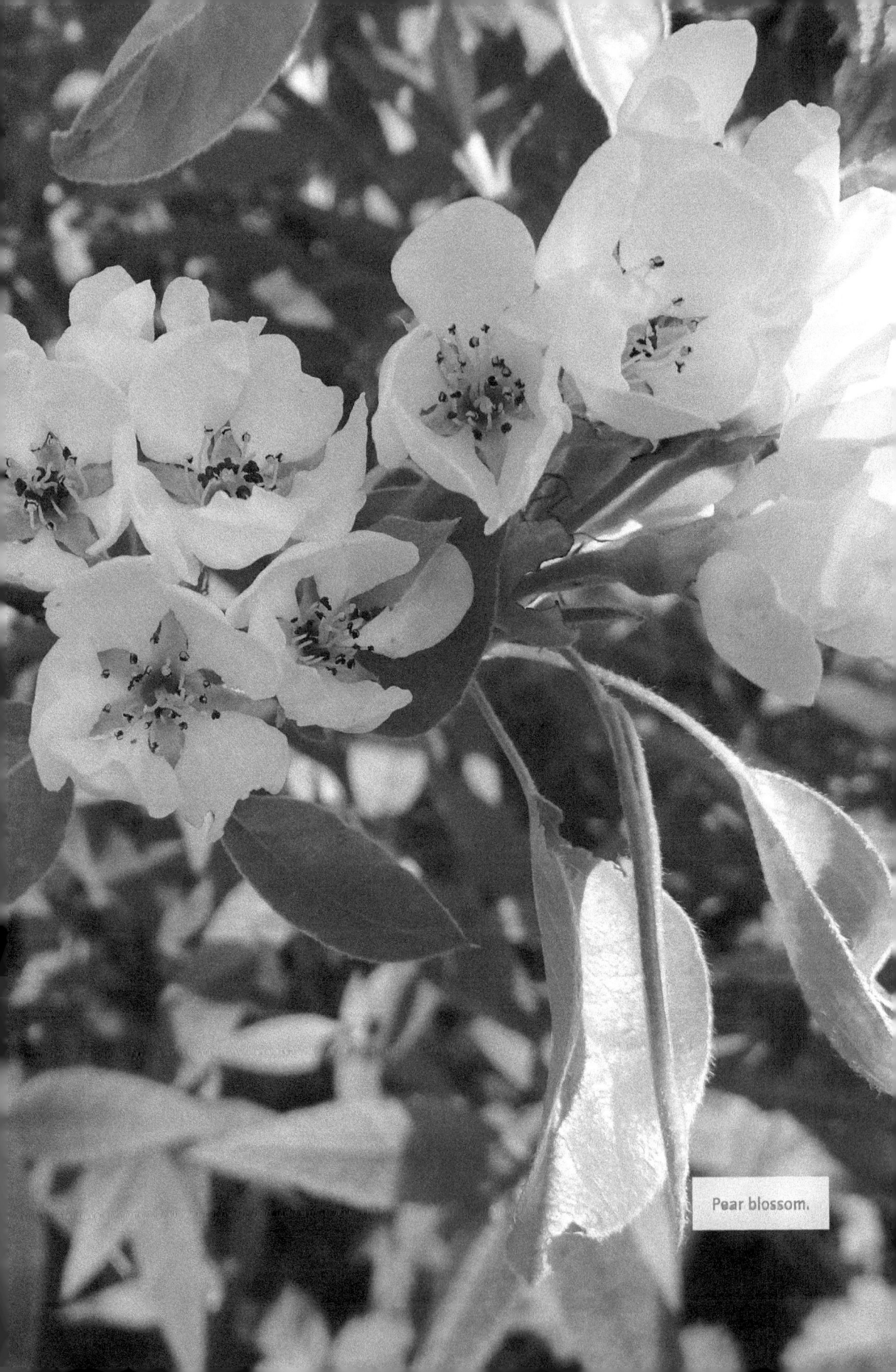

Pear blossom.

Pear

Pyrus communis – Pear – Rosaceae

PEAR – Usefulness – The fruit is well known and liked in cookery, preserves, cider, liqueur, and wine. The fruit, leaves, twigs, and bark have also been used in medicine. The bark of the tree and the leaves offer a good dye. The wood can be turned or small items made from it.

Dangers – Eating unripe raw pears will be likely to cause indigestion.

Getting to Know the Pear Tree – The form of the pear tree is very familiar. In spite of the rising popularity of growing hardier varieties of more exotic fruits, it remains a common fruit tree to grow. Patio trees grown in large pots open the opportunity to a wider public and will not leave the owner with such a large crop that they feel overwhelmed. In our first orchard we planted a Conference pear, which has always been my favourite variety. The sight of the pure white blossom with the five bright green sepals gives perfect contrast appearing as a star in the centre, holding each flower cupped like an open rose and confirming membership of the rose family.

The glossy oval leaves frame the blossom as they hang below gradually unfolding to show the tiny teeth along the edges. When fully open they appear as if lazily relaxed on long stems. The young branches have a reddish tint to the bark that fades to grey with age. Pear blossom time is always precious, as it comes before the apple blossom and therefore is hoped to be a confirmation of spring, although there still may be the danger of frost. Already thoughts of the possible harvest of long, juicy fruits govern the care I give protecting blossom on my small tree with a fine net if frost is forecast. Later in summer there will be a greater danger to the swelling fruit with trees in pots if they are not watered sufficiently.

The fruit can take a long time to ripen if picked unripe and stored. Putting pears in brown paper bags along with an apple may speed this process.

The pear tree that grew wild in Britain before the Romans came is now rare.[1] The Roman occupying military force brought cultivated pears with them and soon the fruit from these being preferred, they became the familiar orchard trees. In England successive monarchs planted all kinds of pears in the Tower gardens and at Westminster, while monastic orchards might be six or seven acres of trees. Those at Manor houses might be half that size but since pears were cooked more than apples they were well represented in all of these areas. The pears that were really appreciated for baking were the Warden pears, and we find recipes specifically for these in fifteenth century cookbooks. One, "Peris in Syrippe" (p.87), involves boiling spiced pears in red wine. This might be served alongside meats or fish. "Peris in Compost" (p.12) also includes a syrup and is coloured with red saunders. In the third recipe, the spiced and sweetened pears are thickened with egg yolks.[2] Pears also went into comfits and were made into cider.

While Sir Hugh Plat had given instructions on drying thin slices of pears without sugar in *Delights for Ladies* 1609, by Eliza Smith's *The Compleat Housewife* of 1739 we have another method suggested, which is to bake them in ale, having made a hole through them from stalk to base with a bodkin, after which they are squeezed flat and drained and then dried in a cool oven.[3] I have to admit I find William Coles' recipe the most attractive, which is to boil the pears in diluted rosewater and honey before draining them and drying in the oven as it cools from baking bread.[4]

There is a belief, which is evidently passed down from the medieval guide to health written at the influential hospital in Salerno, that while cooked pears are restorative, raw pears being often indigestible were seen as a poison only made safe by drinking wine after eating them.[5] The popularity of this idea needs no explanation.

William Coles quotes "a late author" that in 1657 there were 400 or 500 varieties of pear trees. He limits himself to describing fourteen of them. He also tells us of uses of the close-grained, firm pear wood to make blocks for printing for plant illustrations, rulers, and pistol stocks.[4] Green adds more uses for the wood in 1824 and it is made into beautiful items by turners today.

I very much doubt we would be tempted in this day and age to apply sliced pear to reduce inflammation in hot swellings as suggested in the past. Ripe pears remain a welcome cooling fruit in feverish conditions, easing constipation, and acting as a mild antibacterial and diuretic. Perhaps they should be as welcome as grapes at the sickbed.

Legends and Folklore. There is the superstition common with many white flowers, which my grandmother followed, that the white blossom must not be brought into the house or there would be a death in the family. In Worcestershire, a pear tree growing on the site of the Battle of Evesham bearing red blotched fruit was believed to do so to commemorate the dead. A similar tree near Ellesmere was connected in folklore to a murder.[6]

Notes

1. Rackham O. *The History of the Countryside.* (Phoenix Paperback. 1986). 210.
2. Austin T. (ed), *Two Fifteenth Century Cookery Books.* (1888). (Oxford University Press. Reprint 1964). 87, 12,
3. Smith E. *The Compleat Housewife.* (London. 1739). 189.
4. Coles W. *The Paradise of Plants.* (London. 1657). 260, 259.
5. Harrington Sir J. The School of Salernum. *Regimen Sanitatis Salerni.* (Ente Provinciale per Il Turismo. Salerno. Rome. 1957). 42.
6. DeCleene M. & Lejeune M.C. *Compendium of Symbolic and Ritual Plants in Europe.* (Man and Culture Publishers, Ghent. Belgium. 2003). 532.

PEAR TREE – History of Medicinal Use

The evidence for the native status of the now rare wild pear in Britain comes from many charcoal finds dated back to the Neolithic period onwards.[1] Dioscorides writes about all pears binding the bowels when they are eaten raw. Of the wild pear *Pyrus amygdaliformis*, he says that this is more binding than the cultivated varieties and that the leaves were also used in that capacity.[2] Pliny describes drinking decoctions of pear against loose bowels. He specifically recommends the ashes of the wood of the tree as efficacious against poisonous substances in tree fungi.[3]

Cultivars of pears were brought to Britain by the Romans and planted in Villa orchards. By the Anglo-Saxon period Charter documents show pear to be the tenth commonest tree.[1] Chaucer puts the pears alongside apples, quince, and plum trees under the heading homely, or trees well known to him.[4] Pears were popular in the medieval period and a diet for undefined stomach trouble included apples, pears, and peaches with bread in water and salmon.[5] We find cultivars introduced from the Continent to be grown in Cistercian Abbey gardens. One growing in Warden, Bedfordshire was sent from Burgundy and this cultivar took the name Warden and became a popular cultivar for producing cooking pears.[6]

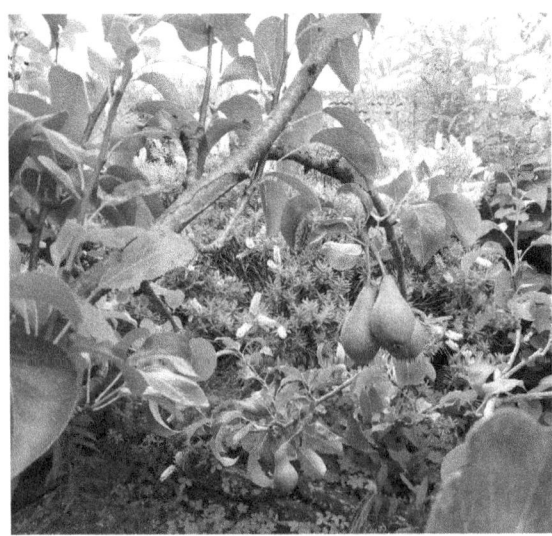

Pear fruits.

The *Regimen Sanitatis Salerni* guide to health has a good deal to say about pears—confirming the belief that wine acted as an antidote to eating raw pears, whereas when the pears were baked they could then be considered medicinal.[7] In the twelfth century, the great length of detail given by Hildegard to the pear tree is indicative of the importance it held at that period. Amongst others, she gives the recipe for a complex electuary, describing it as more precious than gold. This she credits with curing migraine and chest problems, the very things she believed raw pears could produce.[8]

Pears might not only be given internally in medicine but also applied topically. In Gerard's great herbal extended by Johnson and published in 1633, all of the former information on the temperature and good and bad qualities of the pear is repeated. He includes the external use of the leaves. He writes about the wild pear, which he records as growing in woods, the borders of fields, and near to roads.[9]

With Culpeper comes a clear discernment between the actions of the sour pears and the sweeter cultivated ones. Having placed the tree under the dominion of Venus, he states the sweet pears aid the bowels, while sour ones and the leaves bind and constipate. He is also enthusiastic about their ability to cool, bind, and heal new wounds when bound over them. He quotes Galen as finding them to guard against further inflammation. Culpeper repeats that when pears are cooked with mushrooms it makes the fungi safer to eat. Referring to the text of the Regimen Sanitatis from Salerno recommending much wine to be drunk after pears, Culpeper comments "but if a poor man find his stomach oppressed by eating Pears, it is but working hard, and it will do as well as drinking wine" (p.134).[10]

As is often the case, Coles has part of his information almost word for word with that of Culpeper. He adds that when ripe pears are eaten after meat they close the mouth of the stomach and fortify the digestion. He recommends cooked Wardon pears for patients, adding that pears are effective in cooling hot tumours. Coles writes, "The *Perry* that is made of these *Peares* is a speciall *Cordiall*, cheering and reviving the *Spirits*, making the *Heart* glad …. It is also profitable for long life as well as health, for it hath been observed that those that drink *Perry* and *Syder* daily or frequently as their common drink are generally healthy persons, and long lived: It is of speciall use at Sea, in long Voyages to mingle with their fresh-water."(p.260)[11]

Summary. In addition to the pear tree native to Britain, the Romans brought sweeter cultivars. Dioscorides and Pliny were agreed that raw pears and the leaves of the tree were binding to the bowels, while the cooked pears were more wholesome. The Anglo-Saxons planted many trees and they were very popular in the medieval period. Boiled pears were prescribed and the leaves or fruits were applied topically to cool and dry wounds. Culpeper regards wild pears as binding and constipating, while sweet cultivated pears aid the bowels. He repeats the idea held by Dioscorides and Pliny that cooking pears with mushrooms makes the mushrooms safer to eat. Coles has great enthusiasm for the Perry made from pears to cheer and make the heart glad as well as being profitable in giving long life. He writes that it is of special use at sea on long voyages to mix with the store of fresh drinking water.

While Miller records not knowing of any medicinal use of pears in 1722,[12] Ke'ogh in Ireland thirteen years later is still writing about them stopping diarrhoea and being applied to wounds.[13] However, there the trail of pears in medicine ends so far as the herbals are concerned. See Herbalists' Reference for current uses.

Recipe

Extracted from The Paradise of Plants.1657. "Pears applyed outwardly, are effectuall for hot tumors, and greene wounds, if they be laid to at the beginning, and so are the Leaves, for they close and heale new wounds, but more especially Wild Peares, and their Leaves" (p.260).[11]

Notes

1. Rackham O. *The History of the Countryside.* (Phoenix Paperback. 1986). 210.
2. Gunther R.T. (ed), *Dioscorides Greek Herbal.* (Hafner. 1968). 85.
3. Jones W.H.S. (trans), *Pliny Natural History* VI Books XX-XXIII. (Loeb Classical Library. 1989). 491.
4. Harvey J. *Early Nurserymen.* (Phillimore & Co. 1974). 18.
5. Hagen A. *Anglo-Saxon Food and Drink.* (Anglo-Saxon Books. 1995). 117.
6. Campbell-Culver M. *The Origin of Plants.* (Headline Book Publishing. 2001). 57.
7. Harrington Sir J. The School of Salernum. *Regimen Sanitatis Salerni.* (Ente Provinciale per Il Turismo. Salerno. Rome. 1957). 42.
8. Throop P. (trans), *Hildegard von Bingen's Physica.* (Healing Arts Press. 1998). 107/8.
9. Johnson T. (ed), *The Herbal.* John Gerard. (1633 edition). (Dover Publications, New York. 1975). 1457.

10. Culpeper N. *Culpeper's Complete Herbal and English Physician enlarged.* (1652). (London. 1815 edition). 134.
11. Coles W. *The Paradise of Plants.* (London. 1657). 260.
12. Miller J. *Botanicum officinale.* Bell. (London. 1722). 365.
13. Scott M. (ed), *An Irish Herbal.* K'Eogh. (1735). (Aquarian. 1986). 118.

PYRUS COMMUNIS – Herbalists' Reference

The Parts of the Pear Tree Used for Medicine – Fruit.

Dosage and Forms – There is no recommended medicinal dose. Let food be your medicine. Pears can be added to smoothies, eaten alone, or for a feverish cold enjoyed covered with thickened elderberry syrup.

Constituents – Organic acids, vitamin C, arbutin, hydroquinone, beta-carotene, flavonoids, pectin, trace minerals, sulphur.

Actions and Uses – Pears are a useful and enjoyable traditional laxative, eaten in quantity when fully ripe to relieve constipation. They have some astringency, however, and are antibacterial and possibly aphrodisiac. They are one of the foods which are unlikely to cause an intolerance or allergic reaction.[1] I have always recommended them to sufferers of asthma who find them helpful. The arbutin and hydroquinone offer diuretic properties and pears are cooling in fevers. The fruits have

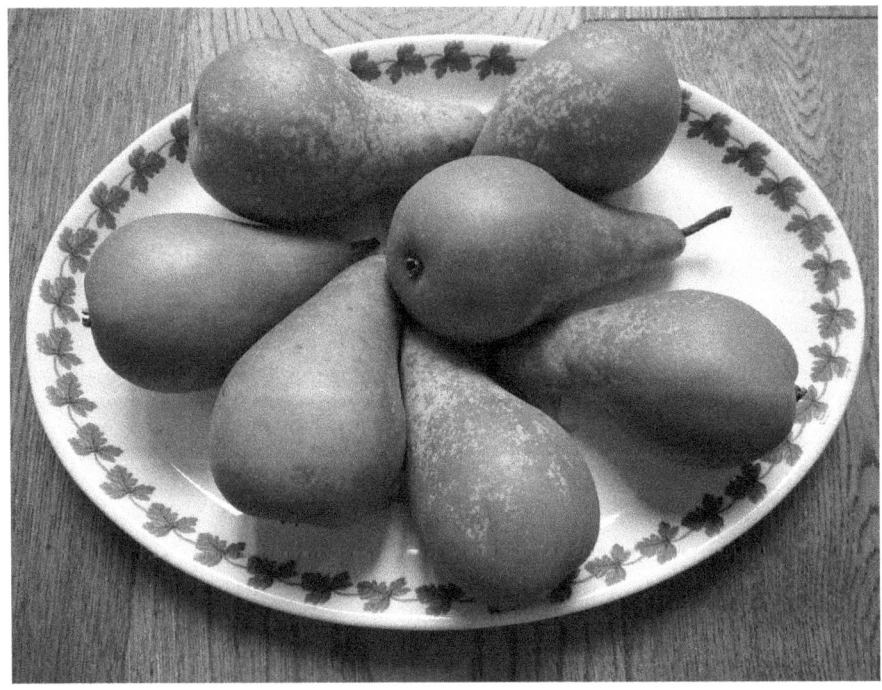

Pears.

additional benefits in relieving dyspepsia. An indication for diabetes has been recorded.[2]

Topical Application – Pears or the leaves of the tree have been used in the past to apply to wounds for a cooling and healing effect.[3]

Contraindications and Precautions – No hazards are known for proper therapeutic dosage but there is no specified dosage either. Too many ripe pears may need an astringent to counteract their laxative effects.

Notes

1. Reader's Digest. *Foods that Harm Foods that Heal.* (Reader's Digest general Books. 1999). 266.
2. Duke J.A. *Handbook of Medicinal Herbs* (CRC Press LLC. 2nd edition. 2002). 560.
3. Coles W. *The Paradise of Plants.* (London. 1657). 260.

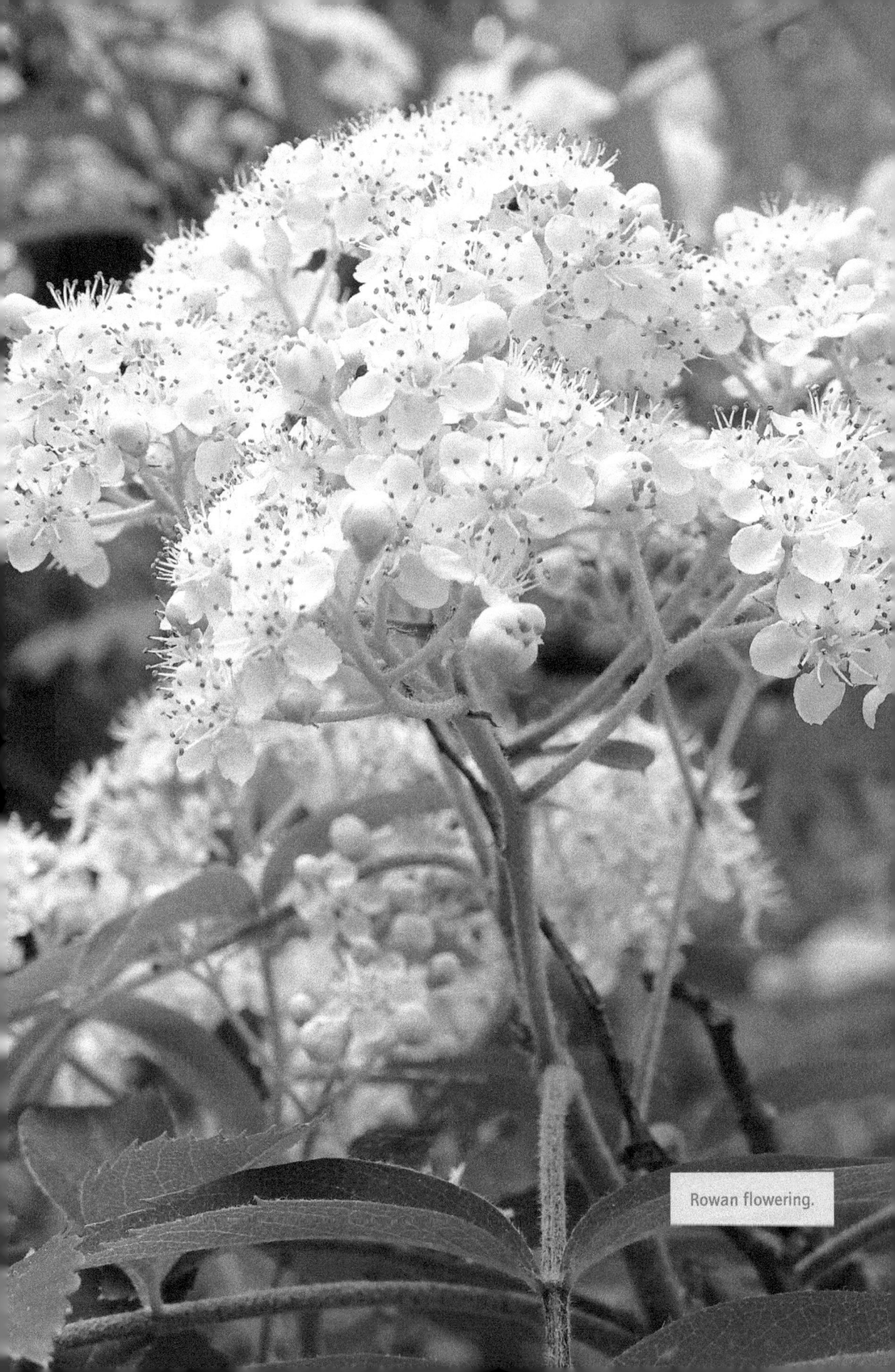
Rowan flowering.

Rowan

Sorbus aucuparia – Rowan – Rosaceae

ROWAN – Usefulness – The fresh flowers, dried fruits, and bark can be used medicinally. The bark has been used as animal feed. The berries can be made into a tart jelly to accompany meat or cheese. Wine can be made from them. The wood can be turned and has been used for beams in houses. The berries provide a dye. Any left on the tree offer welcome food for birds and the tree is ornamental in the garden.

Dangers – It is not recommended to eat the uncooked berries, which may result in indigestion.

Getting to Know the Rowan Tree – While the oak is perhaps the tree most associated with representing England, surely the native rowan carries a similar role of identity with Scotland, Ireland, and Wales. Also called the mountain ash, because of the ash –like pinnate leaves, the tree is actually part of the rose family. It does have an affinity for rocky, mountainous landscapes and is often found in the same areas, which have stone circles. It is largely perceived as a Celtic tree. For all that, the most beautiful rowan tree I have ever seen was on a mountainside in the Swiss Alps, vibrant with life and colour in the clear air and sunshine, it bore many generous clusters of berries.

The delicate white blossom has the typical five petals of the rose family on each of the flowers. These appear to cluster together forming rounded heads and are quite beautiful in May. The scent from them, while resembling elder a little, is slightly sour. An aroma with a touch of honeysuckle and mothballs in the background! Rowan trees may grow to be about eight to nine metres (twenty-seven to thirty feet), although in better soil they may be a little taller. The bark of mature trees is grey, remaining smooth into middle age. The trees may live to be 200 years old. In the south of England, I seem to notice them often brightening car parks with their bright red berries early in the autumn. These give rowan jelly a lovely rich colour and tangy taste, as well as a useful dose of vitamin C ready for the winter. They will be sweeter when gathered after a frost.

Growing in remote places has encouraged as much use as possible to be made of the berries, which can also be dried and pounded to add to flour in hard times. In Scotland they were distilled for a powerful spirit. In Wales they are fermented to make a beer.[1] It seems even birds have a taste of the alcoholic delights of the rowan. Rowan grows wild in Scandinavia, which is on the migratory route of Bohemian waxwings from Russia, as they fly south for the winter. By the time the birds are leaving Scandinavia the berries have been hanging ripe on the trees for some time and have begun to ferment. The birds feed on them and afterwards may crash drunkenly into obstacles in their flight-path. Post-mortems on some found dead beneath the rowan trees have confirmed they had been so drunk they died of liver damage.[2] Waxwings are extremely attractive birds, seen below feeding on berries.

It has long been well known that birds love to eat the berries, which led to rowan berries being included with birch sap or mistletoe berries in some recipes to make bird lime, which was smeared onto trees to catch the birds that found themselves stuck to the mix. *Aucuparia* in the Latin name refers to this practice as it means bird-catching.[3]

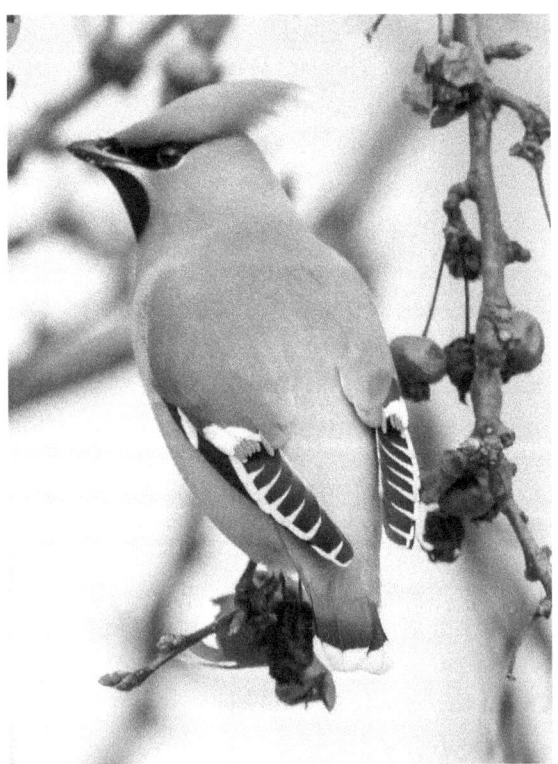

Waxwing feeding on berries. Photo David Papworth.

Legends and Folklore. The tree is sacred to Brigantia and Brigid, which makes it a strongly protective tree, one of the four trees believed to be effective in guarding the garden from evil influences. All manner of household items associated with tasks which might fail from evil influences were made from the wood. This included everything from the cup, dough barrel, butter churn, and spinning wheel, to the yoke for farm animals. The protective qualities of rowan were taken even to the grave with rowan wood included in coffins and the bier for transporting them.[4]

Rowan has not only been associated with protection however, it is also linked to visions and spiritual awakening. The Irish Romance of Fraoth tells of a dragon that guards the magical berries valued through their ability to heal the sick and give longer life.[5]

This story links with the dedication of the rowan to Thor in northern Germany, where legend tells of a rowan saving Thor from drowning as he was able to reach the sapling and pulled himself to the bank.[6] Three supple rowan twigs each tied in a knot are in the care of the Pitts Rivers Museum in Oxford and date back to 1893. These came from Castleton in Yorkshire where they had been ceremoniously attached to house railings and the gateway before the church porch.

Notes

1. Freethy R. *From Agar to Zenry.* (Crowood Press. 1985). 116.
2. Engel C. *Wild Health.* (Houghton Mifflin Co. 1979). 152/3.
3. Adams M. *The Wisdom of Trees.* (Head of Zeus Ltd. 2014). 48.
4. Howkins C. *Rowan Tree of Protection.* (Howkins. 1996). 12.
5. Gifford J. *The Celtic Wisdom of Trees.* (Godsfield Press. 2000). 20.
6. DeCleene M. & Lejeune M.C. *Compendium of Symbolic and Ritual Plants in Europe.* (Man and Culture Publishers, Ghent. Belgium. 2003). 661.

ROWAN - History of Medicinal Use

The rowan tree pollen is distinctive. It has been recognised in plant archaeology from the Neolithic period and appears at Iron Age and later sites. The pollen has been recorded in Northern Ireland as indicating forest regeneration after clearance between 3270–2350 B.C.[1]

We do not have any credible reference from the Roman writers and the only surviving manuscripts for Celtic medicine were not written down until the medieval period and so we come to the Anglo-Saxons for our first evidence of use for the rowan. In Anglo-Saxon recipes, the rowan appears to be referred to as quickbeam. Certainly quickenbeam is a later name for the rowan and this interpretation seems very likely in the light of the names given in Johnson's enlarged version of Gerard's herbal and others. It appears in two recipes in the Leechbook of Bald. The first is a mix of herbs containing five different barks, prepared for just one stage in a complex treatment. In the second recipe the quickbeam bark, or cwicrinde, is given to cure the yellow sickness. In the *Lacnunga*, quickbeam bark is boiled with ash bark and herb in a sweetened drink to reduce inflammation.[2]

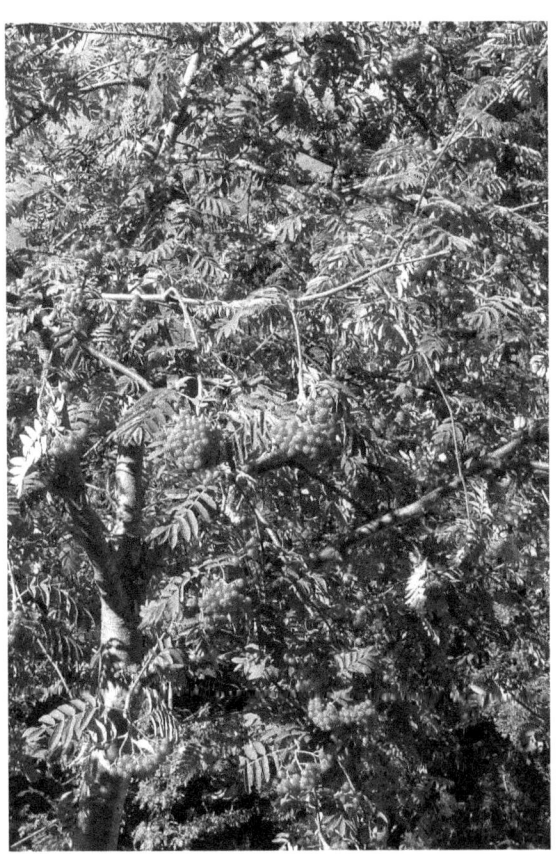

Laden rowan tree.

In the twelfth century, Hildegard of Bingen seems to have little to say about the rowan that is good. She classifies "Spirbaum" as she calls rowan, as hot and dry and goes on to deride the bark, leaves, and sap as of little use.[3] In the medieval period Sorba, which includes the berries of the mountain ash, they are listed as repercussive—that is applied over inflamed, swollen areas of the body. Also regenerative in aiding healing of the wound, with cooling and drying effects.[4]

Johnson's Gerard does not enlighten us on whether the rowan is heating or cooling. He writes that the leaves boiled in wine are good for pains in the sides and the stopping of the liver.[5] Culpeper does not mention the rowan tree. In 1694, Pechey writes of the rowan specifying it is *Sorbus sylvestris* or Quickentree, which ties in with the earlier identification. He clearly likes the flowers, describing them as sweet, but comments that the berries "taste ill." Pechey is more enthusiastic about the acidic juice of the berries, which he notes "purges Water excellently well; and is very good for the Scurvy." He then refers to the "Liquor which drops from the wounded Tree in the Spring,…" Presumably this is the sap he says "cures the Scurvy, and Diseases of the Spleen" (p.172).[6]

Summary. It seems rowan has never played a large part in the history of medicine. Even in the Anglo-Saxon period when the bark occurs in several recipes it was always one among a list of herbal ingredients. Hildegard of Bingen clearly has little respect for the rowan and in the formularies of medieval surgeons again it occupies a minor place together with other herbs offering like actions which were generally preferred. Gerard only gives the leaves in wine for dropsy, pains in the side and stoppings of the liver. He does not mention medicinal use of the berries. Other herbalists are silent, except Pechey writing in 1694 who is enthusiastic about the juice of the berries as a purge and as a valuable source of vitamin C against scurvy. After this date, the rowan vanishes from the herbal scene through two centuries. There are diuretic, anti-inflammatory, laxative, and pectoral effects from the berries, which are largely given as a food. See Herbalists' Reference.

Recipe

Extracted from The Herbal Remedies of the Physicians of Myddfai. "687. For Typhus Fever. Take rue, sage, rosemary, and the inner bark of the mountain ash, a handful of each. Take vinegar, mix the lees, [sediment], and pour upon the herbs in a distillery, so as to extract the spirits by distillation. Drink a spoonful night and morning. Pour some also into your nostrils, and wash your brows, perineum, loins, wrists, soles, pit of stomach, chest, and neck with the same. This will preserve you from every pestilence" (p.108).[7]

Notes

1. Godwin Sir H. *History of the British Flora.* (Cambridge University Press. 2nd edition. 1975). 199/200.
2. Pollington S. *Leechcraft.* (Anglo Saxon Books. 2000). 395. *Bald* (39). 407. *Bald* (72). 211. *Lacnunga* (71).
3. Throop P. (trans), *Hildegard von Bingen's Physica.* (Healing Arts Press. 1998). 113.
4. Rosenman Leonard D. MD. *A Medieval Surgical Pharmacopoeia and Formulary.* 1170–1325. (San Francisco. 1999). 61, 85.
5. Johnson T. (ed), *The Herbal.* John Gerard. (1633 edition). (Dover Publications, New York. 1975). 1473/4.
6. Pechey J. *The English Herbal of Physical Plants.* (London. 1694). 172.
7. Pughe J. (trans), *The Herbal Remedies of the Physicians of Myddfai.* (Llanerch. 1989). 108.

SORBUS AUCUPARIA – Herbalist's Reference

The Parts of Rowan Tree Used for Medicine – Fruits.

Dosage and Forms – Usually given in the form of a jelly, jam, or sauce preserve. Occasionally taken as a juice, also as a syrup or electuary.

Constituents – Organic acids. Flavonoids. Amygdalin, cyanidin, sorbitol, pectin, sugars, and tannins.

Actions and Uses – The anti-inflammatory and pectoral actions of the rowan berries have led to them to be used to treat coughs, catarrh, pharyngitis, tonsillitis, and pneumonia.[1] Additional diuretic and litholytic actions have directed use to urinary stones and inflammation in the urinary tract. Rowan berries are also laxative, helping in constipation and with haemorrhoids. Being generally anti-inflammatory and depurative makes them useful in rheumatism. The astringency is useful in a mouthwash.

Interactions – None.

Contraindications and Precautions – Do not eat large amounts of the raw fruits in which the content of irritant parasorbic acid can cause diarrhoea, vomiting, salivation, and gastric disturbance. The parasorbic acid is destroyed by cooking or drying.[2]

Notes

1. Duke J. A. *Handbook of Medicinal Herbs* (CRC Press LLC. 2nd edition. 2002). 635.
2. Fröhne D. Pfander H. *A Colour Atlas of Poisonous Plants.* (Wolf Science. 1983). 197/8.

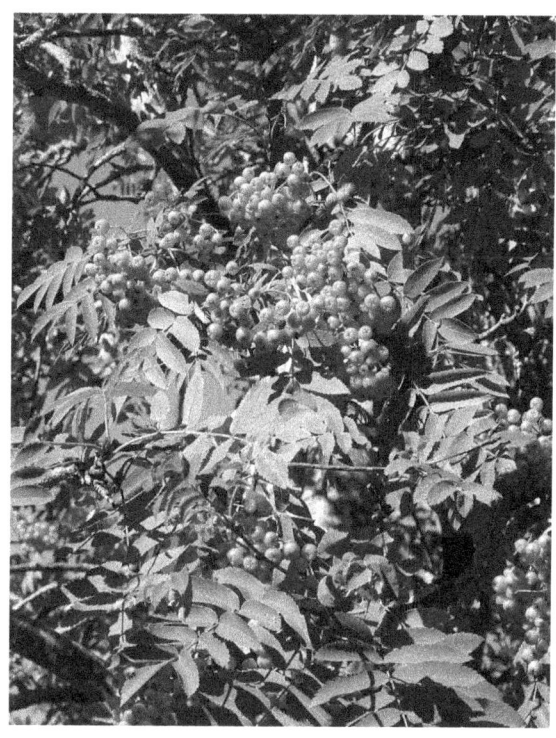

Ripening fruits in autumn.

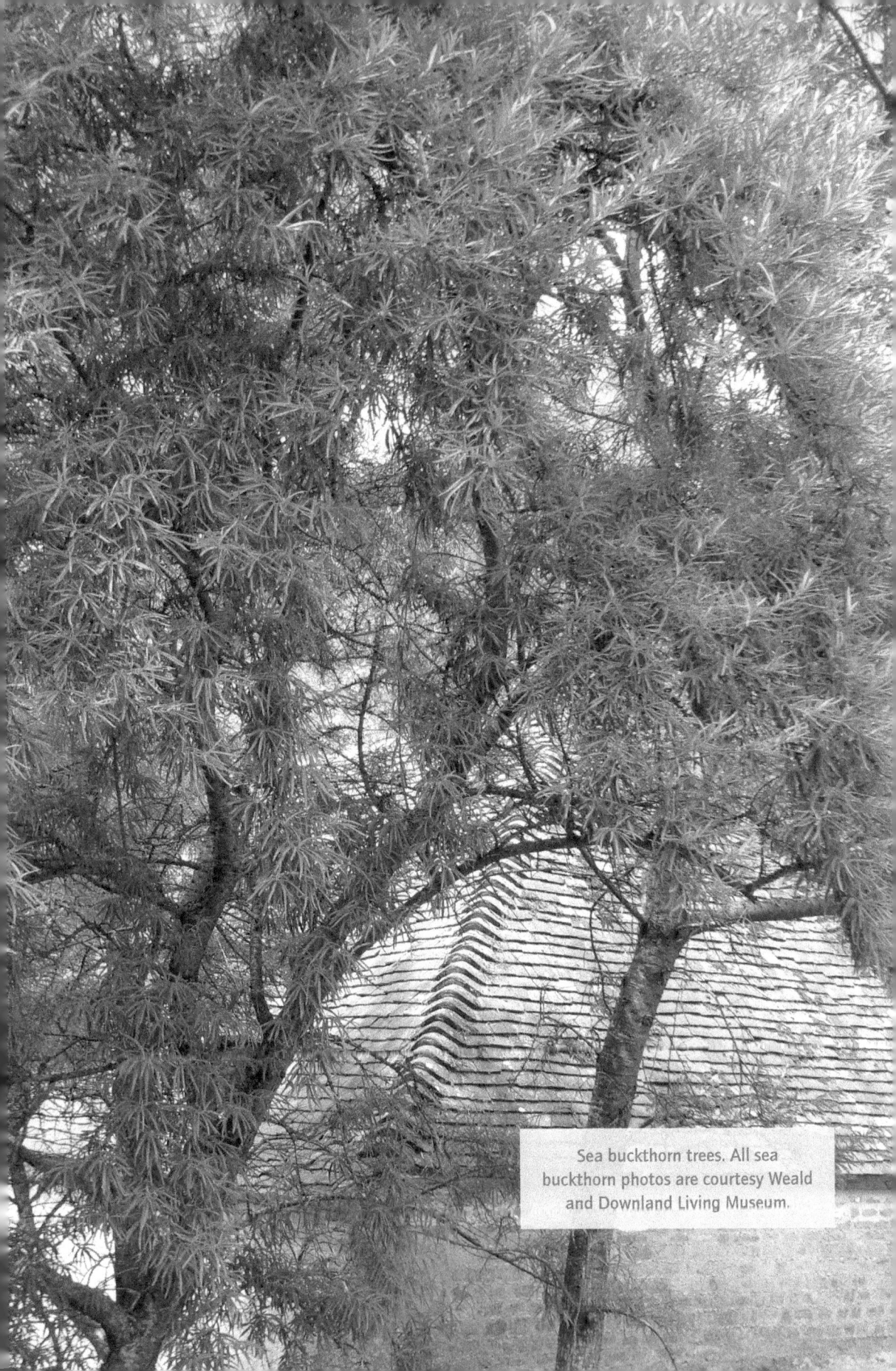

Sea buckthorn trees. All sea buckthorn photos are courtesy Weald and Downland Living Museum.

Sea Buckthorn

Hippophae rhamnoides – Sea Buckthorn – Eleagnaceae

SEA BUCKTHORN – Usefulness – As a food, the berries are rich in Vitamin C. They also have medicinal use, which is currently being enthusiastically researched in several countries. They are eaten by sheep, goats, and horses.[1] Sea buckthorn, which can spread by suckers to form thickets, has often been planted in sand dunes to halt erosion.

Dangers – Care needs to be taken to avoid the thorns when picking berries.

Getting to Know the Sea Buckthorn Tree – The sea buckthorn is native to coasts from Norway to southern Spain, including the coasts of Britain. For over twenty years I have enjoyed seeing the mature trees on my frequent visits to the Weald and Downland Living Museum. I have admired the soft grey of their windswept foliage in early summer and the amazing profusion of bright berries in late autumn and on into winter. At times we have gathered the berries for use in historical herb workshops. In one we were making inks, but the dye that we tried to obtain from the orange berries for this was rather poor, although grown in some sunny situations may be useful for dyeing silk. The leaves or stems are likely to give a stronger colour.

The trees stand next to the lake where they receive the moist air, which seems to suit them well. Their association with the sea coast may have been as much the effect of other trees crowding them out from drier areas inland as a real preference for a site near salt water. Now their common name is witness to their usual habitat either on the coast or by rivers or lakes. In the year the lake was drained for building works at the Museum, the trees did appear to suffer from the dry conditions. Often sea buckthorn can be found growing as bushes right on a shoreline. I have also seen it growing on the shores of Lake Ontario in Canada. It is the ability of the tree to cope with growing in sand and to reach out and spread by suckers that makes it so valuable for holding sand dunes together, safeguarding them from being blown away.

Filled with enthusiasm to use the berries, I planted sea buckthorn in my teaching garden, which was not exactly a wetland habitat, but we did have the brook that turned into a river downstream, right in front of the house. The young tree flourished and I was able to examine the long, drooping leaves, so like willow. It has to be remembered, however, when growing sea buckthorn that you must plant at least one male tree to several female in order to enjoy the harvest of berries. This does unfortunately mean you need a good sized garden to give them the space required. The tiny greenish flowers open in spring on the previous years' growth of twigs. The female drupes are followed by masses of berries, which also cling close to the branches at the bases of the leaf stems.

In the past in Britain, it seems to have been a common misconception that the berries were not edible. A rich source of Vitamin C, they do have an oily bitterness. The dried, powdered berries can be used as a lemon substitute in baking.[2] I have found it is best to mix them with other fruit when making jelly and add cut angelica stem as they are very acidic on their own. The jelly has been eaten with fish in the past, which is a natural partnership arising from their habitat. The name of *Hippophae* seems an extraordinary one to give to this tree but comes from horses eating the berries and their owners being convinced that this helped their eyesight and energy.

In fact, in the present enthusiasm for promoting sea buckthorn as a superfood, which has substantial scientific support,[3] one supplier has developed a veterinary product for horses. Interest in the plant is such that the U.K. Sea Buckthorn Association and Sea Buckthorn Scotland have been founded in recent years and both have informative websites. Both native and imported plants from regions where use of sea buckthorn is better known historically are being harvested. Medicinal use and consequent research from Russia, China, India, and Tibet had already fuelled scientific interest before the tree became valued in Britain. The International Seabuckthorn Association was formed as early as 1998. It has generally been contact with other countries that has led the way to what is perhaps a rediscovery of the value of the berries that have grown on our shores, mainly neglected, for thousands of years.

Sea buckthorn has become highly popular and culinary recipes are easily found on the internet. I first saw sea buckthorn ice cream served in a restaurant in West Sussex a few years ago now and the imaginative recipes that have followed are well worth trying.

Legends and Folklore. Fact or legend I am not sure, but I have heard that Genghis Khan is said to have been so successful because his men fed their horses on sea buckthorn berries.

Notes

1. Green T. *Universal Herbal or Botanical Dictionary.* 2 vols, (Caxton, London. 2nd edition. 1824). Vol. 1. 695.
2. De Sloover J. & Goossens M. *Wild Herbs of Britain and Europe.* (David and Charles. 1994). 17.
3. Zeb A. *Sea Buckthorn: A Functional Food.* (Lambert Academic Publishing. 2014).

SEA BUCKTHORN – History of Medicinal Use

As the Ice Age lifted and the ice retreated so sea buckthorn spread from the ice free areas of Europe to the north, rapidly establishing itself throughout Scandinavia. Pollen records show that it was growing in the British Isles in the interglacial periods. Before woodland gave increasing competition, there were considerable quantities of sea buckthorn growing as scrub rather than trees.[1] It spread throughout northwest Europe and appears to have found considerably more use for food and medicine in the northern areas than in Britain.

Although it seems likely that in prehistory the berries would have been harvested as vitamin rich food, evidence from archaeology is meagre. Sea buckthorn does not feature in herbals and I have not found the berries being used in Britain for medicine in the past. Knowledge of the value of sea buckthorn has come from other countries.

In 1824, Green comments that the berries were "much eaten by the Tartars. They are the principal food of the peasants upon Mount Caucasus." and "The fishermen of the Gulf of Bothnia prepare a rob from them,"(p.695).[2] The rob, it appears, was eaten with fish.[2] Later information simply repeats this. Neither of these references, however, refers to medicine and it would still be many years before this potential was to become known here.

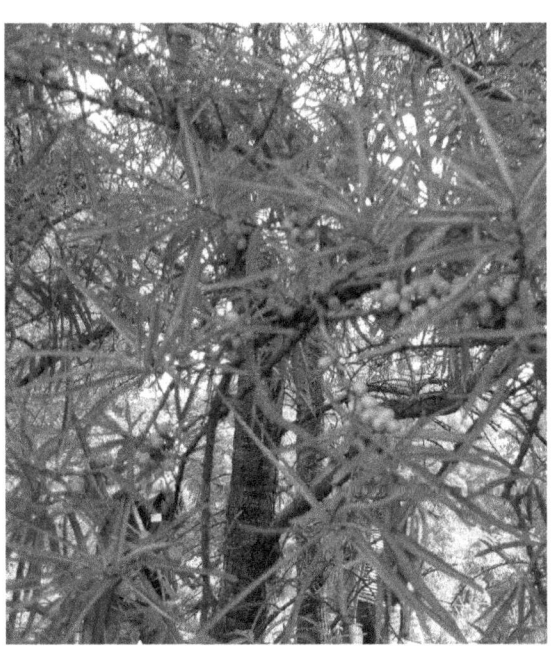
Ripening fruits.

In fact, sea buckthorn grows across northern Europe and seems to have found more use in Scandinavian countries. However, medicinal use has most evidence from the Himalayan regions such as Russia, China, northern India, Pakistan, and Tibet. Across these areas there are various sub-species such as *H. rhamnoides ssp. turkestana* in Pakistan and *H. tibetana* in Tibet.

There, sea buckthorn has had a place in Tibetan medicine since the *Gyud zhi*, written in the eighth century. Referring to Tibetan materia medica based on the Fourfold Medical Tantras,[3] a colleague of mine, Lucy Jones, trained in Tibetan herbal medicine, has shared her knowledge of sea buckthorn with me. As in other cultures, a humoural system of medicine was followed in Tibet. Known as "star bu" or "Tarbu", the sharpness of the sour berries was interpreted as relating to their potency in heating and drying body tissues. The oily nature of their pulp recommended them for treating specific conditions. These were diseases associated with the elements of earth and water, known as "pekén" diseases. It was written that an excess of earth and water can lead to a sluggish, congested state with poor circulation and digestion, and low spirits.

The hot potency and sharpness of "Tarbu" are seen as suitable for helping this congested excess to flow and disperse. In this way it loosens phlegm in the lungs and throat, allowing it to be expectorated and can resolve blood cysts associated with gynaecological disorders by thinning the blood.[4] Herbalist Ben Joffe also says that both the taller form of star bu known as sky tarbu, which grows in ravines, and the shorter earth tarbu offer the first use. It appears a mid-firmament starbu is noted for applying this decongestant property to coagulated blood in the body.

Lucy Jones added, "In Tibetan there is a rich and sophisticated tradition of working with and detoxifying precious metals, 'Tarbu' is one of the many herbs used in the long process of detoxifying Mercury and transforming gold."

Summary. Although sea buckthorn is known to be native to Britain, I have been unable to find evidence for medicinal use. Knowledge of this has travelled here from other countries, particularly Russia, China, and Tibet. Examples of Tibetan use are for treating lung diseases, particularly when there is congestion with phlegm in the lungs or throat, and coagulated blood. More information on medicinal uses can be obtained from Russian and Chinese sources. Having a main focus on medicinal use in Britain means these are beyond the scope of this book.

Notes

1. Godwin Sir H. *History of the British Flora.* (Cambridge University Press. 2nd edition. 1975). 427, 429, 454.
2. Green T. *Universal Herbal or Botanical Dictionary.* 2 vols, (Caxton, London. 2nd edition. 1824). Vol. 1. 695.
3. Doctor Dawa. *A Clear Mirror of Tibetan Medicinal Plants.* (Tibet Domani. 1999). Vol. 1. 86.
4. Pasang Yonten Arya. Dr. *Dictionary of Tibetan Materia Medica.* (Motilal Banarsidass Publishing Delhi. 1998). 25.

HIPPOPHAE RHAMNOIDES – Herbalists' Reference

The Parts of the Sea Buckthorn Tree Used for Medicine – Berries, oils from the berry pulp and seed, berry juice, and leaves.

Dosage and Forms – The berries can be juiced or pulped. Capsules are available of seed or pulp oils or both. Sea buckthorn juice.

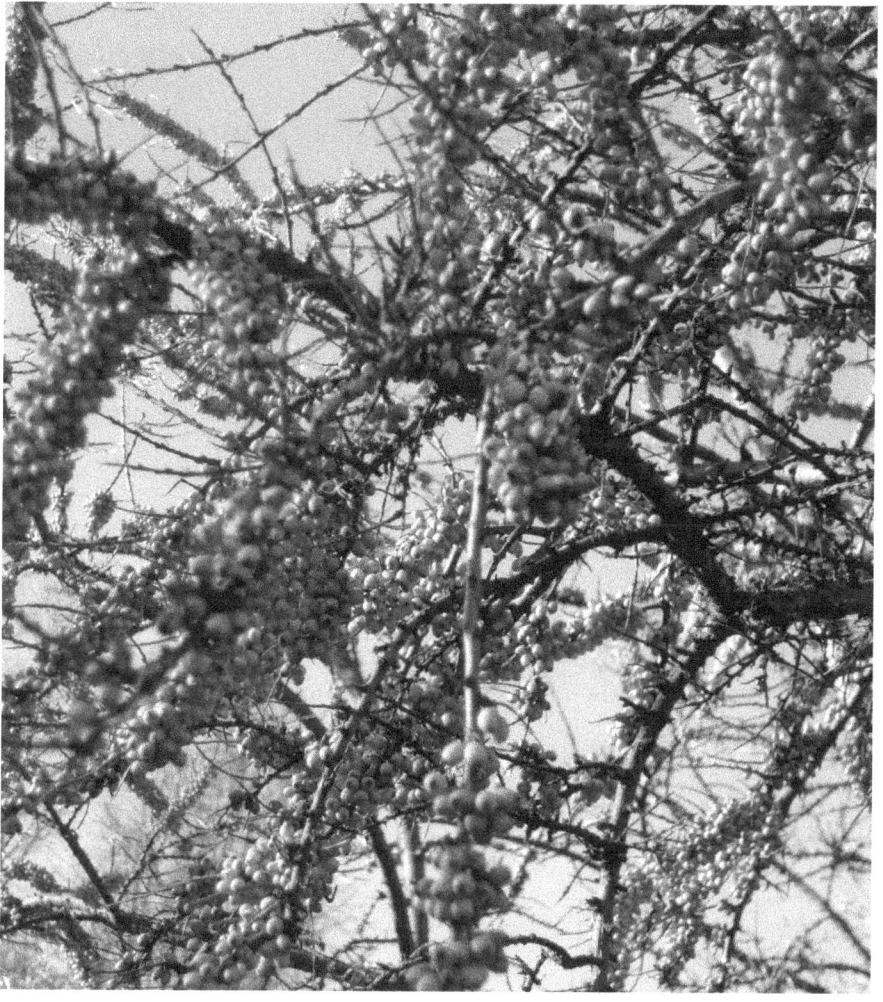

Fruits still available in winter.

Take as directed by the supplier. The tea can hardly be recommended as a drink.

Constituents – There is a fixed oil in both the seeds and the pulp of the fruit. The content of vitamin C, vitamin A, and carotenoid pigments are evident in the brightly coloured berries. Omega 3 and 6 essential fatty acids are high in the seeds. Procyanidins have been isolated from seed extracts. Levels of constituents, including flavonoids, vary from species to species.[1]

Chemoprofiling of seabuckthorn byproducts has found the leaf extract contained significantly the highest amount of total phenols, which are responsible for antioxidant activity. It also confirms that the leaves of sea buckthorn are rich in flavonoids, such as kaempferol glycoside. This supports traditional uses of the leaves in Asia.[2]

Actions and Uses – The high vitamin content renders the berries antioxidant and antiaging. The leaves may also be helpful for encouraging healing in wounds and ulcers. Sea buckthorn is a useful tonic to the heart and support for the eyes, as well as a prophylactic against infection. As an antiaggregant, in the long-term it may help against atherosclerosis. It may also be protective for the liver.[3] Research has included some animal testing on traditional use with gastrointestinal ulcers, cancer therapy and protection from irradiation. Although thousands of scientific reports have been published over recent years, more clinical studies are needed.[1]

Combinations – The berries combine well with rose hips.

Topical Applications – The berries can be crushed and applied to open wounds to stop bleeding.[4] Tea made from the fresh leaves may be applied over wounds.

Contraindications and Precautions – Not known for therapeutic dosages. None found.

Notes

1. Zeb A. *Sea Buckthorn: A Functional Food.* (Lambert Academic Publishing. 2014). 32–35, 39, 44, 48, 50. 51.
2. Ghabru A. *Evaluation of Seabuckthorn byproducts for in vivo in vitro activities.* (Lambert Academic Publishing. 2019). 28.

3. Duke J.A. *Handbook of Medicinal Herbs* (CRC Press LLC. 2nd edition. 2002). 660.
4. Chiej R. *The Macdonald Encyclopedia of Medicinal Plants.* (Macdonald Publishing. London. 1984). 153.

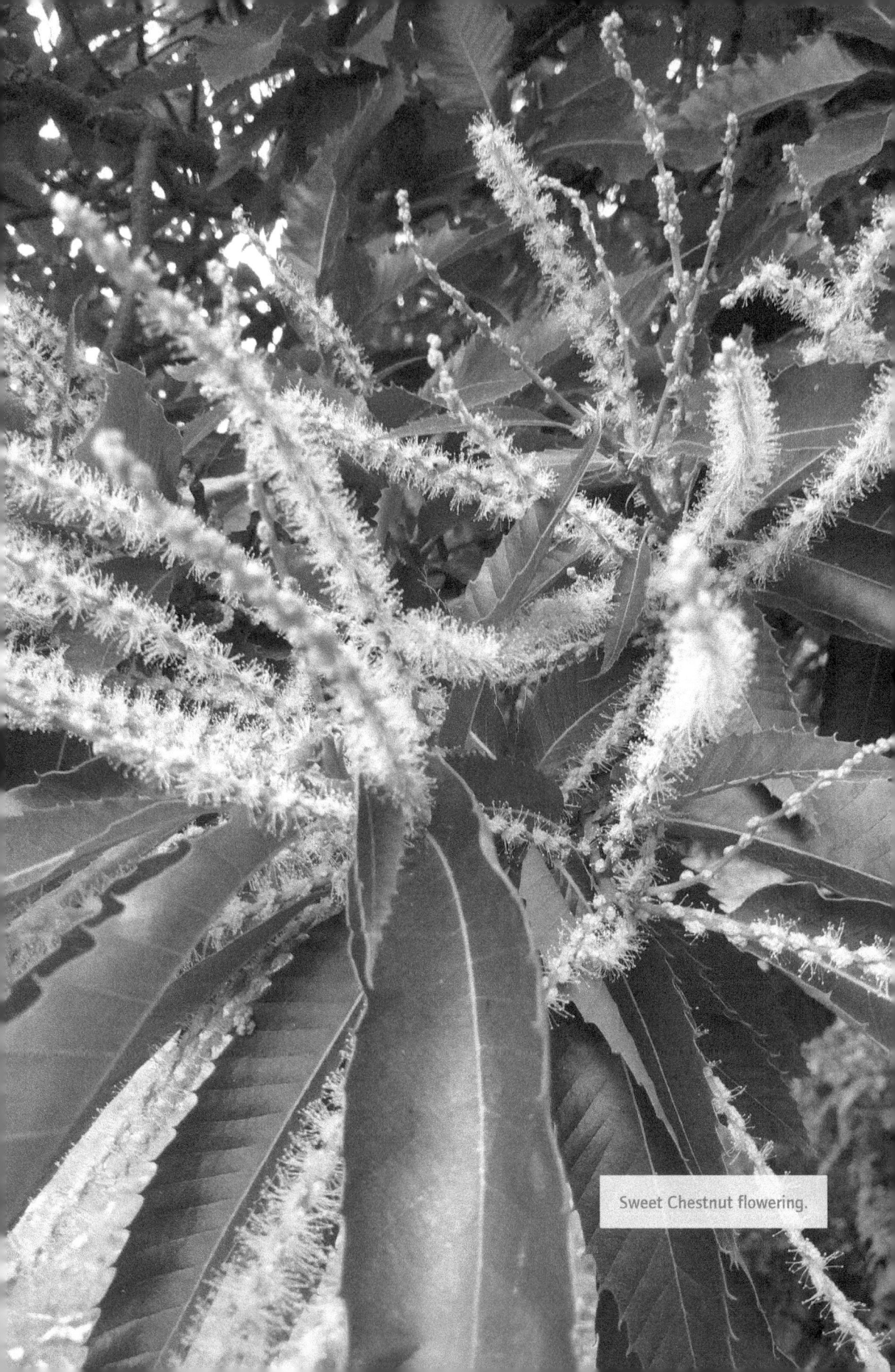

Sweet Chestnut flowering.

Sweet Chestnut

Castanea sativa – Sweet Chestnut – Fagaceae

SWEET CHESTNUT – Usefulness – Chestnuts provide a nourishing protein-rich food. The fruits, leaves, and bark have medicinal properties. Both leaves and chestnut skins can be used in shampoo. The flowers have been included in pipe tobacco. The inner bark is suitable for basketry. The wood can be turned and is especially useful in being water resistant. The bark and twigs produce a dye for wool and silk.

Dangers – None except possible indigestion from eating too many of the fruits.

Getting to Know the Sweet Chestnut Tree – Once my sweet chestnut tree grown from seed reached a size where a very large pot was required. I found it a suitable home elsewhere, for sweet chestnut grows quickly and with a possible height of over thirteen metres (forty-two and a half feet) and spread at the crown of thirty metres (ninety-eight feet), it is hardly a tree for even a large garden.

I came to know the tree more intimately when I attended a class in bark basketry and we were given a choice of branches of sweet chestnut as the starter material. The distinctive outer bark on the trunk is deeply ridged in a spiral pattern and has always fascinated me. On the branches, however, the outer bark was considerably smoother, which was good since our first task was to use a specialist saw blade to remove it. This took time and was hard work. Finally with all the silvery grey bark and green under-layer removed, I was able to saw through the inner bark down to the wood to prepare for stripping. Then I turned to the slow and exciting task of using a wooden tool to carefully peel the bark away. As I did so, I began placing my fingers between the layers. It was the strangest sensation to be touching the inside of a tree, feeling the cool, slippery sap over my hand and breathing in the fresh, cucumber-like smell.

Harvesting bark for basketry or medicine is done in the early spring when the tree is just preparing for new leaves, flowers, growth, and ultimately producing fruits. The slender glossy leaves open first, seeming to spray out drooping in clusters, their edges serrated with spiny tips. These are followed in June by the long creamy coloured catkins, sometimes first brought to your notice by their rich scent. As well as male flowers there are greenish female flowers two or three together at the base of these male dominated catkins. Over the summer, in place of the pollinated female flowers, spiny seedcases develop and inside these are the familiar chestnuts.

Gathering chestnuts in autumn to roast in the embers of the fire was a much-loved part of my childhood in the Kent countryside. Choosing not to eat meat in later years, I spent many hours painstakingly preparing them for nut roasts and other dishes. Now vacuum packed ready to eat chestnuts are available in the shops, which is welcome when in Britain not every year brings a harvest of fruits large enough to be worth the trouble. This year, most from the tree pictured above were tiny. In the warmer climate of southern Europe chestnuts are more dependable as a food. The sweet chestnut is also native to North Africa and South west Asia.

There has been much debate as to whether the chestnut tree was grown here before the Roman occupation, or was introduced by the Romans. In fact, the matter was officially debated by the Royal Society in 1769.[1] This happened even before archaeological excavations resulted in evidence of a possible earlier date. Having visited Oplontis and learned of the finds of the root cavity of a massive chestnut in the internal courtyard of Poppea's luxury villa with evidence of nuts borne at roof height, I can well imagine wealthy Romans wishing to repeat this shade and nut production here as they settled in retirement. In fact, my favourite savoury chestnut dish is one I first adapted from the book of *Apicius* for Roman herb workshops. This was lentils and chestnuts in a cumin and coriander wine sauce. Since that day making it over a brazier in the replica Roman Villa at Butser Ancient Farm, I have repeated the recipe many times. There is never any left at the end of the day.

In the past larger chestnuts were imported from the Continent for the wealthy, the price at the time of Queen Eleanor in the thirteenth century was two pennies for 100.[2] The poor living in forested areas would have gathered from the wild. English chestnuts, at the time called "castaynes", might be eaten raw or roasted. The nuts could also be ground and made into flour as they still are today. Chestnut flour is a tasty gluten-free substitute for wheat, which mixes well with other flours.

When editing *The Receipt Book of Lady Anne Blencowe* from 1694, I found a note against her version of caramelised oranges that roasted chestnuts can be caramelised in the same way. Today they are sold as Marrons Glacé. Her cookery is always elegantly presented and I could just imagine both dishes set on a laden table at Christmas parties.

The sweet chestnut is not only about food however, over the centuries much use has been made of the inner skin separated from the nut before it is fully ripe and dried for the astringency in stopping bleeding. This might be taken in wine. The pounded fruits were given for coughing up blood and an emulsion of chestnuts in a decoction of liquorish had a few poppy seeds added and was given for coughs and urinary infections.[3] Chestnuts have also been prepared in honey for the liver and digestion. William Langham in his *Garden of Health*, written at a time when there was great interest in health advice to lengthen life, even suggested chestnuts could stir up lust![4] By the First World War the leaves began to be used in herbal medicine and new research on this is promising.

Legends and Folklore. In Italy, chestnuts were eaten on Hallowe'en, also known as All Soul's Day Eve. It was customary to leave a few nuts for the dead to enjoy during the night. Chestnuts have been carried in pockets as a charm against rheumatism in several countries.[5] In England, I have always understood it would be necessary to borrow the chestnut or receive it as a gift first for it to be effective.

Notes

1. Rackham O. *The History of the Countryside.* (Phoenix Paperback. 1986). 54.
2. Harvey J. *Mediaeval Gardens.* (Batsford. 1981). 84.
3. Pechey J. *The English Herbal of Physical Plants.* (London. 1694). 45.
4. Coles W. *The Paradise of Plants.* (London. 1657). 43.
5. DeCleene M. & Lejeune M.C. *Compendium of Symbolic and Ritual Plants in Europe.* (Man and Culture Publishers, Ghent. Belgium. 2003). 677.

CHESTNUT TREE – History of Medicinal Use

There has been some debate as to whether the Sweet Chestnut grew in Britain before the arrival of the Romans, whether they introduced the tree, or it came later. The tree is native to southern Europe, North Africa, and South West Asia. No pollen has been found to verify sweet chestnut, but there was a questionable find for chestnut in the Neolithic layer recorded by Godwin. Chestnuts were part of the staple diet of Roman legionaries based here and the introduction of the tree is generally attributed to the Roman invasion. However, the chestnut that has naturalised here over the centuries is not a variety that was specially grown for nuts in Italy.

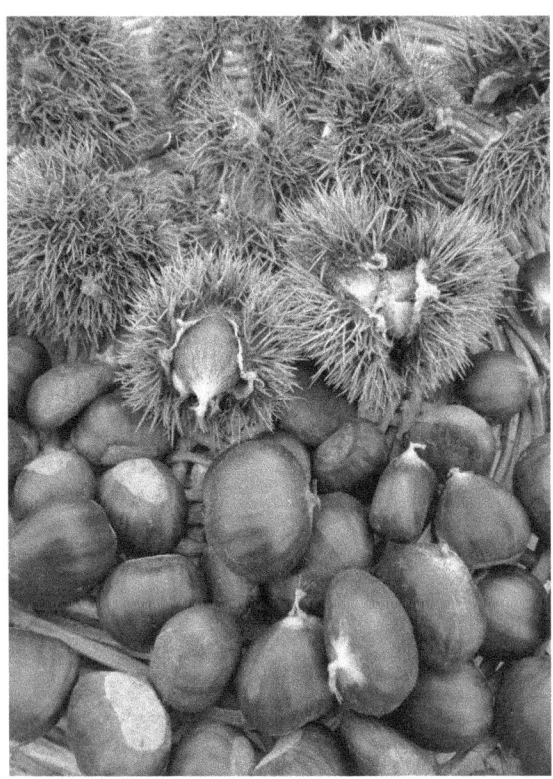

Sweet chestnuts.

Dioscorides calls chestnuts *Castanea vesca* "Juppiter's Acornes" he remarks that their medicinal effects are like those of the oak in binding tissues.[1] In the early Medieval period we find references to chestnut as cistenbeam and the timber is recorded in Anglo-Danish York in the tenth century. In the monastery orchard garden plan of St Gall, along with the fig, hazel, almond, quince, medlar, apple and pear, it was clearly regarded as a necessary nut tree. Anglo-Norman recipes, which may have followed on from Anglo-Saxon, include a spiced paste with chestnuts, hard-boiled eggs and pork liver.[2]

In the twelfth century, Hildegard prescribes the nuts in honey for the liver and chestnut with liquorice to purge the stomach and strengthen digestion.³ I feel she is really depending upon the liquorice here as chestnuts are consistently viewed by others as constipating. William Turner wrote in 1551 that chestnut trees grew plenteously in Kent in fields and gardens. He quotes Symeon Sethy who agrees with Hildegard that they are hot and dry in the first (lowest) degree and very nourishing. This remark was made despite the caution that followed on affirming they were full of wind and by taking a long time to be digested, caused stoppage. He advises drying or cooking them to lessen this effect.⁴

At this period, many trees were being planted in parks and large gardens. Culpeper does not include the chestnut tree but in 1657. Coles brings a new slant on the properties of the nuts. He writes "It is not ordinarily delivered, that this Nut should stir up *Venery*; onely *Langham* in his Garden of Health mentioneth it for this purpose, which is more than probable, if the much nourishment they afford, and the windiness going along with them (both which qualities are very conducible hereunto) be considered"(p.43).⁵ To the recipe for an electuary with honey directed to treat a cough, especially when bloody phlegm is produced, he adds that a decoction of the powdered inner skin taken in wine or water is helpful for bleeding. He not only applies the powdered kernels with barley meal and vinegar to swellings of the breasts, but recommends them pounded with honey and salt for the bite of a mad dog.⁵

At the end of the eighteenth century Pechey gives us a way of telling the good nuts from bad. He floats them in water noting that if sound they sink, while if they float they can be discarded. He offers a new recipe amongst those familiar for coughs. This is an emulsion of Chestnuts, in a decoction of liquorish with a few seeds of the opium poppy added. It was a treatment for "Heat of Urine" (p.47).⁶

In 1722 Joseph Miller set out to reveal all manner of deceptions, whether of identification or uses of herbs. He grants that chestnuts are binding, but adds, "especially the inward Skin, which some pretend to be good for all kind of Fluxes, either of Blood or Humors"(p.123)⁷

The thin skin of the kernel continues to be used in medicine through the nineteenth century. Brook in his herbal directs that the thin skin covering the kernel or nut is to be separated from the nut before it becomes fully ripe and dried to use as an astringent.[8] Not until 1916 in the instructions for gathering herbs during the First World War when supplies were cut from Germany do we find the statement, "It is the leaves, however, which are used in herbalist medicine"(p.174).[9]

Summary. Chestnuts were recommended by Dioscorides and Pliny for encouraging peristalsis and stopping bleeding in the gut. In spite of the recommendations for the digestive system, there is a constant undercurrent of comment on eating chestnuts producing constipation. Others stating that they not only give good nourishment but produce wind. In 1657, Coles states that he can see why Langham recommends chestnuts for stirring up lust, as in his opinion nourishment and windiness support this!

The astringent uses, particularly of the powdered inner skin are consistent for stopping bleeding and Gerard recommends the powdered kernels in honey for coughing up blood. It is not until the First World War that we find the statement that the leaves are used in herbal medicine. To find out why, read Herbalists' Reference.

Recipe

Extracted from Culpeper The Complete Herbal and English Physician Enlarged. "If you dry Chesnuts, (only the kernels I mean) both the barks being taken away, beat them into powder, and make the powder up into an electuary with honey, so have you an admirable remedy for the cough and spitting of blood" (p.47).[10] The electuary consists of the chestnut powder mixed with honey to a consistency which is not too stiff to swallow but sufficiently stiff for the powder and honey not to separate.

Notes

1. Gunther R.T. (ed), *Dioscorides Greek Herbal.* (Hafner. 1968). 77.
2. Hagen A. *A Handbook of Anglo-Saxon Food.* (Anglo-Saxon books. 1992). 62.
3. Throop P. (trans), *Hildegard von Bingen's Physica.* (Healing Arts Press. 1998). 115.
4. Chapman G. & Tweddle M. (ed), *A New Herball.* William Turner (1551.) (Carcanet Press. 1989). 265.

5. Coles W. *The Paradise of Plants.* (London. 1657). 43.
6. Pechey J. *The English Herbal of Physical Plants.* (London. 1694). 46/7.
7. Miller J. *Botanicum officinale.* Bell. (London. 1722). 122.
8. Brook R. *Brook's Family Herbal.* (J.A. Brook, Richardson & Co. London. Revised edition. 1876). 301.
9. Teetgen A.B. *Profitable Herb-Growing and Collecting.* (London. 1916). 174.
10. Culpeper N. *Culpeper's Complete Herbal and English Physician enlarged.* (1652). (London. 1815 edition). 47.

CASTANEA SATIVA – C VULGARIS – FAGUS CASTANEA – Herbalist's Reference

The Parts of the Sweet Chestnut tree Used for Medicine – Leaves and fruit.

Dosage and Forms – 2 teaspoons of dried shredded leaf per cup of water. Bring to the boil and decoct for 5 minutes. ½–1 cup as needed. 1:1 in 25% alcohol. Dose 1–4ml three times daily.

Constituents – Hammamelitannin, flavonoids, calcium, and iron.

Actions and Uses – The tannins have astringent and healing applications. The leaves are expectorant and the infusion is used as a gargle for sore throats and given in cases of bronchial catarrh, tracheitis, and whooping cough. The leaves may be helpful as an anti-rheumatic sedative to ease pain of lumbago and muscular rheumatism. The bark is more suited to treating diarrhoea and fevers. Nervous conditions and insomnia have also been treated with the leaves.

Specific Indication – Paroxysmal cough.

Combinations – With wild cherry for whooping cough. Or with Apium, Cimicifuga, Menyanthes, and Filipendula for muscular rheumatism.[1]

Topical Application – A compress of the cold, wet leaves against the burn and a cloth soaked in the leaf tea to cover is recommended as a traditional remedy to cool burns and prevent scar tissue.[2]

Contraindications and Precautions – None given for recommended dosage.[3] Large doses should be avoided due to the tannin content.

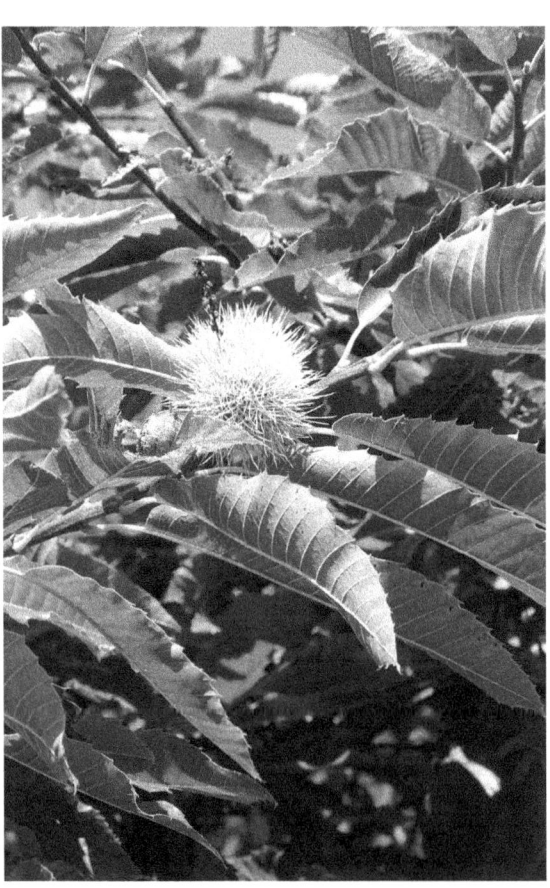

Sweet chestnut case and leaves.

Notes

1. *British Herbal Pharmacopoeia.* (British Herbal Medicine Association. 1983). 52.
2. De Bairacli-Levy J. *The Illustrated Herbal Handbook for Everyone.* (Faber and Faber. London. 1991). 188.
3. Duke J.A. *Handbook of Medicinal Herbs* (CRC Press LLC. 2nd edition. 2002). 687.

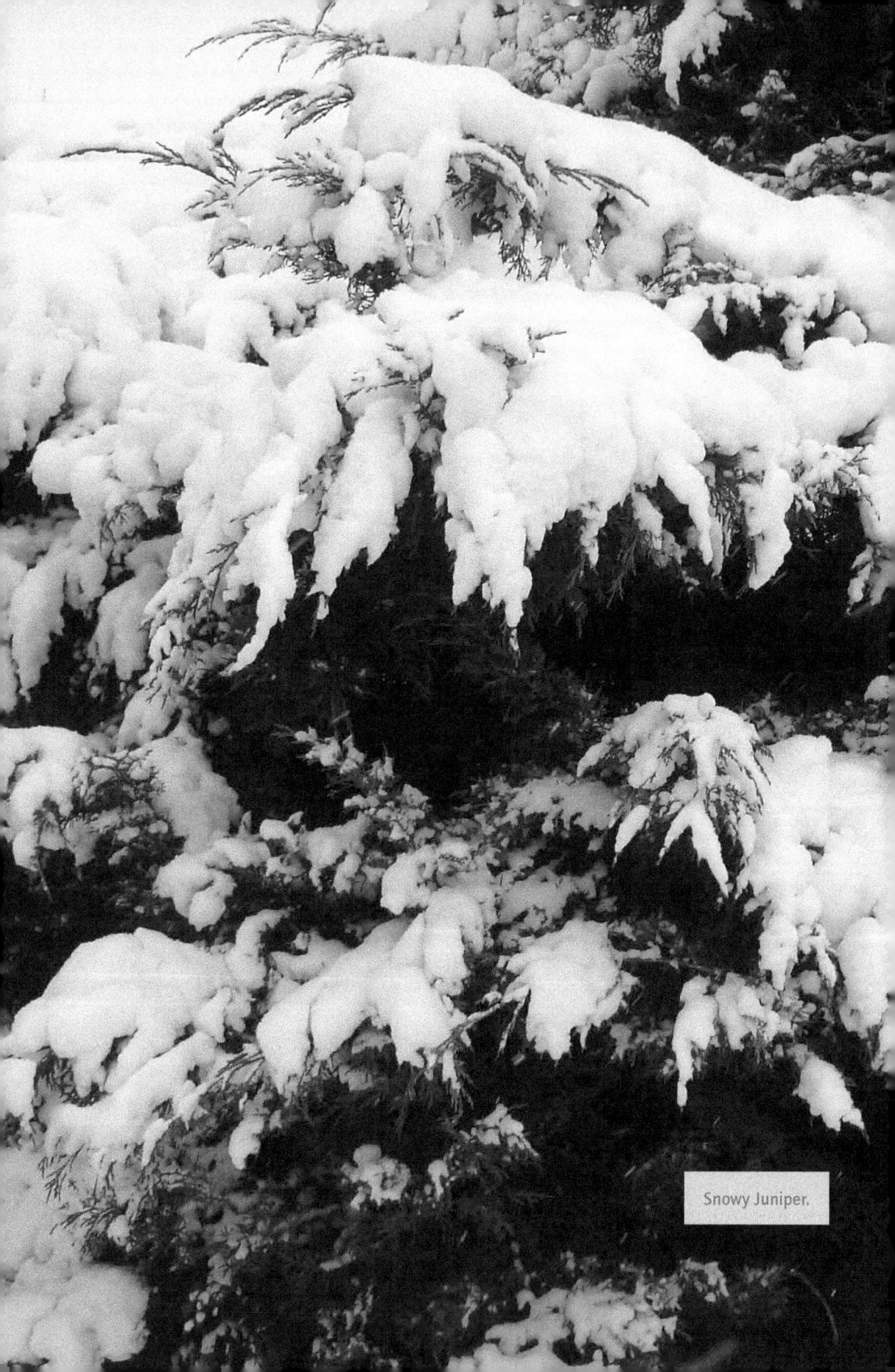
Snowy Juniper.

WINTER

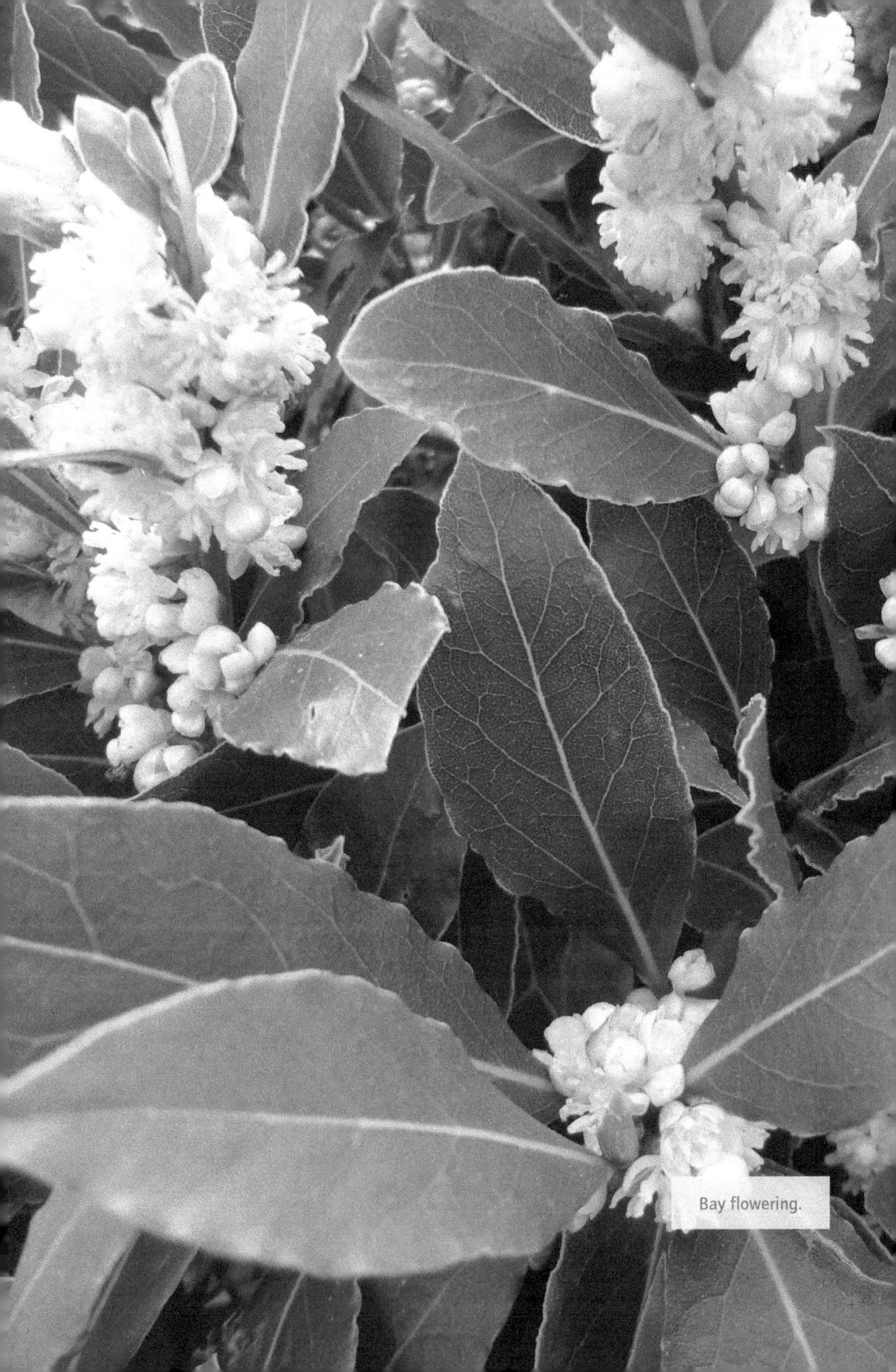

Bay flowering.

Bay

Laurus nobilis – Bay – Lauraceae

BAY – Usefulness – The smooth glossy foliage has a special value enlivening the garden in winter. Stems can be brought in at Christmas and New Year for decorations. Bay leaves are a valued digestive flavouring in foods. The leaves are helpful against muscular and neuralgic pain in topical applications. Young stems can be used in basketry. The wood can be turned.

Dangers – Bay leaves can be very sharp even when cooked and if large pieces are swallowed with food they may seriously damage the intestines. Always remove as the food is served.[1] A possible consequence of handling the oil may be contact dermatitis.

Getting to Know the Bay Tree – A sunny, sheltered location is needed for bay to thrive since it originally came from the warmer climate of the Mediterranean and North Africa. Culpeper classed it as a tree of the sun under the sign of Leo, which feels exactly right. While living in the cold north-east of England I took my bay tree inside for the winter. Having moved south, it was planted in the garden and over the next twenty years grew to be a sizeable tree over six metres (twenty feet) tall. However, try as I did with three successive young bays they did not survive in a spot just three metres (ten feet) away, which was more open to frost. Clearly location can be all important and it is wise to protect young trees from bitter cold.

Each year I gave the tree an iron tonic in spring, using home-made nettle liquid fertiliser.[2] Cuttings taken in early autumn remained in pots for two years for special attention and then received fresh compost annually. As the tree matured, it bore dense clusters of creamy coloured flowers, the males appeared almost spiky with eight to twelve yellow stamens. The female flowers looked simpler, with ovary, style, and stigma. These are followed by large purplish-black berries. The name bay is actually an old English term meaning berry, which tells us how much this part of the tree was valued in the past. The berries come ripe in January.

As time passed, I took bay fresh from the tree for seasoning foods as it is a digestive tonic as well as an antibacterial seasoning. The scent from sprays of the leaves is strong and enjoyable and I had the idea of weaving young growth into a flat, oval platter for serving bread. Young stems and old leaf have the highest content of essential oil. Although leaves are left on around the edge more can be freshly inserted into the weave before use, so that warm bread served on their surface takes on the flavour and scent of bay. Tear into the edge of each leaf to release the oil. If you hold a leaf up to the light as you are working with it you can see the many glands amongst the prominent veins on the paler underside of the leaf, which produce the scented oil as you bruise the plant. Leaves destined to stay on the platter for some time need to finish drying with a weight on top to stop them curling.

I planted a crescent of purple sage around the base of the tree and laid a bark path next to it. I had no thought of growing another tree from seed but the path offered moisture retention and warmth for any falling berries. Three weeks before we were to move away I was weeding the path and came upon a tiny bay sapling growing amongst the bark. It felt as though the tree had deliberately given me its young to look after and gratefully I potted it up. That tree is healthy and several feet tall now, giving me harvests.

As it is a bitter herb, bay seasoning aids the flow of bile from the liver and lowers blood glucose, helping the body to use insulin more effectively.[3] Bay herb helps to relieve wind as it passes through the intestines, is useful against worms in children, and to balance gut flora. It is, therefore, both food and medicine. The wood is used for smoking meat and cheese, adding aroma and flavour. Bay leaves and berries are ingredients in liqueurs.

The aroma of bay is strong and refreshing and ensured it was a popular ingredient in scented waters made by ladies in their stillrooms in the seventeenth and eighteenth centuries. Aromatic distilled water may be used as a last rinse after a shampoo, or added to bathwater. Alternatively a tea made from crushed leaves may be added to a pain-relieving hot bath. Oil from the berries is included in soaps. The leaves can be burned on the fire to appreciate their properties as a fumigant, sweetening the air. As the oil glands burst open they will hiss and crackle. The insecticidal qualities make bay suited for inclusion in anti-mosquito creams. Finally, bay is an ingredient in toothpastes as it may help to prevent dental decay.[3]

Legends and Folklore. In ancient Greece, bay was dedicated to Apollo and Artemis and the leaves were connected with the ability to see into the future and make prophesies.[4] Long viewed as a symbol of victory, wreaths were worn by Roman Emperors and bay was associated with Roman palaces and Temples. In the Temples leaves were used in purification rituals. Sprays of bay were hung over doorways to greet the New Year, being seen as protection from death and evil spirits.[5] We may not still believe that bay can protect us against lightning, witchcraft, and devils, as came to be accepted much later in England, but this is a custom we can still enjoy. The smooth leaves, with added dried orange slices and spices make perfect welcome wreaths. Small bay trees also appear as lovely miniature Christmas table decorations when light ornaments are added.

The so-called magic of bay was in evidence at other times of year too. Greek papyri tell of magical charms written on bay leaves. Laurel branches were also used to sweep the paving at the Temple of Delphi.[6]

Notes

1. Duke J.A. *Handbook of Medicinal Herbs* (CRC Press LLC. 2nd edition. 2002). 65.
2. Stapley C. *Herb Sufficient.* (Heartsease Books.1994). 36.
3. Kelly W.J. (ed. director). *Nursing Herbal Medicine Handbook.* (Springhouse Corporation. 2001). 43.
4. Coats A.M. *Garden Shrubs and their Histories.* (Vista Books. London. 1963). 192.
5. Stapley C. *Herbcraft Naturally.* (Heartsease Books. 1994). 194.
6. Moncrieff A.R. Hope. *Classical Mythology.* (Senate. 1994). 174.

BAY – History of Medicinal Use

Although some authorities view the introduction of bay to this country as being in 1562, it would seem highly likely that the Romans imported bay trees during their occupation of Britain 2000 years ago. McLean tells us that in 1538 after closure of the monasteries the King's Commissioners took bays and other evergreens growing in the London Charterhouse gardens at Spitalcroft to Hampton Court.[1] Proof that the bay was already established here then.

Roman writers give a long list of medicinal preparations of the leaves, berries, and bark to treat a great variety of conditions. In treating lethargy, Celsus instructs the head to be fomented with a decoction of laurel in vinegar, as the first step of the treatment. In treating severe liver disease the berries might be given sparingly in internal medicine. Oil from the berries was used in a plaster and was seen as useful to draw collections of unwanted matter to the surface.[2]

After the many ways in which the Romans enthusiastically prepared parts of bay to treat the body, the ninth century *Macer Floridus* gives us a rather daunting entry for the herb. The berries are set forth in a "noble potion" (p.191)[3] as a purge that works by the nether parts of man purging all the inner parts of man's body! This evacuation of the bowels apparently helps and heals whatever ails the stomach, bowel or lungs. Then we have the caution if any great or grievous cause of the problem means it does not help, it is no wonder, as all may not

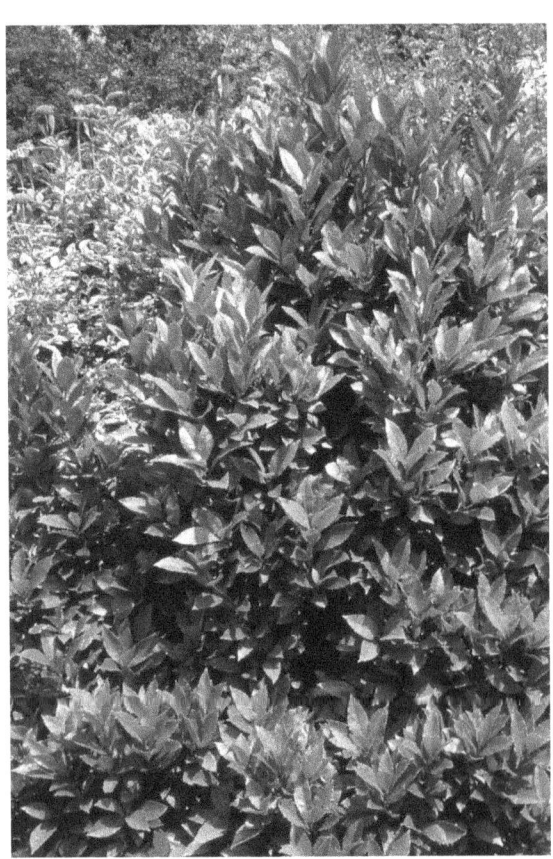

Mature bay.

be known and sickness does not affect all men alike. This was sound advice. Nevertheless the entry states this potion would not harm.[3] In the Anglo-Saxon Leechbook of the *Lacnunga* the berries are included in salve recipes for the eyes, inflammation and asthma.[4]

Hildegard in the twelfth century uses bay berries as a substitute for rue, and the bark and leaves together as a purge.[5] Medieval medicine used bay in treating sciatica and gout as might be expected, and in powders for the stomach together with spices. In the fifteenth century applications of resin, wax and turpentine for covering wounds were tempered with oil of bay to soften them for use. Gout was viewed as either hot or cold in nature and oil of bay heated alone was a treatment for cold gout.

Inevitably through its digestive properties, bay was included in a number of powders for the stomach, as well as those with more general applications. We can also relate to its use for sciatica.

It was 200 years later that Culpeper described the powers of the Leonine bay as resisting witchcraft and evil. Of the bark of the root he said it is less sharp, but more bitter than other parts. He viewed it as effective in breaking the stone, and to open obstructions in the liver and spleen which produce jaundice and dropsy. He saw it to be also "effectuall" (p.18), against all poison of venomous creatures and infectious diseases. The long list of benefits from the berries included aids to menstruation and childbirth, expelling wind, killing worms, for old coughs, and the megrim (migraine). Culpeper further recommended the oil from the berries for the joints and nerves, to dissolve bruising, and aid in convulsions and palsies.[6]

Pechey in his herbal of 1694 prefers a decoction of the bark, berries, and leaves together to be used in a bath for the womb and bladder. He singles out the berries against poisons and bee stings, and for use in the plague and gives a recipe for a clyster (enema) containing the berry powder.[7] A considerable collection of recipes published fifty years later has only two containing bay for physic and both of these are complex. "*An Incomparable* Ointment *for a* Strain, Weakness, *or* Shrinking *in the* Nerves" (p.127)[8] is so unusual and interesting I have made it on herb workshops.

In 1790, the surgeon Meyrick administered a simple infusion of the leaves for strengthening the stomach and nervous disorders.

This it seems from his herbal is also good if continued for paralytic disorders, creating appetite etc. The oil is still used for bruising, cramps, and ear-ache.[9] Herbalists in the nineteenth century repeat what has gone before until in the First World War bay is confirmed as still on the list of herbs to be gathered for medicine, the leaves selling at three pence per pound.[10]

Summary. Bay has always been regarded as a heating herb for cold conditions. We have seen recipes using the root bark, berries, the oil from the berries, and leaves. The most consistent recommendations have been for bay as an analgesic in easing joint or nerve pain. Culpeper and Coles specified bay as a treatment for migraine, whereas from the first century onwards others recommended bay for headaches. A further use, which is repeated over the centuries, is prescribing oil of the berries as ear-drops for pain or deafness. Other, secondary uses have been for aiding recovery in palsies and treating the digestion. The only warning note was given in the *Macer Floridus* on using the berries as a purge. Root bark also had purgative properties and is no longer used. See Herbalists' Reference for the modern view of bay in herbal medicine.

Recipe

Extracted from A Collection of Recipes. 1746. "*An Incomparable* Ointment *for a* Strain, Weakness, *or* Shrinking *in the* Nerves. Take Sweet-marjoram, Penny-royal, Rosemary-tops, Camomile-flowers, Lavender-flowers, Sage, and young Bay-leaves, of each a large Handful; a very large Nutmeg, and its Weight in Mace; the Rind of four Lemons, and as many Oranges: Stamp all very fine, and boil it in a quarter of a Pint of rich *Malaga* Wine, and half a Pound of unsalted Butter; let it boil till the Wine is wasted; press it through a fine Sieve, and keep it cool for Use. Rub it Morning and Night before the Fire, on the Part affected" (p.127).[8]

Notes

1. McLean T. *Medieval English Gardens.* (Barrie & Jenkins. 1989). 52.
2. Spencer W.G. (trans), *Celsus De Medicina* 1 Books 1–1V. (Loeb Classical Library. 1971). 311, 415.

Spencer W.G. (trans), *Celsus De Medicina* 1 Books V-V1. (Loeb Classical Library. 1989). 11.
3. Frisk G. (ed), *A Middle English translation of Macer Floridus de Viribus Herbarum.* (Harvard University Press Cambridge, Mass. 1949). 191.
4. Pollington S. *Leechcraft.* (Anglo Saxon Books. 2000). 193, 197. *Lacnunga* (30, 37).
5. Throop P. (trans), *Hildegard von Bingen's Physica.* (Healing Arts Press. 1998). 38.
6. Culpeper N. *Culpeper's Complete Herbal and English Physician enlarged.* (1652). (London. 1815 edition). 18.
7. Pechey J. *The English Herbal of Physical Plants.* (London. 1694). 15/16.
8. Anon. *A Collection of Receipts.* (Printed for the Executrix of Mary Kettilby. 1746). 127.
9. Meyrick R. *The New Family Herbal.* (Birmingham. 1790). 32.
10. Teetgen A.B. *Profitable Herb-Growing and Collecting.* (London. 1916). 175.

LAURUS NOBILIS - Herbalists' Reference

The Parts of the Bay Tree Used for Medicine – Medicinal use of bay has traditionally included recipes containing the root bark, but these have been discontinued. Today the leaves, berries, and seed oil are used. Essential oil and aromatic water are distilled from the leaves.

Dosage and forms – The leaves are decocted by adding 25g (1oz) of crushed leaves to 600ml (1 pint) of water, bring this to the boil and simmer for twenty minutes, reducing the volume slightly. Dose half a cup three times daily. Bay leaves are also ingredients in ointments and creams. The aromatic water is used topically as a wash or might be added to a hand-bath or footbath.

Constituents – Those seen as important are compounds, such as parthenolides and santamarin, also present in feverfew, which may help to prevent migraine. Also bactericidal 1.8 cineol. Eugenol in the yellow volatile oil is seen as anti-inflammatory. The flavonoids quercetin and rutin, helpful to blood vessel walls, are among other meaningful constituents. Volatile oils are present in both the leaves and berries.

Actions and Uses—In herbal medicine, bay may be prescribed to support a weak digestive system when appetite is poor and insulin activity is low. As a stimulant bitter, bay has a tonic effect on both the stomach and the liver. It aids the flow of bile, assisting with digestion of fats and in helping the body to use insulin effectively, can lower blood glucose. A carminative herb, bay helps to relieve gut spasms, indigestion, and colic.

While the antibacterial properties can be applied against urinary

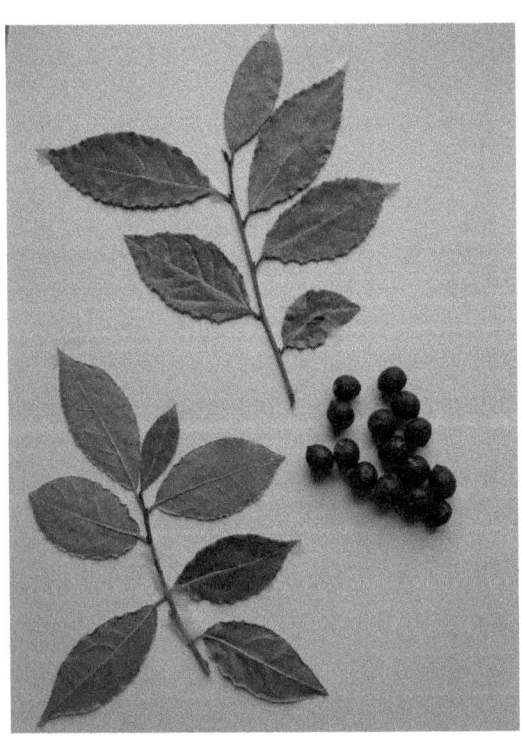

Herbarium specimen for Bay.

infections by taking a decoction of the leaves, for chest infections preparations of the berries are used. The oil has antibacterial and anti-fungal properties. In addition to the volatile oil, the berries yield fatty oil which can be used to prepare warming and analgesic ointments for relieving rheumatic pain. Anti-dandruff and alopecia treatments may contain bay.

Topical Applications – Torn bay leaves are a helpful ointment constituent when teamed with rosemary and calendula or birch and ginger for treating rheumatic or muscular pain. For occasional symptomatic relief two or three torn bay leaves may be hung under the hot tap while running a pain-relieving bath. Tied together in muslin they can also be floated in the bathwater. An alternative is to take baths of comfortably hot water with either the decoction or the aromatic water of bay added. Do not use in a full-body bath without testing on a small area of skin.

Contraindications and Precautions – It should be noted that bay encourages menstrual flow and is therefore not to be taken in medicinal quantity when pregnant. Contact dermatitis may sometimes occur as a reaction to handling the oil which is active against insects and parasites.[1]

Note

1. Duke J. A. *Handbook of Medicinal Herbs* (CRC Press LLC. 2nd edition. 2002). 65.

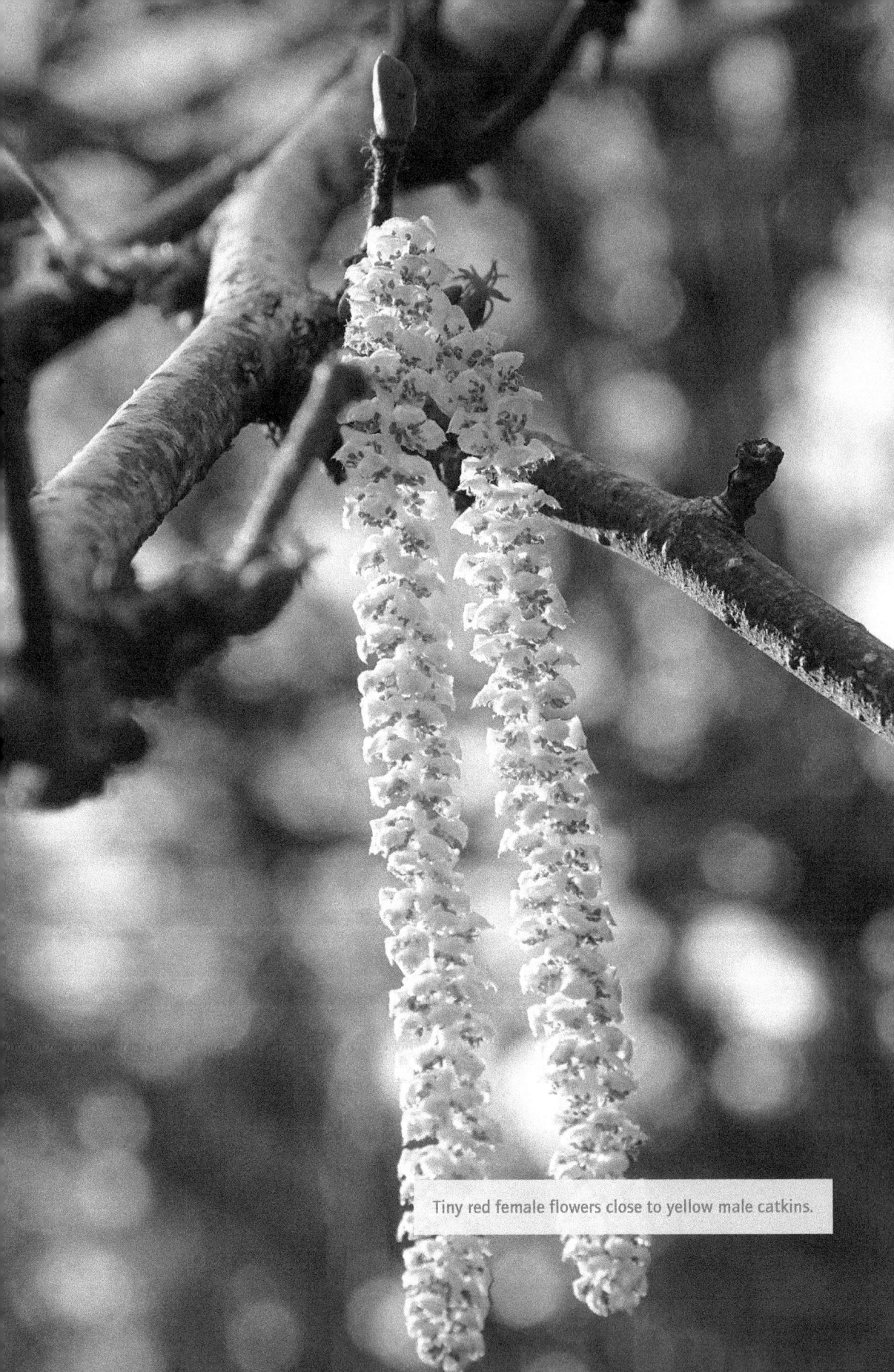
Tiny red female flowers close to yellow male catkins.

Hazel

Corylus avellana – Hazel, Filbert – Betulaceae

Hazel – Usefulness – The nuts provide a nutritious food for man and wildlife, such as squirrels. Hazelnut milk and hazelnut oil are popular foods, both have also been included in historical medical recipes. The milk was formerly recommended for bringing down fevers and the oil given against threadworm and pinworms. Stakes and weavers cut from young growth are suitable for everything from wattle hurdles and ornamental garden structures to baskets. The nut shells and catkins produce dyes. Flour made from the nuts has cosmetic uses.[1] Hazel bark appears in recipes to thicken hair growth.[2]

Dangers – Many people are allergic to hazel pollen, which is produced profusely.

Getting to Know the Hazel Tree – There are few sights more welcome than the bright tassels of male hazel catkins announcing the end of winter and coming of spring. They have of course been on the tree since the previous late summer; slowly developing and turning from green to yellow once they are fully grown. Not many people, however, appreciate the tiny, delicate beauty of the female flowers. Just as the showy male catkins dangle like abandoned Christmas decorations on the branches, the minute, round female flowers hug the upper parts of the branch closely. They are included in the future bud with a tuft of bright red styles at the tip. The small round germen at the centre becomes the nut. Trees of the filbert sub-species stand more erect than the common hazel and I can always tell their fallen nuts from those of the other hazels in my garden as they are considerably larger.

At this time of year I harvest the male catkins, which with their golden load of pollen dye silk quite beautifully. It will be late summer before I begin patrolling my garden in an attempt to beat the squirrels to collecting the fallen nuts. These are held from one to five together, often there are three, each in a "frilly" green case. They remind me of three heads wearing old-fashioned bonnets with lacy trims, touching, but each looking in a different direction.

The cases, later russet brown, like the branches and leaves of the hazel feel soft and hairy to touch. Though they are actually stiff and maintain shape after the nuts have fallen out. Hazel nuts should not be picked until they begin to fall from the tree. If some are still in their cases when they fall, they are better stored in this condition in order to retain moisture in the nut.

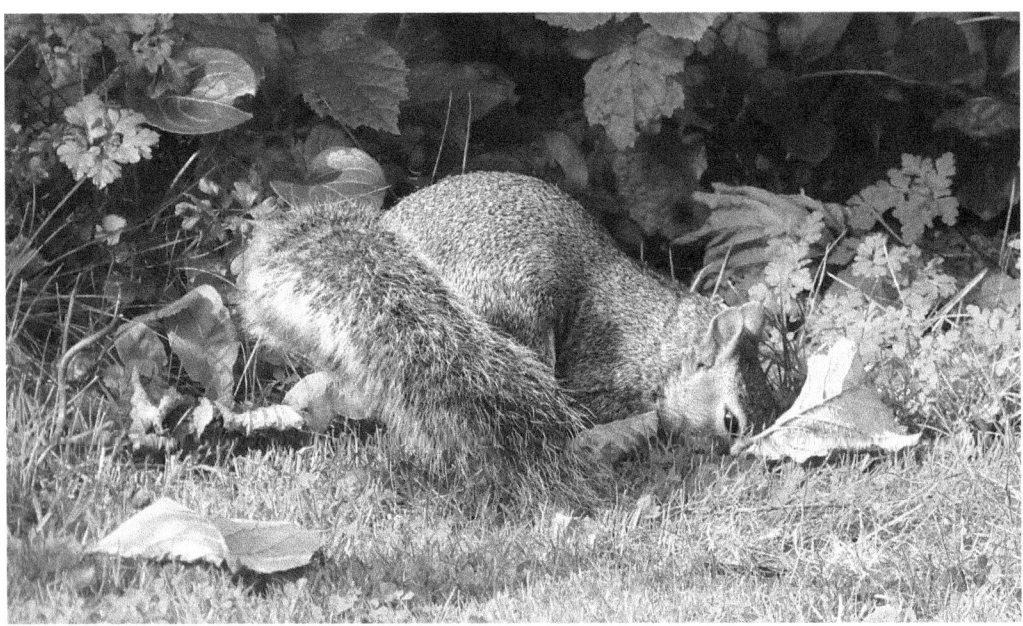

Sam squirrel hiding his hazelnuts.

Hazel nuts can be sown in February and should you require a tree without the help of squirrels, then it would be wise to store and then sow the nut under cover. In my garden the squirrels make an excellent job of propagation, unfortunately, often in the lawn. As a result I have named my house Hazel Impyard. (Impyard was the medieval name for a tree nursery). Alternatively, a sucker or branch may be laid down, pegged and left to grow roots to produce a new tree.

Over the years, in addition to enjoying eating hazelnuts in savoury and sweet dishes and as tasty snacks, I have appreciated hazelnut milk. This milk, fairly recent on supermarket shelves, has a history going back centuries. It is made in the same way as almond milk. During the spring 2020 lockdown due to Covid-19 flour became scarce and I was glad of my store of home grown hazelnuts. Mixing ground hazelnut with other flours adds enjoyable flavour to cakes and nut loaves. Having cracked twenty-six ounces of them in one session to raise funds for charity, I also made hazelnut milk and invented a tasty and nourishing drink using a concentrate of ground hazelnuts, honey and 100 percent chocolate.

At Butser Ancient Farm and other pre-Roman sites where I have taught hedgerow basketry, we have looked upon hazel as one of the important sources of stakes and handles for sturdy baskets, as part of sessions on herbs in Celtic life. The young rods bend willingly and hazel found great use in the past being coppiced to produce straight flexible rods. Perhaps the most fascinating and instructive find from pre-history was that of the body of a man released by a melting glacier in the Alps. Freezing had preserved not only his body from some 5,000 years ago, but also his backpack and quiver with arrows. Both containers had inner supports made of bent hazel rods.[3] In fact, hazel is so pliable that after soaking, a length can be bent and then tied in a loop sufficiently strong and tight to be used as a nutcracker.

I also have a stout forked hazel thumb stick provided ready–formed by the tree, the perfect height for me. This tall pole or stick has a wide natural fork at the top, which provides a comfortable place to grip and rest my hand as I walk along. It is just right for outings in search of elder and hawthorn during autumn harvesting. Hazel that has not been coppiced often grows with a forked top, something that led Tusser in his sixteenth century rhyming husbandry instructions to write that hazel should be saved for making forks.[4] Hazel walking sticks have been favourites over the centuries. A particularly popular form has been the twisted rod produced by ivy or honeysuckle winding around the shoot as it was growing. The plain bark with its white touches is attractive in its own right.

Since pre-history, the hazel has always been cultivated for the convenience of harvest. We have enjoyed a close relationship with hazel due to its many uses supplying everything from wattle fencing and wall supports, basketry materials and fishing rods, to besom broom handles, thatching spars, hop poles, barrel hoops, bird and animal cages, firewood, charcoal, and even a constituent in gunpowder.[5] The bark and leaves meanwhile offer sufficient tannins for tanning leather.

Legends and Folklore. The hazel has long been rich in folklore. It has been seen as a tree of knowledge by the Celts. The hazel has distinguished connections with the old gods of other cultures too. It has been linked to Hermes and the tree is ruled by Mercury. The hazel rod with two snakes entwined around it facing each other, was the caduceus symbol. This stood not only for power to heal, but also for divination.[6]

More recently the nuts have been carried against rheumatism. Twin nuts have been especially prized for their healing properties. In Scotland it was believed that a twin nut could protect you from witchcraft.[7] Hazel, bay, rowan, and elder are the four protective trees traditionally planted one in each corner of the garden against bad influences. It has always been the preferred wood for divining rods used to find water. Philips records that for this purpose the rod should be cut on St. John's Day (24th June) or Good Friday, to work best.[8]

Notes

1. Chiej R. *The Macdonald Encyclopedia of Medicinal Plants*. (Macdonald Publishing. London. 1984). 98.
2. Anon. *A Collection of Receipts*. (Printed for the Executrix of Mary Kettilby. 1746). 268.
3. Spindler K. *The Man in the Ice*. (Weidenfeld & Nicolson. 1994). 234.
4. Tusser T. *Five Hundred Points of Good Husbandry*. (Original 1573). (Oxford University Press. 1984). 98.

5. Warren P. *British Native Trees, past and present uses.* (Wildeye. 2006). 39/40.
6. Gifford J. *The Celtic Wisdom of Trees.* (Godsfield Press. 2000). 92.
7. Grigson G. *The Englishman's Flora.* (The Folio Society. 1987). 247/8.
8. Phillips R. *Wild Food.* (Pan Books. 1983). 138.

HAZEL – History of Medicinal Use

Hazel nuts and wood are well preserved by water-logged conditions, and so we have plentiful evidence for the presence and use of hazel from as long ago as 2,000 B.C. and earlier in Britain. The pollen has been found in greater abundance from the Neolithic period as men started to clear forest for farming.[1] Evidence of large areas of hazel being deliberately coppiced has been uncovered on hillsides in Somerset. The straight shoots were laid down together with other wood as a base for building early track-ways in the nearby Somerset Levels. Hazel wattle was also standard within house walls.[2] More uses are weaving animal traps and hazel handles of tools and weapons. A main harvest must have been for food, since hazel nuts provide good nutrition in winter and can even be ground into flour to make bread. Hazel could also have been grown to provide animal fodder for sheep and goats.

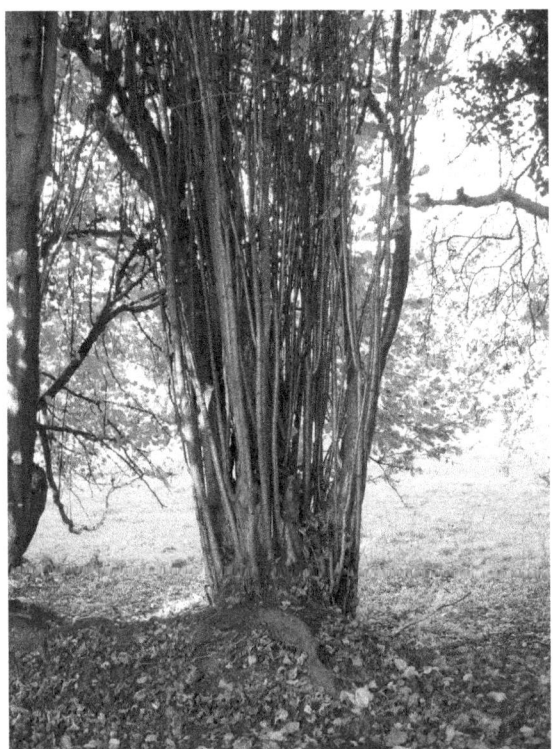
Coppiced Hazel.

In the first century, hazel has already entered medicine in Melicrate, a honeyed drink to cure a cough. Dioscorides also gives an interesting recipe consisting of burning whole hazelnuts and then pounding what remained with bears grease as a hair restorative.[3] Pliny wrote that eating hazelnuts caused headaches and flatulence and further, resulted in a surprising amount of weight gain.[4] No doubt this property would have recommended them to prehistoric man. They do in fact contain some protein as well as fat, and carbohydrates.

Hazel flour appears in the Anglo-Saxon Leechdoms and we find it included in three salves.[5] In the twelfth century, Hildegard is apparently as unimpressed with hazel in medicine, as the Romans. Condemning hazel as a symbol of lasciviousness, she includes the nuts in a recipe for a man whose semen is not potent.[6] Arguments for or against the hazel in medicine aside, the tree found a place in medieval orchards, by providing a welcome harvest for the kitchen. By the thirteenth century young hazels were being sold by garden nurseries.[7] In Gerard's herbal we find the first reference to hazelnut milk, used for the properties of the tannins in stopping bleeding and diarrhoea. These are problems he notes that may be caused by the nuts. He recommends the milk also for reducing fevers.[8] It would be interesting to see whether the hazelnut milk now readily available might have this effect.

Culpeper places hazel nuts under the dominion of mercury and takes a determined stand supporting them against the former accusations, reminding us that tradition can be "a friend to error". He enlightens us with "If any part of the Hazel Nut be stopping, it is the husks and shells, and no one is so mad as to eat them, unless physically; and the red skin which covers the kernel, you may easily pull off. And so thus I have made an apology for Nuts, which cannot speak for themselves" (p.89).[9]

A few years later, William Coles, often at odds with Culpeper, recommends the red skins to be taken in wine to lessen menstrual bleeding and adds that the shells can also be taken in red wine for the same result. He extends medicinal use to the catkins, and a decoction of the inner rind of the branches in small ale for the strangury. This is the frequent and unsuccessful urge to empty the bladder, due to a blockage or swelling. For those wishing to eat a large quantity of the nuts he recommends eating them with raisins to counteract their dryness—something snacking packs offer to us today.[10]

An Irish herbal of 1735 repeats an old idea of eating the nuts roasted with pepper for catarrh and to relieve runny eyes. Then John Ke'ogh adds a twist to the Roman alopecia recipe. In his version, the burnt nuts are mixed with hogs lard rather than bears grease and applied to cure a scald.[11]

The recipe for alopecia also appears to have inspired the first recipe given below. This is to make hair grow thick.[12]

Summary. Although medicinal applications for the common hazel are found in the Greek and Roman herbals and continued to be noted for over a thousand years, they were always accompanied by criticisms. These mainly related to digestive upset or weight problems caused by eating too many. Meanwhile, the medicinal uses seem to rely mostly on the presence of tannins, which can be found in many herbs. Evidently during the eighteenth century hazel recipes lost favour both in medicine and use for cosmetic purposes in encouraging hair growth. Even *The Toilet of Flora* with numerous such recipes, published in 1784, does not include hazel in the ingredients. By 1790 Meyrick and all herbals from there on omit the tree and the medicinal role passes into folklore. Mention of hazelnut milk reducing fevers is intriguing but not something modern herbal medicine has yet researched.

Recipes

Extracted from A Collection of Receipts. 1746. "*To make the* Hair *grow thick.* Take Rosemary, Maiden-hair, Southern-wood, Myrtle-Berries, Hazel-Bark, of each two Ounces; burn these to Ashes on a clean Hearth, or in an Oven; put these Ashes in White-wine, to make a strong Lye, and wash the Hair daily at the Root; keep it cut pretty short: It kills the Worm which is at the Root, and is more effectual than Bears Grease, or any Sort of Pomatum, which rather feeds than destroys that Enemy to the Hair" (p.268).[12]

Extracted from Culpeper The Complete Herbal and English Physician Enlarged. "*Oil of Hazel Nuts.* College. It is made of the Kernels, cleansed, bruised, and beat, and pressed like Oil of sweet Almonds. Culpeper.] You must put them in a vessel (viz. a glass, or some such thing) and stop them close that the water come not to them when you put them into the bath. The oil is good for cold afflictions of the nerves, the gout in the joints, &c" (p.353).[9]

Notes

1. Godwin Sir H. *History of the British Flora.* (Cambridge University Press. 2nd edition. 1975). 267, 269.
2. Rackham O. *The History of the Countryside.* (Phoenix Paperback. 1986). 73, 87.
3. Gunther R.T. (ed), *Dioscorides Greek Herbal.* (Hafner. 1968). 88. (179).

4. Jones W.H.S. (trans), *Pliny Natural History* VI Books XX–XXIII. (Loeb Classical Library. 1989). 517.
5. Pollington S. *Leechcraft*. (Anglo Saxon Books. 2000). 189, 195, *Lacnunga*. (15, 31, 33).
6. Throop P. (trans), *Hildegard von Bingen's Physica*. (Healing Arts Press. 1998). 114.
7. Harvey J. *Mediaeval Gardens*. (Batsford. 1981). 86.
8. Johnson T. (ed), *The Herbal*. John Gerard. (1633 edition). (Dover Publications, New York. 1975). 1440.
9. Culpeper N. *Culpeper's Complete Herbal and English Physician enlarged*. (1652). (London. 1815 edition). 89, 353.
10. Coles W. *The Paradise of Plants*. (London. 1657). 569.
11. Scott. M. (ed), *An Irish Herbal*. K'Eogh. (1735). (Aquarian. 1986). 79.
12. Anon. *The Toilet of Flora*. (London. 1784). 268.

CORYLUS AVELLANA – Herbalists' Reference

The Parts of Hazel Used for Medicine – The bark, catkins, leaves and fruit have all played a part in medicine as well as the fixed oil.

Dosage and Forms – Decoctions or infusions may be made from parts of the hazel tree. Nut oil and tincture may also be given or applied.

Constituents – As a nutritious food the nuts are rich in minerals, including iron and selenium. They also contain protein, carbohydrates, and fat. Further medicinal benefits come from the presence of tannins, resin, and flavonoids in other parts of the tree.

Actions and Uses – As we left the history section it seemed we had heard the last of hazel in medicine, but not so. In the late 1990s, paclitaxel

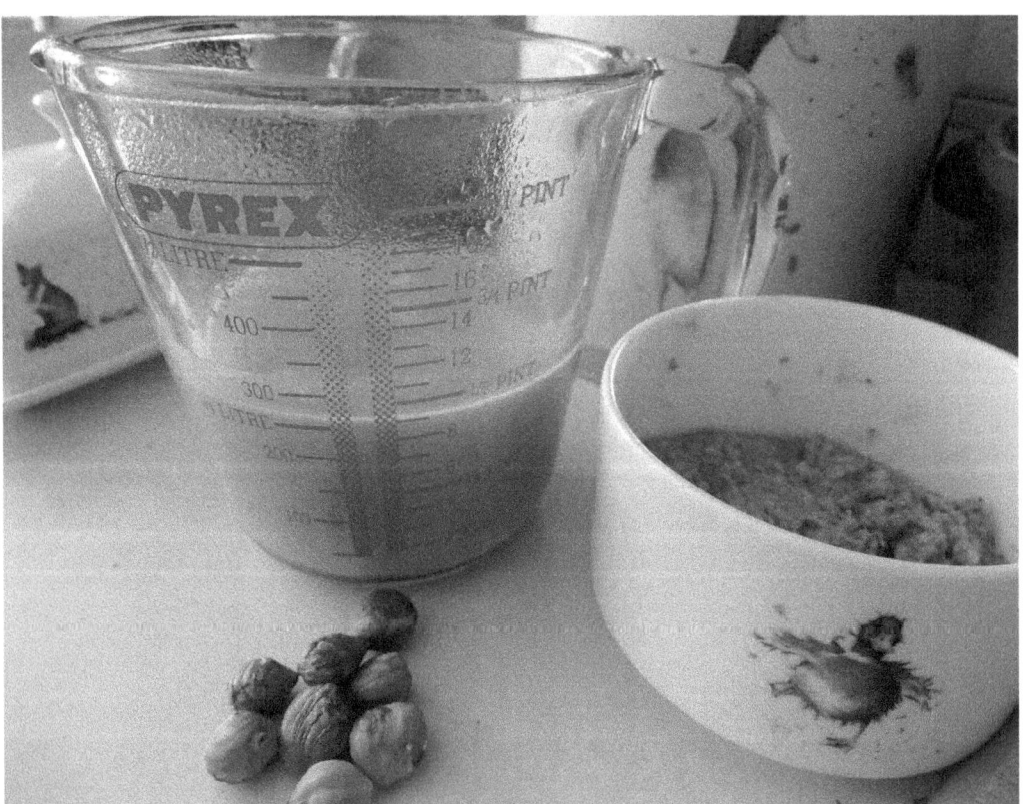

Hazelnut milk and spread.

and other similar substances were discovered in trees other than the yew. The nuts, branches, and shells of the hazel nuts were found to contain this chemotherapy substance. Chemists have since synthesised similar compounds to produce the drug Taxotere.[1] Knowledge of hazel in this role might be added to those medicinal properties appreciated in the past. These are largely from their astringent tannins, stopping bleeding, treating mouth conditions and diarrhoea. Reducing fevers with a diaphoretic effect and re-mineralising depleted patients have been other uses.

Oil from the nuts has been looked upon as a gentle and effective treatment for threadworm and pinworm in children.[2] The American witch hazel has overshadowed our native tree over the past hundred years. However, the astringent constituents, and minerals, have ensured the common hazel deserves a place amongst medicinal trees.

Precautions and Contraindications. **None found.**

Notes

1. Lewington A. *Plants for People.* (Eden Project Books. 2003). 230.
2. Chiej R. *The Macdonald Encyclopedia of Medicinal Plants.* (Macdonald Publishing London. 1984). (98).

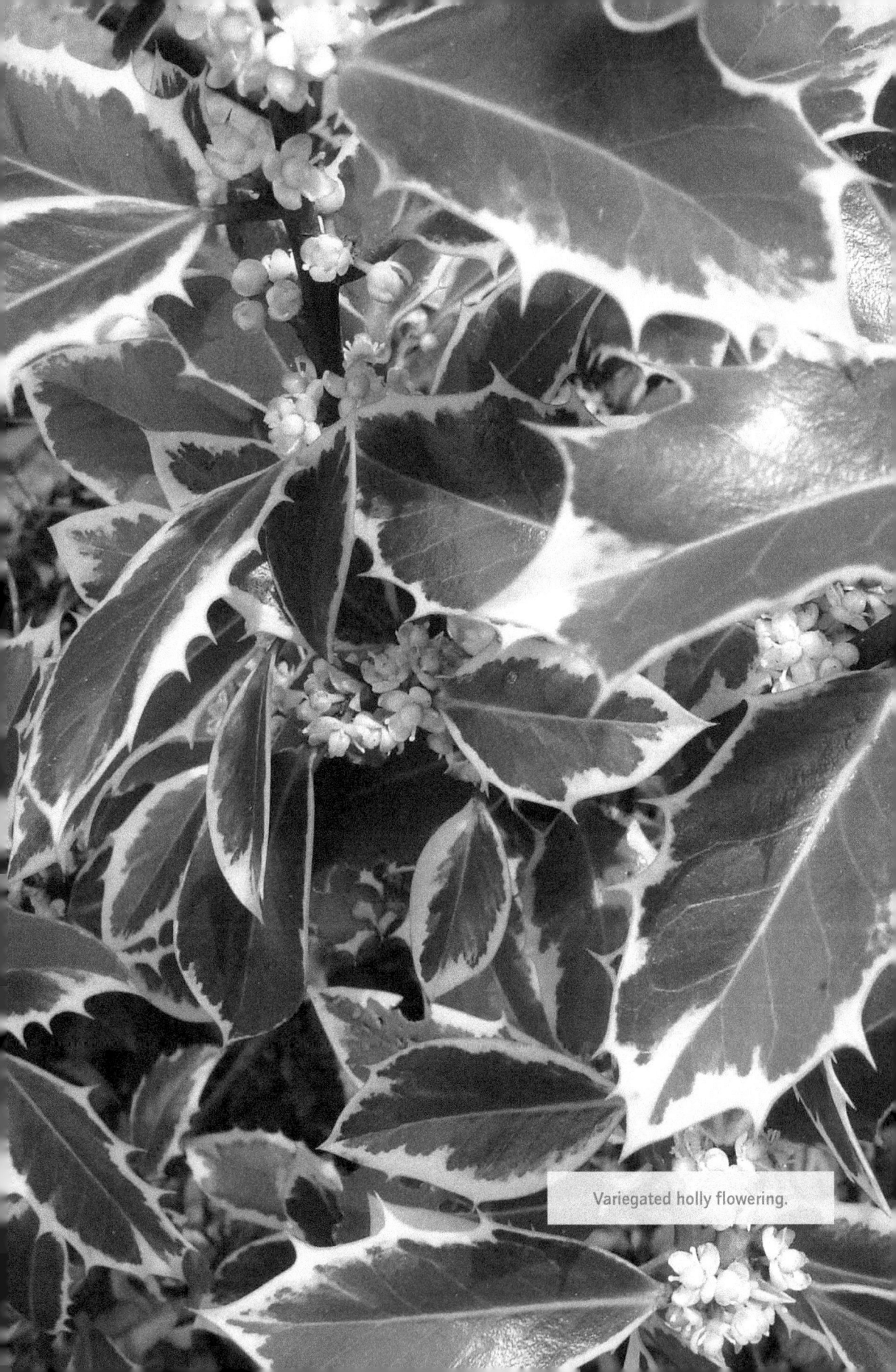
Variegated holly flowering.

Holly

Ilex aquifolium – Holly – Aquifoliaceae

HOLLY – *Usefulness* – As an ornamental evergreen, holly brightens the winter garden. The berried branches are a traditional Christmas decoration. The berries provide food for garden birds and the flowers attract the aptly named holly blue butterfly as the buds are food for the larvae.

Dangers – Sharp prickles on the leaves mean gloves are required when pruning. Berries are toxic when eaten in large quantity.[1]

Getting to Know the Holly Tree – The flowers are white and quite small, often passing unnoticed. The first time I became aware of their beauty was in the New Forest. Holly is an under-storey tree in woodland and this was a small copse of beech with holly growing in the shade. It was a sunny day in May when I caught a waft of the most beautiful perfume. On my search to find the source, their scent led me to look closely in the axils of the dark leaves. There were clusters of small white waxy flowers, each with four petals. The male and female flowers are borne on different trees, although sometimes they can be bisexual, and it is the male flowers which are fragrant. I was enchanted and now eagerly watch for the flowers opening in my garden each year. I had noticed the holly blue butterflies near the holly before and was reminded that their first brood of larvae feed on the flower buds. Of course it is not only butterflies that are attracted to holly flowers, the bees love them also and work to carry pollen from the male flowers to the female.

In the garden and countryside, holly is more than just a decorative evergreen. It is a valuable tree in supporting wildlife. The fleshy scarlet berries each containing three to five seeds are loved by the birds. It can be hard to keep a berried branch or two on the bushes in my garden through the colder days of November, as they are very popular with the resident blackbirds. In my former garden, a thrush guarded them. Berries that are not eaten seem quite often to germinate in the second year beside the tree or wherever a bird drops them. Tiny holly trees growing naturally in the garden have always been welcomed.

Whether the natural or variegated holly is planted it will be slow to grow, and in my experience when planted out takes a year to establish itself before any sort of a growth spurt. There are few really tall trees in gardens due to the popularity of gardeners' preference for encouraging holly to form a dense evergreen hedge. Once established this will be less work than most to keep trim. A height of around six metres (twenty feet) seems the limit of general experience but holly can grow to be fifteen metres (fifty feet).[2] I remember reading that one was noted in the seventeenth century to have grown in an orchard to such a size that the owner had coffins made from the wood for both himself and his wife. An aside to this story was that they were both corpulent, which required a good width to the planks. Many years ago a friend turned a bud vase for me in the creamy coloured dense wood, which has also been a favourite material with woodcarvers.

Evergreens bearing berries were brought in at the darkest time of the year even before Christians adopted holly as a Christmas decoration. The glint of firelight on the glossy, leathery leaves and bright red berries adds welcome colour and contrast to the scene. It seems extraordinary when you think of how prickly holly leaves are, but the foliage has been encouraged from early times as fodder for animals. Holly has been pollarded to serve this purpose for sheep on the Stiperstones in Shropshire close to a frequent walk of ours when my family lived nearby. Deer also enjoy holly and in the New Forest the height that the wild ponies can reach for grazing is evident. Smaller animals, such as rabbits, also benefit from nibbling on holly wood, which acts as a tonic.[3]

Holly berries are generally thought of as being poisonous and eaten in sufficient quantity they are. However, quite a large number are required before serious symptoms are produced. In smaller doses they act as a purgative producing vomiting and diarrhoea.[1] Culpeper puts holly under the influence of Saturn and as he remarks elsewhere "Saturn loves his bones" (p.99). Unlike those in Maté tea, which comes from South American holly, the leaves from trees growing in Europe do not contain caffeine but only traces of theobromine.[1] Both substances are found in varying amounts in coffee, tea, and chocolate. Their leaves also contain saponins.

A product once made from holly in quantity was birdlime. This was made in early times by burying holly bark in a moist hole in the ground, covering it with tree branches and then a layer of earth. It was left there to rot for approaching two weeks before pounding the now thick and sticky remains with a little nut oil. Paste from the soaked inner bark has been laid over the broken limbs of animals and hardened as a plaster cast.[4] The main use for it was to trap small birds. It would be spread on the branches of trees so that as the bird landed the gluey nature of the birdlime would hold it fast. Birdlime has also previously been exported to the East Indies, this time for catching destructive insects.[5]

Legends and Folklore. The tree itself has been referred to as representing the male in contrast to the female nature of the ivy in the woodlands. Returning to thoughts of Christmas, holly has gathered a mass of superstition around when it is to be put up, when taken down, and even how you dispose of it afterwards. It was traditional to put the berried greenery up on Adam and Eve's day, known to us now as Christmas Eve. In centuries past, doing so earlier could have meant you were celebrating the Roman Saturnalia, which runs from the seventeenth of December for the next seven days.

In large halls great interlocking hoops would be decorated with sprays of holly and hung above the feast. I have seen how wonderfully effective this is when at the Weald and Downland Living Museum at Christmas. If gathering your own holly you will notice that some leaves are far less spiny at the edges and these came to be known as "she" holly as opposed to the pricklier "he" holly. There is a belief that whichever you choose for your decorations will decide whether he or she rules the house for the coming year.

Both kinds of leaves can be found on the same tree and it has been suggested that changes in climate as the leaves are formed may account for it. "She" holly leaves were understandably chosen for the love spells to have the initials of possible future husbands pricked into them and be placed under the pillow to give a dream of the right one.[6] Sewing nine leaves onto her nightdress in another method with the same aim, the young girl would see the man of her heart in a vision—sleep was hardly likely! Nowadays we take down decorations by the sixth of January, long ago in some areas the holly ring stayed up until Candlemas Eve, which is February the first.

Notes

1. Fröhne D. Pfander H. *A Colour Atlas of Poisonous Plants.* (Wolf Science. 1983). 50.
2. Sterry P. *Collins Complete Guide to British Trees.* (Harper Collins. 2007). 278.
3. Grieve. M. *A Modern Herbal.* (1st published 1934 Jonathan Cape. Saavas. 1984). 406.
4. De Bairacli-Levy J. *The Complete Herbal Handbook for Farm and Stable.* (Faber and Faber, London. 1991). 85.
5. Freethy R. *From Agar to Zenry.* (Crowood Press. 1985). 75.
6. Grigson G. *The Englishman's Flora.* (The Folio Society. 1987). 115.

HOLLY – History of Medicinal Use

Holly wood and charcoal have been the commonest finds from archaeological sites from the Iron Age onwards.[1] Small poles of holly and other woods were used in building the raised Sweet Track across the marsh near Shapwick 4,000 years ago.[2] The first mention of holly in medicine comes from the Anglo-Saxon period with holly bark heated in goat's milk to treat asthma.[3] In the medieval period, holly was referred to as holm and the spiny leaves with their accompanying red berries were already symbolic of the Christian crown of thorns. The wood was valued for carving. Since nowadays two holly berries are recorded as likely to produce vomiting,[4] the dose of ten or twelve of them to treat colic in the seventeenth century makes one concerned for the patient.

Culpeper also values ripe berries for treating the colic and dried berries as a powder were given to stop diarrhoea. Holly root bark and leaves meanwhile were applied as hot fomentations to fractures and dislocations.[5] Coles regards the berries as having both a heating and drying action within the body. He ventures that the hardness of the seed shows by the doctrine of signatures that it is good for urinary stones. For this the berries were boiled in ale. The prickly edges of the leaves were also seen as significant and powdered leaves with their prickles removed were given for "stitch" (p.386)[6] or pricking pains in the side. There seems to be no similar explanation for gathering the sap, which oozed out of the wood when it was burning on the fire and using this for ear-drops to restore hearing to the deaf.[6]

After first mentioning the berries, Pechey comes up with what sounds to be a safer treatment for colic by boiling the prickles of the leaves in a posset, in his 1694 herbal. This was a comforting drink containing wine and milk. He writes a gentlewoman cured herself with this when nothing else

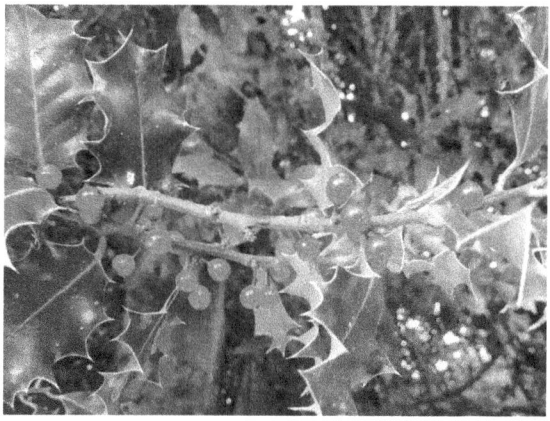

Berries on Ilex aquifolium.

worked.[7] A century later the young surgeon Meyrick records a person known for his success in treating rheumatism would boil young holly buds or leaves in water and sweetened this with sugar. In both of these last remedies, the spines and leaf would have been strained out before the drink was administered to the patient snug in bed to make them sleepy. It seems large amounts with plenty of fluids were given until there was relief from pain. This appears to be the first mention of such a prescription[8] and it is repeated by Mrs. Grieve.

Just when it seemed doses of the heating, purgative berries were becoming less, we see in Brook's herbal the number of them has been raised to fifteen to twenty. He also brings a treatise written by Dr. Rousseau on the value of holly leaves in treating fevers to our notice. He describes the effects as superior to Jesuits bark (cinchona). It appears Dr. Rousseau extracted a bitter principle, ilicine, from the leaves, which he viewed as the active ingredient.[9] Mrs Grieves unfortunately does not give her sources for the use of holly tea for removing catarrh or the leaf juice to treat jaundice. These appear to be new ideas.[10] In the twentieth century Juliette de Bairacli-Levy, who collected much folk herbal knowledge, recommends a paste from the soaked inner bark to be laid over the broken limbs of animals so that it hardens as a plaster cast to aid healing.[11] This was a use which may have survived from Culpeper.

Summary. Although holly has appeared in medicine over several centuries, it has generally been other properties of the tree that have attracted the most attention. Namely the characteristics of the wood for turning and the production of birdlime from holly bark. Most treatments seem to have related either to the purgative properties of the berries, or ideas that have originated in the doctrine of signatures. This is illustrated by using the prickles cut from the leaves and prepared for a cure for pricking pain. Also by the practice of giving the berries to treat urinary stones, which had been suggested from the hardness of the seed. Holly is rarely included in herbal medicine in Britain but has been more regarded in France. See Herbalists' Reference.

Recipes

Extracted from Leechcraft. The Lacnunga Manuscript. "121. Against asthma: boil holly-bark in goat's milk and sip it warm, having fasted" p.225.[3]

Extracted from A Manual of Materia Medica and Pharmacy. 1829. "*wine of holly* prepared by infusing, during twelve hours, one drachm of pulverized leaves of holly, in a tumbler of white wine." To be given two or three hours before the paroxysm in intermittent fevers. Attributed to Dr. L. Rousseau p.148.[12]

Notes

1. Godwin Sir H. *History of the British Flora.* (Cambridge University Press. 2nd edition. 1975). 172.
2. Rackham O. *The History of the Countryside.* (Phoenix Paperback. 1986). 73.
3. Pollington S. *Leechcraft.* (Anglo Saxon Books. 2000). 225. *Lacnunga* (121).
4. Fröhne D. Pfander H. *A Colour Atlas of Poisonous Plants.* (Wolf Science. 1983). 50.
5. Culpeper N. *Culpeper's Complete Herbal and English Physician enlarged.* (1652). (London. 1815 edition). 99.
6. Coles W. *The Paradise of Plants.* (London. 1657). 385.
7. Pechey J. *The English Herbal of Physical Plants.* (London. 1694). 103.
8. Meyrick R. *The New Family Herbal.* (Birmingham. 1790). 228.
9. Brook R. *Brook's Family Herbal.* (J.A. Brook, Richardson & Co. London. Revised edition. 1876). 39.
10. Grieve. M. *A Modern Herbal.* (1st published 1934 Jonathan Cape. Saavas. 1984). 407.
11. De Bairacli-Levy J. *The Complete Herbal Handbook for Farm and Stable.* (Faber and Faber, London. 1991). 85.
12. Togno J. Durand E. (trans) *A Manual of Materia Medica and Pharmacy.* (Philadelphia. 1829). 148.

ILEX AQUIFOLIUM – Herbalists' Reference

The Parts of the Holly Tree Used for Medicine – Fresh or dried leaves can be used throughout the year. Holly leaves remain on the tree for a long time and so it is preferable to search out young leaves. Bark should be harvested from branches in spring before the sap thickens. Berries have been used but their emetic and purgative action is no longer likely to be appreciated.

Dosage and Forms – An infusion, decoction, powder or tincture. 30g (1oz) dried leaves should be brought to the boil in 1 litre (2 pints) water and simmered for 10 minutes. The berries may act as an emetic even in small doses.

Constituents – Unlike *Ilex paraguariensis*, which provides Maté tea, the leaves of European holly contain only traces of theobromine. Saponin is also present in the leaves as well as tannin and ilicin. Small amounts of triterpene compounds have been isolated from the berries with apparent digitalis-like action.[1]

Actions and Uses – Tannins in the leaves have an astringent effect. This has been used in treatments for diarrhoea. The berries on the other hand act as a purgative. Use of the leaves is recorded for treating rheumatism and as a febrifuge and anti-tussive in bronchitis and influenza.[2]

Contraindications and Precautions – It really is wisest not to use the berries. Among sixty four calls to the Zurich Poison Centre between 1973–9 slight symptoms were noted in only nine of the reports.[1] The current web poison control site offers a report of an infant eating perhaps 2 berries, again the only symptom was loose stools.[3] However, serious symptoms of poisoning are supported on eating a larger quantity.[1]

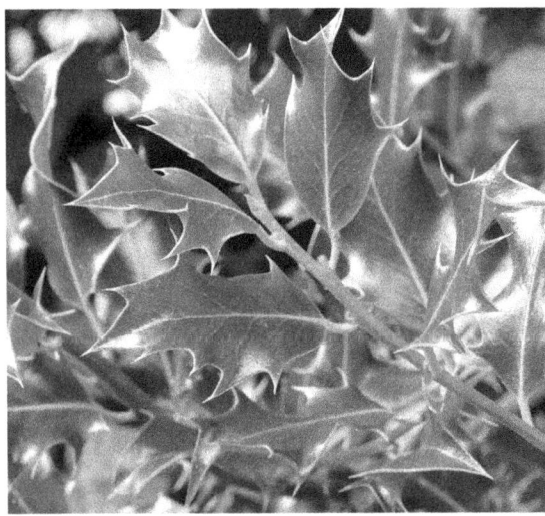

Holly leaves.

Notes

1. Fröhne D. Pfander H. *A Colour Atlas of Poisonous Plants.* (Wolf Science. 1983). (Guse, P: Zur Mikroskopie gesundheits-schädlicher Früchte verschiedener botanischer Artzugehöorigkeit, Dissertation, Hamburg, 1977). 50.
2. Barker J. *The Medicinal Flora of Britain and Northwestern Europe.* (Winter Press. 2001). (178).
3. https://www.webpoisoncontrol.org/articles/2014-dec/holly-berries? Accessed 15/2/2019.

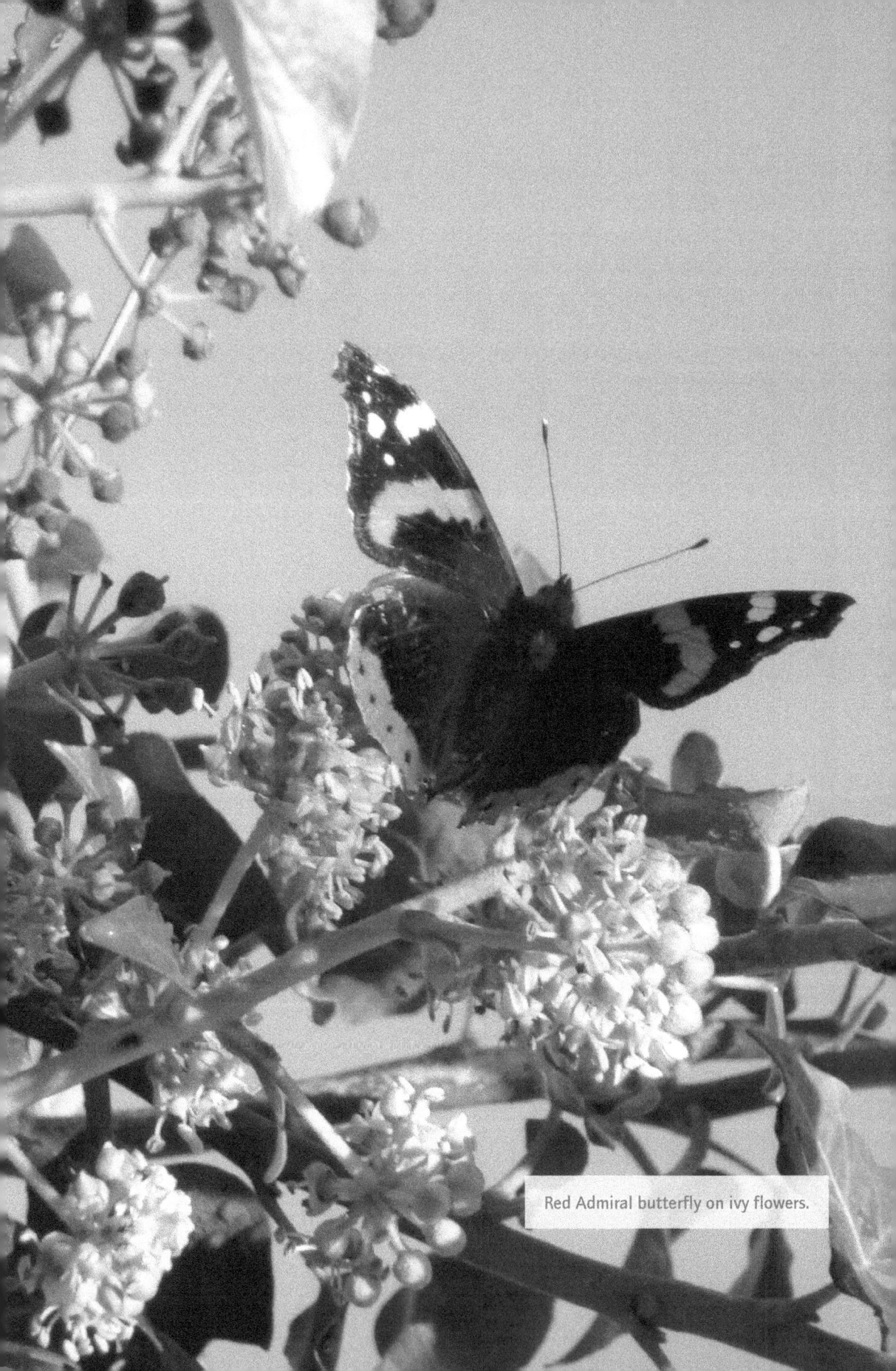

Red Admiral butterfly on ivy flowers.

Ivy

Hedera Helix – IVY – Araliaceae

IVY – Usefulness – Ivy flowers attract and feed insects including many butterflies, wasps, and bees. The berries feed birds. Leaves provide a tonic feed for sheep, goats, cows, and horses.[1] Ivy leaves are also medicinally valued for coughs, treating skin conditions etc. Creeping stems can be used for basketry, wreaths, and ties. Thick trunks of ivy wood are perfect for turning. Leaves and berries give dyes, and ivy leaves have been recommended for dry cleaning some fabrics.

Dangers – If left unchecked ivy will eventually smother trees, sometimes ring barking them with damaging climbing suckers. It is, however, not a parasite and does not feed on tree sap. The saponins in the berries and especially the seeds are toxic. Historical accounts of fatalities should, however, be viewed with scepticism. Ivy can cause contact dermatitis in sensitive people. Repeated contact may cause reactions up to forty-eight hours later.[2]

Getting to know Ivy – Ivy is the only member of the tropical *Araliaceae* family to grow as a naturalised plant in Britain. Over thousands of years it has proved itself surprisingly adaptable to climate change as evidence of its presence has been found from at least two interglacial periods. It qualifies then as a semi-native, yet formerly tropical, plant. It may be suggested that this is why it flowers so late in our year. To most people ivy is not a tree but a pest that damages trees, walls, and fences. Due to the understandable attitude towards this climber, it is rarely left for the possible lifespan of 500 years. Climbing a tree it may reach as high as thirty metres (100 feet), growing at about forty-eight centimetres (eighteen inches) a year; it may live to produce a trunk that can be thirty centimetres (twelve inches) in diameter, occasionally larger.[3] The supporting tree is unlikely to outlive it.

Thick ivy trunks can be seen ascending trees and then dividing, only for the narrower branches to cross and weave again further up. Occasionally, thick stems can also be found hanging loose from the supporting tree. In shade the plant remains a mass of dark green, hairless, shiny leaves on spreading stems. The leaves vary in shape according to their situation and manner of growth. Unlike other plants as ivy grows it turns away from the light to find a crevice in rocks or wall, or a shady tree and support. After twelve years or so when it has climbed out of the shade the stem turns back towards the light and flowers appear.

The tiny yellow-green flowers sit like round balls on stalks in open umbels and form in late autumn, so that they may still be visited by insects in November or even December. Many wasps visit them. I am not concerned at their presence when I am gathering as they do not sting. I love to watch the butterflies still out on warm autumn days alighting on the nectar-rich flowers. The painted lady, tortoiseshell, in some areas, delicate holly blue and, if you are lucky, red admirals may be seen on ivy flowers. Sometimes I have counted as many as ten butterflies on a single plant.

A long hedge clothed in ivy not far from my present home is a joy to see, as it offers many flowers at slightly different stages of development over an extended period. Ivy will be more likely to flourish in younger woodland, rather than the really ancient. On reaching a tree, in order to climb it, the stem puts out sucker feet at regular intervals and clings tenaciously with the aid

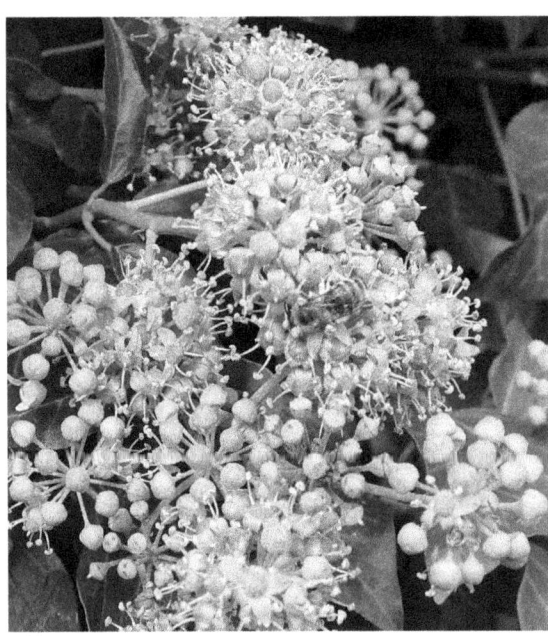

Bee on ivy flowers.

of a sticky substance. It is damage caused by this penetration of the bark that is dangerous to the host. Additionally, in time, the foliage spreads at the top of the tree and smothers it. The berries, first green and then darkening to black, ripen during December to February depending on weather and their situation. The round berries with the remainder of the calyx showing on the top of the ovary, black when ripe, are looked upon as poisonous and would certainly be no fun to eat.

I have used ivy in hedgerow basketry classes and for making swags and wreath bases for Christmas workshops for many years. There is something very satisfying in December dragging the best lengths across the garden to plait them as a rich-looking swag for the base to carry colourful ornaments and bags of spices. In our old cottage, these looked wonderful hung along the dark beams. I have also picked the berries and leaves for dyeing days using wool and silk.

During historical workshops, we have explored the value of the leaves in the Victorian period for renewing black on silk, as tiny white dots were apt to appear with natural blacks. A decoction from the leaves was also used in the past to take the greasy shine from suit lapels and cuffs and school gymslips.

Medicinal use has entered my historical workshops from the "do not do this at home" category when talking about ivy juice in anaesthetics during Medieval workshops. When it comes to ointments and applications for sunburn and skin problems, this is much safer territory and these and other uses appear in various historical periods.

One of my favourite turned items is a cup of ivy wood. Years ago I was giving a talk on folklore and telling the audience about the tradition of giving children their milk from a cup of turned ivy wood in order to cure whooping cough. I said I had never seen an ivy cup and would like to. A gentleman stood up and said he knew of some really thick ivy and offered to make one for me. A year later he brought me an elegant light-coloured goblet, which I have treasured ever since. The traditional use of the cup is interesting, considering ivy extracts are used today in herbal medicine to liquefy bronchial phlegm in whooping cough.[4]

Ivy then is a welcome "weed" in parts of my garden, offering harvests and bringing a range of autumn insects, including many butterflies and bees. Later, hungry birds arrive in the coldest months of winter; pigeons, in particular, just love to feast on the berries. A friend who farms sheep also looks upon ivy as helpful for the health of ewes after lambing. She therefore wants them to have access to feed on it as a cleanser at that time.

Legends and Folklore. In ancient Egypt, ivy was sacred to the god Osiris, while in Greece and Rome it was dedicated to the god Bacchus, also known as Dionysius, god of wine. Just as Moses was reputed to have been found as a baby in the bulrushes, legend has it that the young Bacchus was found amongst ivy. As a reminder, the sceptre he carried was wreathed with ivy. From this connection early taverns were often known by a bunch of ivy hanging on a pole outside and we still see public houses known as the Ivy House.

It was also believed in earlier centuries that ivy cups could absorb alcohol from liquor so that you could drink as much as you liked without becoming drunk. Culpeper dates this belief back to Cato. The leaves in wine similar to that drunk the night before, (presumably not from an ivy cup), were recommended by Culpeper as a cure for "the morning after feeling").[5] Another "do not try this at home" recipe.

Notes

1. De Bairacli-Levy J. *The Complete Herbal Handbook for Farm and Stable.* (Faber and Faber, London. 1991). 92.
2. Blumenthal et al. *Herbal Medicine. Expanded Commission E monographs.* (Integrative Medicine Commission. 2000). 216.
3. Freethy R. *From Agar to Zenry.* (Crowood Press. 1985). 76.
4. Bartram T. *Bartram's Encyclopedia of Herbal Medicine.* (Robinson. 1998). 255.
5. Culpeper N. *Culpeper's Complete Herbal and English Physician enlarged.* (1652). (London. 1815 edition). 100.

IVY – History of Medicinal Use

Although ivy is part of a tropical family and not a native plant of the British Isles, evidence has been found of the herb growing here in two interglacial periods.[1] It seems probable then that Neolithic man was familiar with ivy leaves as an acceptable fodder. Sheep and goats will eat it eagerly after giving birth. We can only reflect on possible Celtic use of ivy in medicine, but Roman medicine contains plentiful evidence. Pliny lists twenty kinds of ivy, crediting them all with medicinal uses. Celsus lists ivy with other cooling herbs, such as laurel and quince. In a recipe for treating ulcerations, he uses the black ivy in particular.

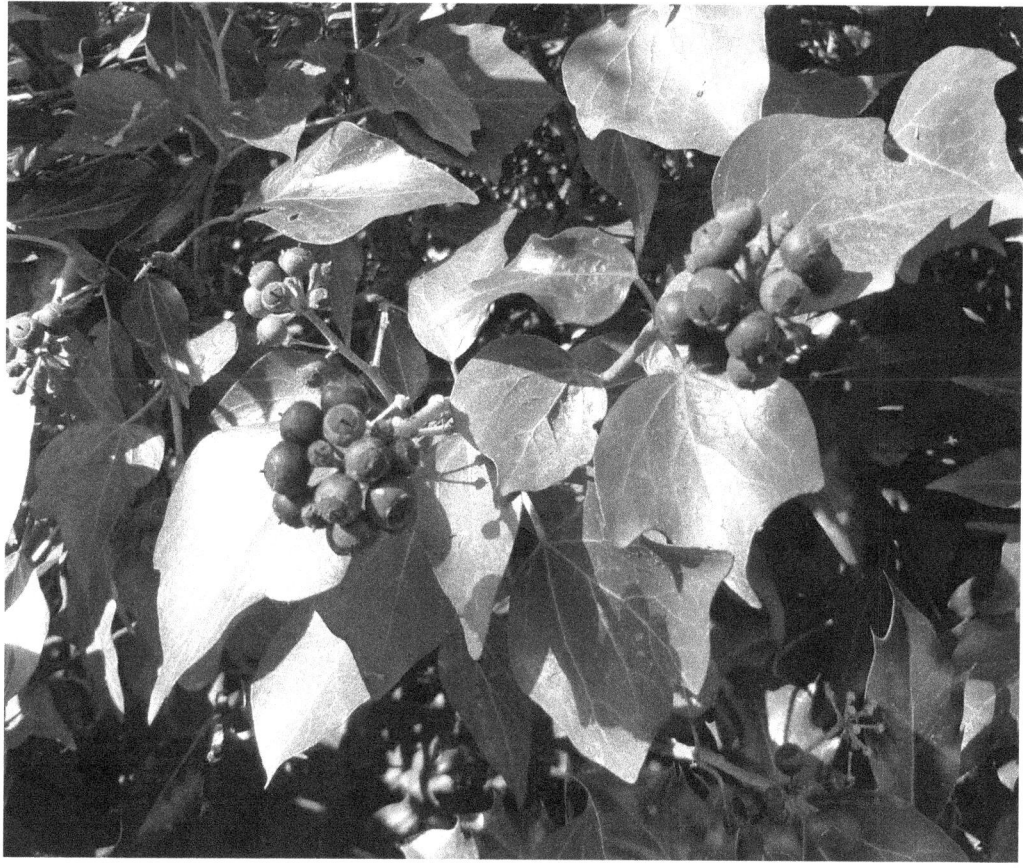

Ivy berries early in January.

To remove a decayed tooth, an ivy berry with the tegument removed is packed into the cavity. Apparently this will result in the tooth splitting and falling out.[2]

In the Anglo-Saxon period, the Leechbooks refer to the anti-inflammatory actions of ivy. In the Anglo-Saxon *Lacnunga* and the *Leechbook of Bald*, ivy growing on a stone is used with other herbs for general inflammation. In the *Olde English Herbarium* there is a recipe for the golden berried ivy seeds in wine to treat a urinary disorder.[3] Hildegard of Bingen recommends the cold quality of ivy for slowing unwanted menstrual bleeding.[4]

The medieval period offers one of the most interesting uses of ivy in the soporific sponge. This recipe was the first to prescribe an inhaled anaesthetic in order to give a deep sleep to enable pain-free surgery. A number of anaesthetic blends appear from different sources and in these, at first sight—witches brews; the recipe may include an alarming mix of ivy juice with opium and other powerful herbs such as henbane, hemlock, or mandrake. Where the reduced decoction was absorbed into a sponge it would then be dried. The efficacy returned with later soaking in hot water, after which it would be applied to the patient's nostrils until they lost consciousness. No modern pharmacist or herbalist would dare to prescribe such a mixture but skilled surgeons evidently made it for patients, some of whom survived. In a Leechbook of 1443 we find Roman influence evident in a gentler dental application, treatment for gout, and inclusion in a plaster to treat sores.[5]

Ivy as an external soother is a use that continues. In the sixteenth and seventeenth centuries, Books of Secrets became popular with well-to-do ladies responsible for healthcare of their households, and in the case of the charitable, their tenants as well. In one of these, translated from the original Italian, drinking powdered berries in wine was used to make the patient sweat to be rid of infectious fevers.[6] Do not try this at home! Also in the seventeenth century, James Primerose published his Latin treatise on women's diseases. In this he picks up another thread of knowledge from Roman and Greek medicine in recording the action of powdered English ivy in a drink to cause sterility.[7] We find ivy in different countries used both for contraception and abortion.

Culpeper confirms the cold nature of ivy, putting it under the dominion of Saturn. Coles, a contemporary and great critic of Culpeper, states that the coldness of ivy is removed by drying the herb, leaving the heat which is also in its nature, to wreak damage. It is then, he writes "it causeth berrenness in Man or Woman, if they should take too often thereof, and procureth a weakness and trouble in the Brain and Senses" (p.56).[8]

After writing of various cures he brings us to another interesting facet of ivy, this time concerning the wood. The idea was that drinking from a cup made of the wood had healing properties. He recommends it for problems with the spleen. He also quotes the Roman writer Cato who wrote of the antipathy between water and wine, which meant that if wine were placed in a porous ivy cup the wine would pass through, leaving only water. This was followed by a drink from ivy leaves in the same wine as the cure for a hangover, presumably for those without an ivy cup.[8]

In the eighteenth century, the Ivy Tree appears in herbals with the familiar uses of cooling inflammations, burns, and ulcers and purging the head. K'Eogh, from Ireland, adds a new treatment of taking a decoction of the flowers to stop dysentery.[9] Caustic ivy gum is often mentioned as in earlier times, for clearing the face of freckles and unwanted marks, but this is not obtained from English ivy. In Flora's Toilette (1784), a cosmetic compendium of recipes, we find reference to this and a recipe for hair dye described as darkening the colour by simple means, when it is actually really elaborate. Ivy berries are among some twenty ingredients.[10]

One hundred years later, Brooks' Herbal records little use of the leaves and berries, although it lists a decoction of the leaves to destroy lice and nits and heal the soreness they cause. He regards the purging effects of the berries as beneficial, writing "they are an excellent remedy in rheumatisms and pains of all kinds." (p.66).[11] Meanwhile Green's encyclopaedic work of 1824 states that the common people apply ivy leaves to their corns, and the berries to infective "issues" (p.657) to increase the discharge.[12]

Summary. Several uses of the herb are consistent throughout the 2,000 year period. The strongly cooling nature of the herb saw it ranked alongside other herbs that are potentially toxic, through slowing or cooling body processes, as in the Soporific Sponge. Such cooling herbs may be valued as ivy has been, against feverish conditions and phlegm, and ivy has seen these uses from the beginning. As an anti-inflammatory herb, ivy is used for applications to the skin treating burns and ulcers and from the earliest time onwards for various forms of rheumatic pain, especially gout. Use as either a contraceptive or abortive herb has been widespread. Today ivy still has a well-deserved and researched place in herbal medicine—see Herbalists' Reference.

Recipe

Extracted from The Receipt Book of Lady Anne Blencowe. 1694. "For ye stone. Take unsett Leeks, parsley roots, Bettany & Ivy Berrys. Braiz them all together, & temper them with white wine, & drink it first & last & it will break ye stone. In proof, lay a flint stone in ye medicine & it will break in 24 hours" (p.124).[13]

The parsley will be parsley piert (*Aphanes arvensis*), also known as parsley break-stone. The test makes the internal effects of the medicine sound quite alarming.

Notes

1. Godwin Sir H. *History of the British Flora.* (Cambridge University Press. 2nd edition. 1975). 219.
2. Spencer W.G. (trans), *Celsus De Medicina* 1 Books 1–1V. (Loeb Classical Library. 1971). 213.
   Spencer W.G. (trans), *Celsus De Medicina* 1 Books V–V1. (Loeb Classical Library. 1989). 139, 251.
3. Pollington S. *Leechcraft.* (Anglo Saxon Books. 2000). 213. *Lacnunga* (76). 391. *Bald* (30). 343. *Old English Herbarium.* 121.
4. Throop P. (trans), *Hildegard von Dingen's Physica.* (Healing Arts Press. 1998). 71.
5. Dawson W. (ed), *A Leechbook of the XVth Century.* (Macmillan & Co. 1934). 25, (31), 213, (674), 315. (1036)].
6. Warde W. & Anglosse R. (trans), *The Secretes of Maister Alexis of Piemont.* (Atenar. 2000). 64.

7. Riddle J.M. *Eve's Herbs*. (Harvard University Press. 1997). 151.
8. Coles W. *The Paradise of Plants*. (London. 1657). 56.
9. Scott. M. (ed), *An Irish Herbal*. K'Eogh. (1735). (Aquarian. 1986). 87.
10. Anon. *The Toilet of Flora*. (London. 1784). 11, 82.
11. Brook R. *Brook's Family Herbal*. (J.A. Brook, Richardson & Co. Revised edition. London. 1876). 66.
12. Green T. *Universal Herbal or Botanical Dictionary*. 2 vols. (Caxton, 2nd edition. London. 1824). Vol. 1. 657.
13. Stapley C. (ed), *The Receipt Book of Lady Anne Blencowe*. (Heartsease Books. 2004). 124.

HEDERA HELIX – Herbalists' Reference

The Part of Ivy Used for Medicine – Only the leaves of ivy are used in modern herbal medicine. These are best freshly gathered in late summer, August and September, before flowering.

Dosage – 0.3g per day of cut herb. Tincture 1:5. 1.5ml three times daily. Extracts in drug products with a daily dose equal to 0.3g of crude drug.

Constituents – The leaves contain about 5–8% of saponins, flavonoids, anti-oxidants, and falcarinol.

Actions and Uses – There are numerous studies on actions of the constituents of ivy herb, as well as some double-blind placebo controlled studies. This is an area to watch for a greater understanding of wider treatments. Commission E approved the use of ivy in treating both acute and chronic inflammation in the respiratory tract.[1] Helping to liquefy bronchial phlegm and acting as a stimulating expectorant have made ivy a popular herb for these conditions. However the level of chronic toxicity needs to be borne in mind when prescribing.[2]

The saponins have astringent properties, which are vasoconstrictive while the flavonoids improve the circulation. Having vasoprotective properties from inhibition of elastase and hyaluronidase means the herb has potential for treating venous insufficiency. Anthelmintic and molluscicidal activities have been reported.[3] The saponins are

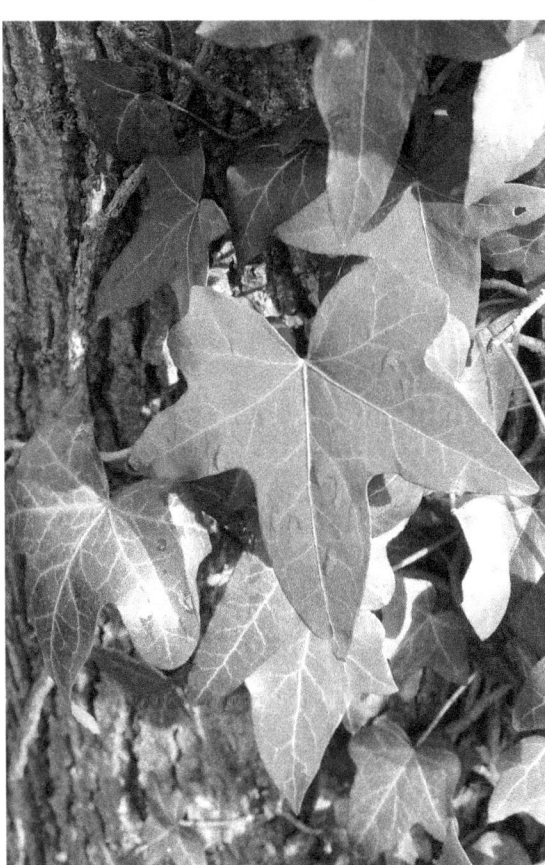

Ivy foliage.

only fully extracted by 60% alcohol. Ivy is recommended for treating cellulitis.

Topical Preparations – Suitable applications of poultices, compresses, or ointments of the herb may be applied to cellulitis, neuralgia, calluses, corns, warts, or impetigo. The pain-relieving and antimycotic properties will be useful in these situations so long as the patient has shown no sensitivity to contact with the herb. An infusion may be used as a scalp application.

Precautions and Contraindications – A test on a small area of undamaged skin is advisable before adding the infusion or leaves to hot baths, or applying poultices, compresses etc. Repeated use may cause contact dermatitis due to the falcarinol. This may appear up to 48 hours after contact with the ivy. Allow this amount of time to elapse before the test is seen as negative.

Notes

1. Blumenthal et al. *Herbal Medicine. Expanded Commission E monographs.* (Integrative Medicine Commission. 2000). 216.
2. Holmes P. *The Energetics of Western Herbs.* Vol. 1&2. (Snow Press. Boulder. Revised 3rd edition. 1989). Vol. 2. 514.
3. Burlando B. et al. *Herbal principles in Cosmetics.* (CRC Press. 2010). 146.

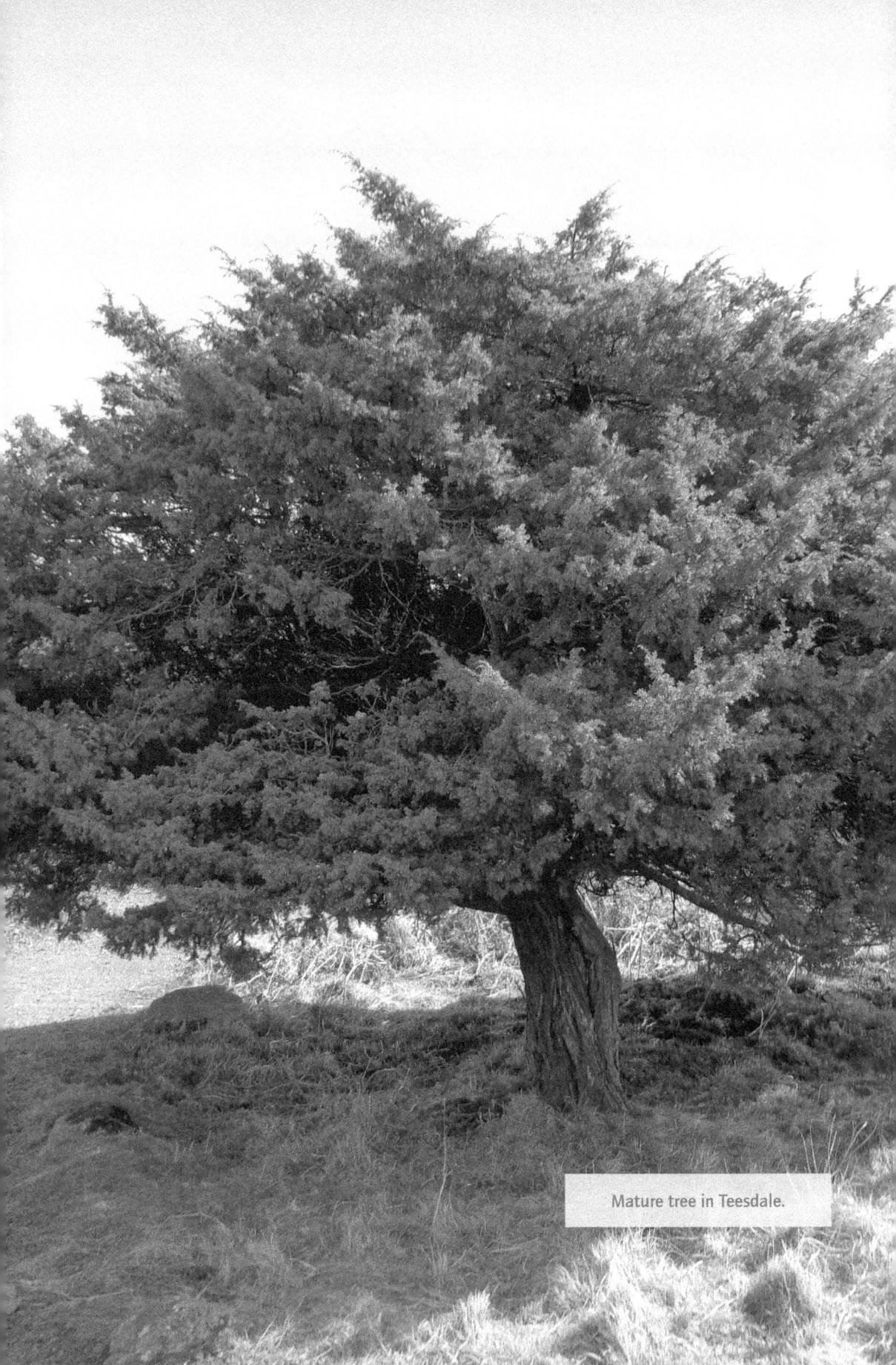
Mature tree in Teesdale.

Juniper

Juniperus communis – Juniper – Cupressaceae

JUNIPER – Usefulness – In cookery juniper berries are an antibacterial and flavoursome seasoning. The wood is used to smoke meats. The berries are an essential ingredient in gin and are also added to spiced wines and ales. All parts of the tree have been used in medicines. Juniper is a diuretic, which is considered to be specific for treating rheumatic diseases. Juniper oil is an ingredient in perfumes, scented beads, and fumigants. In the garden it provides safe nesting for birds.

Dangers – The leaves rubbed the wrong way are extremely sharp. There is a possibility of allergic reactions from contact with the oil. Juniper is not to be taken medicinally in pregnancy as the berries can cause abortion. In large doses or with prolonged usage juniper may cause kidney damage.[1]

Getting to Know the Juniper Tree – Juniper grows in a temperate climate in Europe, Asia, and America. It is an evergreen tree that I had always associated with bleak, inaccessible places, perhaps because for years I had lived close to an ancient juniper forest in Teesdale above the stunning High Force waterfall. This is a wild, magical area I have always loved.

After our move south I decided to grow juniper in my teaching herb garden. To start from berries did not feel like an option. They need to be newly ripe so that their three seeds still retain supporting resinous sap in a tiny bladder within the berry, and I would be waiting perhaps two years for them to appear above ground. Since both sexes are required for a harvest of berries, I planted a male and female in neighbouring beds in the area dedicated to herbs for wines and liqueurs. This was in Hampshire, in an area of chalky, flint scattered soil in the valley bottom. Birch and willow, wild companions of juniper, also thrived in the garden. Juniper has been the pioneer of future woodland in the past, protecting birch and willow until as they form a wood around it, the juniper dies away. The role of juniper as a prickly protector was certainly appreciated by the nesting birds in my garden. Trimmings can also be laid on newly-dug beds to keep cats away.

I expected my trees to grow to about two metres (six feet), unlike the height of some in Sweden and Norway where they can grow as tall as ten to eleven metres (thirty to thirty-six feet) and live for hundreds of years.[2] As time passed, I came to know my two junipers well. Although I planted them only a few feet apart, the form of their slow growth was very different. The male took on a bowed appearance, as if hunched beneath a weight, while the female towered above him with spreading shoulders and an air of elegance. It was tempting to think that she dominated him.

In 1997, the year I planted them, Oliver Rackham's *History of the Countryside* was published. He gave the figure of 80,000 junipers then left in lowland England, half of them in Wiltshire. As their numbers continue to diminish it is hard to imagine the huge quantities of berries exported from Scotland to Holland to make gin in the nineteenth century. The present popularity of gin, however, is seeing some harvesting of Wiltshire berries by local small distilleries.

The flowers resemble tiny catkins in the axils of the leaves and are easily overlooked. Even with the trees just outside my door I completely missed the miniature flowers in May at the stage of pollen release. Whilst on holiday in Scotland where many junipers were growing wild, this was much more obvious, as shown in the photograph. A breath of wind or the slightest touch sent clouds of pollen flying into the air. The presence of identifiable stems, fruits, seeds, and even galls caused by a gnat specific to juniper, from before the last Ice Age, has enabled archaeologists to confirm juniper as an indigenous tree.[3]

I was not expecting a huge harvest, nor was I planning to make gin. I was interested at the time in another use. This was laying sprays of juniper in the bottom of a wine or ale bin to catch and preserve settling yeast from the fermentation. The coated juniper was to be hung dried for use as a new starter in the next batch. This experiment would be useful research for my Celtic workshops. The trees were also often seen over the years hung with drying wool, silk, or paper that I had dyed, hung there so that I did not have to worry about staining the washing line.

I also wanted the berries for cookery, and when sufficiently matured, medicine as well. A couple of years after planting the young trees, I watched eagerly as berries were formed by three whorls of fleshy bracts growing together to become each fruit. These remained a full year, green on the tree. It takes another one or two years for them to mature, turning purple and finally black. The mixture of green and fully ripe berries as years pass makes picking even more exacting. I soon found the harvesting was too delicate an operation to wear the thick gloves you might wish to put between your skin and the prickles. Stroked downwards, the branches are relatively forgiving but push your fingers up to take hold of the berries and you soon experience the sharp nature of the leaf spikes. There must be an easier way.

One winter we had a sudden fall of very heavy snow and icy temperatures following. This taught me to appreciate the amazing resilience of juniper—no doubt the reason for its survival for hundreds of years in such cold environments as within the Arctic Circle. I walked out of the cottage the next morning to see everything shrouded in snow. The female juniper, then about six feet

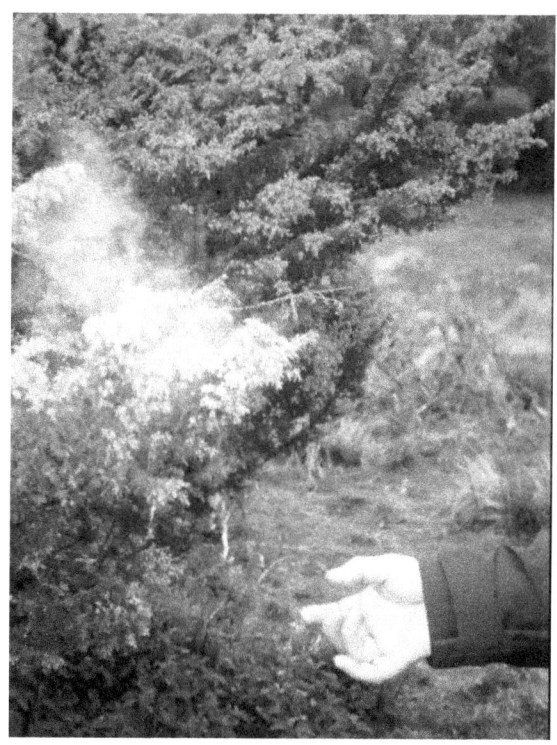

Juniper pollen release in Scotland.

tall, had been uprooted by the weight and lay with the roots iced over in the bitter air. I did not think any tree could survive such an experience but swept the snow from the tree, removed the ice as best I could and wrapped the bare roots in sacking. It was several days before the ground was thawed sufficiently to re-plant the tree. I did this with care, staking it while it re-established itself. My juniper not only survived but continued to thrive, producing berries still.

The main danger to survival of junipers has been fire, and burning of heaths has been responsible for some decline in numbers. In the ancient juniper forest in Teesdale and in other countries, a new danger threatens. The disease is called *Phytophthora austrocedrae*. It is spread on footwear and by animals. Antibacterial footbaths were mandatory on entering and departing the Teesdale forest when last I visited. It is hoped the disease can be controlled.

Legends and Folklore. In Scotland the juniper, sometimes known as the mountain yew, was believed to be protective against evil spirits. Juniper wood was sufficiently trusted to be carved into teething rings for protection. At Hallowe'en branches were burned at the threshold of the barn.[4] In Wales, juniper was looked upon as a tree to be respected.[5] On the Continent also, the aromatic branches were burned at Yule to purify the air and were hung in stables. Juniper burns with little smoke but a sweet scent. In Germany, juniper branches were used for cremations to give aromatic purification and protection against demons.[6]

Notes

1. Blumenthal et al. *Herbal Medicine. Expanded Commission E monographs.* (Integrative Medicine Commission. 2000). 218.
2. Flückiger & Hanbury. *A History of Drugs.* (Macmillan & Co. 2nd edition. 1879). 625.
3. Godwin Sir H. *History of the British Flora.* (Cambridge University Press. 2nd edition. 1975). 111.
4. Darwin T. *The Scots Herbal.* (Mercat Press. 1996). 62.
5. Vickery R. *Oxford Dictionary of Plant-Lore.* (Oxford University Press. 1997). 207.
6. DeCleene M. & Lejeune M.C. *Compendium of Symbolic and Ritual Plants in Europe.* (Man and Culture Publishers, Ghent. Belgium. 2003). 365.

JUNIPER – History of Medicinal Use

Although growing only in the temperate regions of Europe, Asia, and America, juniper berries were imported for use in ancient Egyptian medicine. The Ebers Papyrus recipes use juniper for treating urinary problems, tapeworm, to give aid in giving birth and offer cooling pain relief.[1] Juniper was associated with the process of mummification and the berries were an ingredient in the Egyptian perfume Kyphi, made with wine, raisins, aromatic herbs and resins.[2] Herbals in what was once known as the dark ages, the *Macer Floridus*, *Vitex Agnus Castus* and the Anglo-Saxon Leechbooks, concentrate on the more powerful

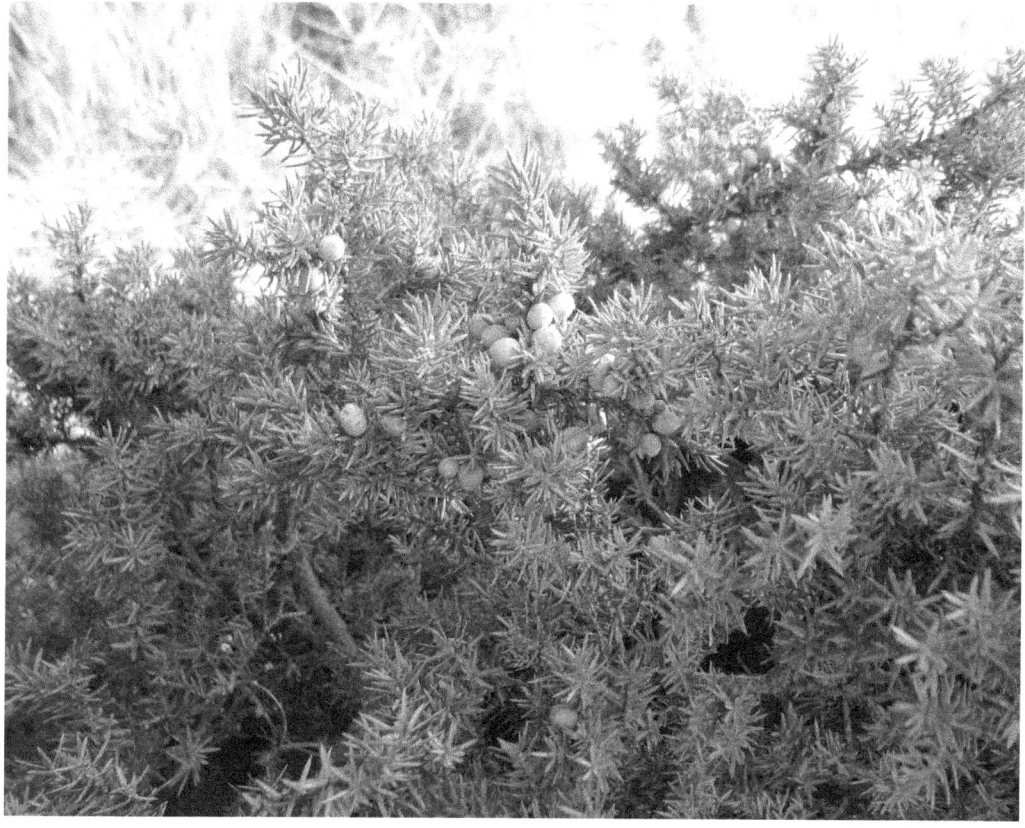

Berries of various ages.

Juniperus sabina. Hildegard appears to refer to *J. communis* when she gives a recipe for spiced wine containing the berries for chest, lungs, or liver. She also suggests a sauna using juniper.[3]

In the recipes of Maister Alexis published in England in 1558, juniper berries have a place in sweet balls.[4] Having made this recipe, I feel with quite a heavy content of resins in addition to fragrant herb flowers that they hardly need their final coating of a little musk to maintain a delightful perfume. Predictably, since juniper burns with a sweet scent but little smoke, and is seen as a long-lived and protective tree, it has been burned as a fumigant in times of plague. Plague recipes often contain multiple highly antibacterial herbs.

Juniper was still being used to purify the air in sickrooms of those with fevers and infections in the nineteenth century.[5] I have been told that burning juniper berries on hot coals took place in Swiss schoolhouses to disinfect the air. Since the herb has been shown to be active against numerous bacteria including *Staphylococcus aureus, Streptococcus spp., Escherichia coli,* and *Salmonella spp* it could be presumed this may have been effective.[6]

Culpeper declares the berries to be hot in the third degree and dry in the first, supporting Pliny and Gerard in recommending juniper as a counter-poison, and adding that the berries strengthen the brain and memory and are taken for convulsions among other symptoms. He gives our first dose of ten to twelve ripe berries taken in the morning fasting. Use of the ashes has widened from removing scurf on the scalp to treating many skin conditions and is suggested in the form of a lye in baths for scabs and leprosy.[7]

In 1657 William Coles writes about using the "Chimicall Oyle" (p.388),[8] four to five drops in broth or beer, or eating twelve berries a day. He also tells us the berries strengthen the brain and memory, the optic nerves, other senses and heart. While recommending the powdered gum in wine as an anti emetic, he explains the gum only occurs in hotter countries. Coles gives a wonderful picture of either fumigating the head and nightcap with juniper smoke to treat catarrh, or taking the fumes through a funnel into the mouth to cure toothache.[8]

By 1694 Pechey confirms the oil of juniper is commonly used against tooth-ache in drop doses in "a proper Vehicle". He tells us succinctly that "The Berries are good for a cold Stomach, and are good against

Wind and Gripes: They provoke Urine, and expel Poyson, and are good in Diseases of the head and Nerves"(p.110).[9]

Around this same year Anne, Lady Blencowe, copied a number of recipes given to her by friends and family into her stillroom book. Five contain juniper berries. Her cousins' recipe for treating dropsy with small ale in which juniper berries, the ashes of burnt juniper and broom, elder, a sprig of wormwood and raisins have been steeped, gives us evidence of powerful recipes in home use.[10]

Similar recipes appear elsewhere. Smith also includes a frightening dose of thirty to thirty-five drops of the oil in a glass of sack to bring away the afterbirth.[11] Ensuring the afterbirth is expelled, remains a post-delivery necessity of concern to every midwife. Juniper berries had long been known to be dangerous when taken in pregnancy and in ancient Egypt were included in a vaginal suppository to induce childbirth.[2] Juniper berries appear in Dioscorides herbal in the first century as a contraceptive when applied to the genitals before intercourse. Do not try this at home![12]

In a lesser dose they appear with other herbs in pills to ease the birth of a living foetus, while reducing labour pains. This recipe, together with others, appears in *The Byrth of Mankynde,* or *Woman's Boke* which was first published in 1540 and remained popular for over a century.[13] Use for stimulating the uterus appears again in Victorian times with adverts clearly marketing juniper as a cure for lack of a menstrual period. The advert asks pointedly, "Late? Worried? Take Juno Juniper Pills" (p.207).[14]

In 1751 Hill gives a different warning, "In all Cases where Inflammation is to be fear'd, either in the *Primae viae* or in the Kidneys, the Use of Juniper Berries is to be avoided"(p.487).[15] He comments that only the essential oil is sold in the Apothecary Shops, the Juniper Water having been discontinued due to the vulgar finding it a pleasant dram. In consequence it is now made by the distiller as *Geneva.*[15] In 1790 Woodville notes that the fresh berries yield, on expression, a rich sweet honey-like aromatic juice. "the decoction, inspissated to the consistence of a rob or extract, has a pleasant, balsamic, sweet taste, with a greater or less degree of bitterness."(p.260).[16] In 1810 Thornton prefers berries from Italy[17] and in 1879 sources are given as the south of France, Austria and Italy, the latter producing the largest supplies.[18]

In the nineteenth century juniper was valued for treating chronic catarrhs of the bladder and urethra, atonic affections of the digestive system, loss of periods for other reasons than pregnancy, and some skin diseases. It had been noted that a strong decoction cleared scabies from the hands. Also, where juniper was not sufficiently powerful alone it could be given alongside foxglove and squill.[19] In the twentieth century, we find juniper's diuretic properties continue to be extolled as an adjunct to other medicines for rheumatism, sciatica, and lumbago. This was alongside earlier recommendations, including for mucus discharges from the bladder.[20]

Summary. For well over 2,000 years, juniper has been associated with treatments involving water retention and the urinary organs. As understanding of the human physiology has grown, the importance of the cleansing role of juniper has extended this use to cover skin diseases and rheumatic conditions, both of which require diuresis.

The strongly antibacterial qualities of juniper when taken or used as a fumigant have found numerous applications over the centuries and are upheld by modern research. Just as consistently the berries have been known for their abortive and contraceptive applications, as well as aiding the birth process. That juniper can irritate the kidneys and is not suitable in some conditions has been understood for almost 300 years. See Herbalists' Reference for modern uses in herbal medicine.

Recipes

Extracted from A Book of Simples. 1700–1750. "13. *For the Giddiness in the Head.* TAKE an ounce of comming (cumin) Seed and Steep it in white wine all night as much wine as will cover it and then you must dry it in an oven after the bread is drawn and dry with it an ounce of Juniper berrys & a handfull of rue then you must beat all these together to a fine powder and when you use it take as much of the powder as will lay on a Sixpence in a Spoonfull of honey well mixed together or in a Spoonfull of Sugar and take it dry" (p.6).[21]

Extracted from Bates Dispensatory. 1794. "Juniper-berry Comfits. Bate. [*They are made by sprinkling choice Juniper-berries ibj. with Mallaga Sack; then strewing over them trebble refined Sugar in fine Pouder ʒiv through a Sieve, and drying them with a gentle heat* ... Salmon.] They remove Stoppages in the Reins, Ureters and Bladder, provoke Urine, and are good against Sand, Gravel and Stone ... this I know, they expel Wind admirably and are a powerful Anticolick." (p.801).[22]

Notes

1. Nunn J.F. *Ancient Egyptian Medicine.* (British Museum Press. 2000). 72, 160, 195.
2. Manniche L. *An Ancient Egyptian Herbal.* (British Museum Press. 1989). 57. 112.
3. Throop P. (trans), *Hildegard von Bingen's Physica.* (Healing Arts Press. 1998). 128.
4. Warde W. & Anglosse R. (trans), *The Secretes of Maister Alexis of Piemont.* (Atenar. 2000). 104.
5. Waller J. *Waller's New British Domestic Herbal.* Cox & Son. (London. 1822). 212.
6. Buhner S.H. *Herbal Antibiotics.* (Storey Books. 1999). 50.
7. Culpeper N. *Culpeper's Complete Herbal and English Physician enlarged.* (1652). (London. 1815 edition). 100/101.
8. Coles W. *The Paradise of Plants.* (London. 1657). 387.
9. Pechey J. *The English Herbal of Physical Plants.* (London. 1694). 110/111.
10. Stapley C. (ed), *The Receipt Book of Lady Anne Blencowe.* (Heartsease Books. 2004). 117.
11. Smith E. *The Compleat Housewife.* (London. 1739). 291.
12. Gunther R.T. (ed), *Dioscorides Greek Herbal.* (Hafner. 1968). 57.
13. Hobby E. (ed), *The Birth of Mankind.* (1560). (Ashgate. 2009). 121.
14. Vickery R. *Oxford Dictionary of Plant-Lore.* (Oxford University Press. 1997). 207.
15. Hill J. M.D. *A History of the Materia Medica.* (London. 1751). 487.
16. Woodville W. *Medical Botany.* 3 vols + Supplement. (London. 1790). Vol. 2. 260.
17. Thornton R.J. *A New Family Herbal.* (London. 1810). 845/6.
18. Flückiger & Hanbury. *A History of Drugs.* (Macmillan & Co. 2nd edition. 1879). 626.
19. Thomson A.T. M.D. F.L.S. *The London Dispensatory.* (London. 4th edition. 1826). 378.

20. Scurrah J.W. F.N.A.M.H. *The National Botanic Pharmacopoeia.* (Bradford. 1905). 51.
21. Lewer H.W. (ed), *A Book of Simples.* [1700–1750]. (Sampson Low, Marston & Co. Ltd. 1908). 6.
22. Salmon W. *Comment on Bates Dispensatory.* (1794). 801.

JUNIPERUS COMMUNIS – Herbalists' Reference

The Parts of Juniper Used for Medicine – The ripe, bluish purple fruit, which will by then have been on the tree for 2–3 years, and the needle-like leaves, which can be gathered at any time. The roots, heartwood of the tree, and the bark also contain active constituents and may be used externally for treating skin infections.[1] If the berries are examined carefully the large oleoresin glands in the hard testa of each seed are evident.

Dosage and Forms – Tea: ½–1 teaspoon of crushed berries to each cup of boiling water, infuse 30 mins. ½–1 cup three times daily. Or use as inhalation or wash. Tincture of the berries 1:5 45% alcohol 1–2ml three times daily. 1:1 2–3ml three times daily.

Constituents – The volatile oil from the berries contains some sixty constituents. They include terpene hydrocarbons, such as pinene, thujone, and limonene. Also, caryophyllene and 4-terpinol. Resin-and-wax-containing compounds. Oil obtained from the leaves is similar. Juniper berries also contain sugars, tannins minerals, flavonoids, and vitamins B and C.

Actions and Uses – Juniper has "a powerful personality" and is not to be used lightly. Flushing through the system, it aids in removing toxins which cause joint and muscle pain— uric and lactic acid. The prickliness

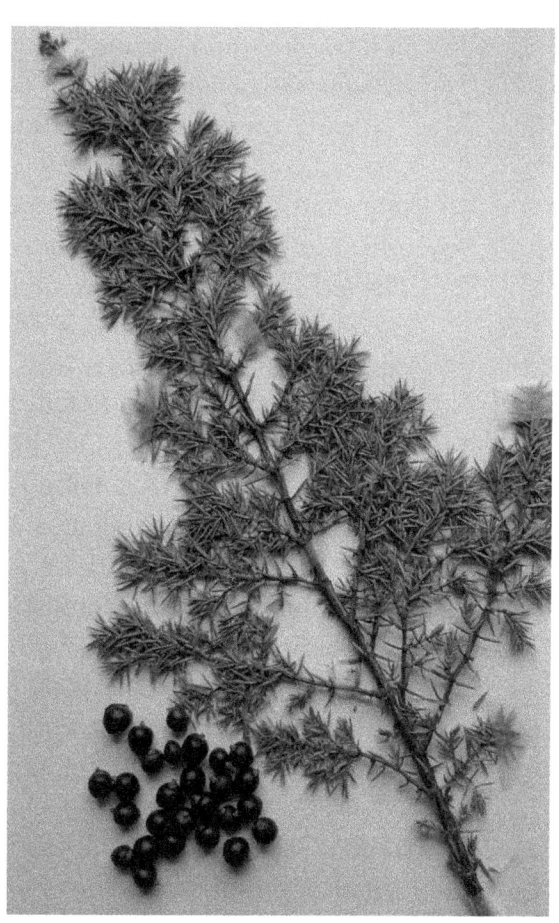

Juniper Herbarium specimen.

of the leaves warns of the way the terpinen-4-ol acts in the body, irritating the kidneys into working harder. Tradition supports juniper as an aid in dissolving gravel and stones in the urinary system. Thomas Bartram recommended a combination of juniper with wild carrot and *Hydrangea arborescens* in this situation. Unlike many diuretics the herb produces an aquaretic effect, which is to say there is greater loss of fluid without a corresponding increase in loss of electrolytes. Meanwhile an increased glomerular filtration rate has been recorded.[2]

In the bloodstream, juniper acts as an arterial stimulant believed to aid in reducing the build-up of cholesterol on the artery walls. Aiding circulation further supports the role of juniper for treating rheumatic pain, particularly gout. This combined with diuresis is not only useful in water retention, cystitis, and urinary gravel but also helpful in detoxifying to the benefit of skin health in eczema and psoriasis.

Clearly these properties will be well suited to treating a patient who tends to have a cold, slow constitution where stagnation leads to infections.[3] Juniper oil is powerful against many bacterial, microbial, and fungal infections, *Pseudomonas, Streptococcus spp., Escherichia coli*, and *Candida albicans*. When the herb is taken internally the essential oil is excreted in the urine and is able to act against the antibiotic-resistant bacteria that cause urinary tract infections. In vitro studies have shown strong activity against antibiotic-resistant bacteria, especially *Staphylococcus aureus*.[1]

Juniper also contains tannins, which reduce catarrh and other discharges. Although acting as a diuretic, juniper relieves incontinence, since it tones the urinary organs, enabling them to work more efficiently. In addition to stimulating the circulation generally, the herb promotes digestion, acting both as a carminative herb, relieving flatulence and heartburn, and increasing appetite. This makes it a good supportive aid for the older person if their circulation within the digestive system may be impaired. Juniper has been given in painful labour.

Topical Applications – 3–6 drops of essential oil in 2 teaspoons of almond oil or other base for application. The oil can be added to boiling water for an inhalation.

Precautions and Contraindications. Due to the irritant nature of the herb within the urinary system it is best administered alongside demulcents, such as Althea or *Zea mays*. It should not be given internally without a break for more than 6 weeks.[3] It is contraindicated in chronic renal insufficiency.[4] Needles of juniper contain high levels of isocupressic fatty acid, which exhibits pronounced abortifacient activity by causing decreased uterine blood flow.[5] Clearly it must not be taken during pregnancy.

Notes

1. Buhner S.H. *Herbal Antibiotics.* (Storey Books. 1999). 51.
2. Kelly W.J. (ed. director). *Nursing Herbal Medicine Handbook.* (Springhouse Corporation. 2001). 247.
3. Holmes P. *The Energetics of Western Herbs.* Vol. 1&2. (Snow Press. Boulder. Revised 3rd edition. 1989). Vol. 1. 352/3. 229.
4. Weiss R.F. M.D. *Herbal Medicine.* (Thieme. 2nd edition revised and expanded. 2000). 229.
5. Mills S. & Bone K. *The Essential Guide to Herbal Safety.* (Elsevier Churchill Livingstone. 2005). 100.

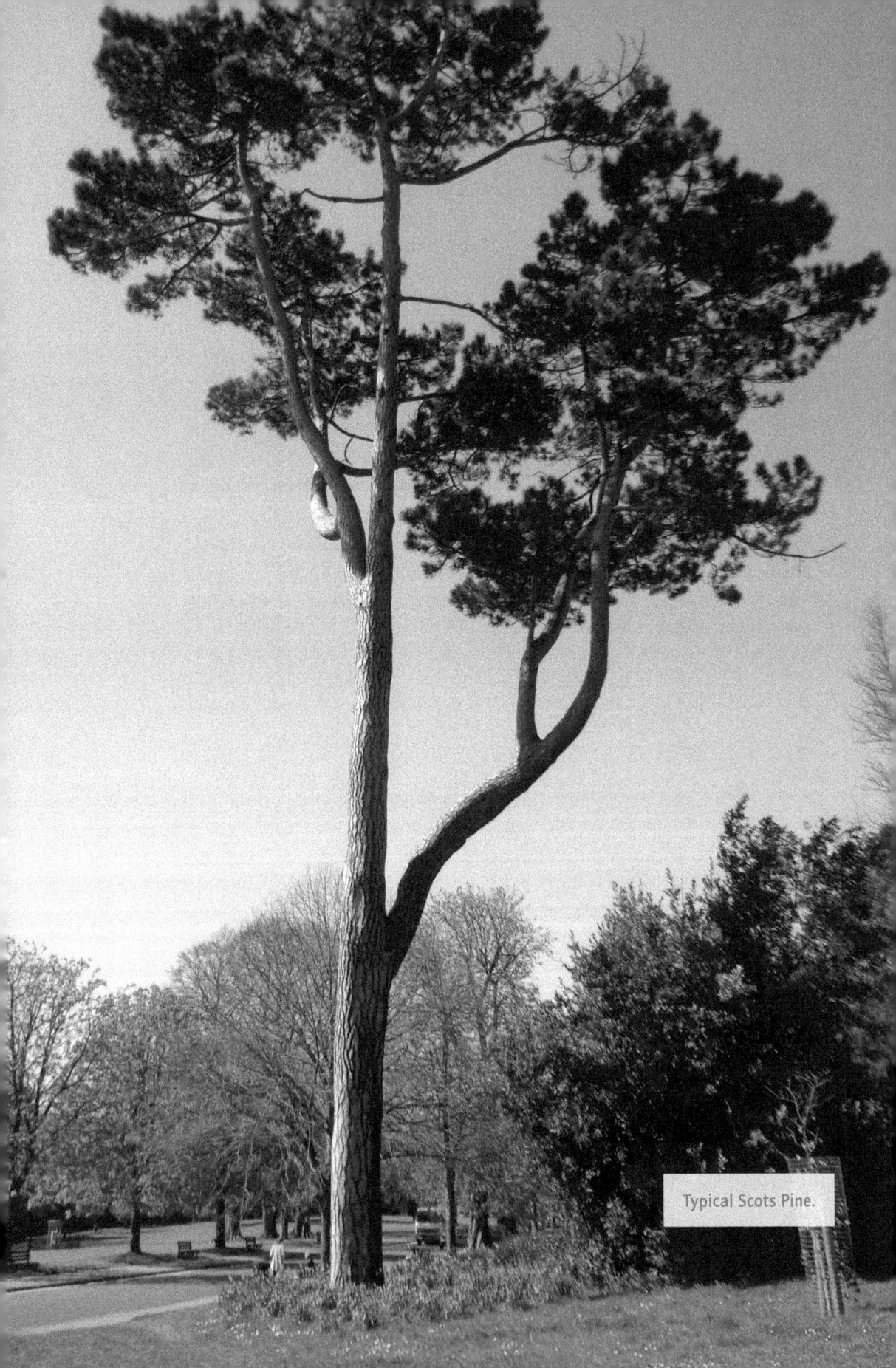
Typical Scots Pine.

Scots Pine

Pinus sylvestris – Scots Pine, Christmas tree – Pinaceae

SCOTS PINE – Usefulness – There is medicinal use for parts of the tree in veterinary and human medicine. The resin is added to varnishes and paints. Bast fibres from the bark have been used for rope and basket-making. The tree gives dyes, wood for telegraph poles, ship's masts, boat building etc. The seeds provide food for wildlife. The essential oil can be used to protect plants from snails.

Dangers – All parts of the tree are readily combustible due to the resin content.

Getting to Know the Scots Pine Tree – Originally native to much, possibly almost all, of Britain, Scots pine has been re-introduced in the south and is regarded as native in Scotland. Known there simply as pine, *Pinus sylvestris* also grows throughout Scandinavia and across Europe to Siberia and Turkey. In northern America it is introduced. The straight nature of growth of the trunk and sheer height of the tree, up to thirty six metres (118 feet) can be breathtaking and recommended it to be used as a windbreak in small plantations. It has also led to the wood, known as red deal, being used for telegraph poles and pit props. The lower bark is grey and rough, appearing on older trees to have raised plates, which are left as the bark splits, as islands raised above a purplish base. Higher up the tree the bark tends towards a reddish colouring.

The scent of pine resin from the needles in a forest is both enjoyable and refreshing. The needles are used to fill soothing scented pillows to ease coughs and colds. On the Scots pine, needles grow in pairs, on other pines they grow in odd-numbered groups.

The tree flowers in late spring, the yellow male flowers hanging in clusters from the previous years' growth to shed their pollen, while the red female flowers grow at the tips of new growth. As the female germen ripens through summer they gradually turn brown and remain until the following year when they become larger as green cones ripening to greyish brown in winter. This cycle ends in the following spring as they shed their seeds and fall.

The cones produce many seeds tucked well inside their scales. Extracting these poses a problem for most birds, to the extent that some have developed crossed bills to use as tools to gain access. In Scotland in the Caledonian Forest the Scots pine supports the Scottish crossbill, a bird unique to this environment. It has a specially adapted bill for extracting seeds from the pine cones as food.[1] Further south in England there are fewer Scots pines together in one place, but a slightly different crossbill feeds on seeds of the Scots pine and spruce there. A friend who is a keen birdwatcher was lucky enough to have both male and female crossbills visit his Hampshire garden. He took the photo of the male crossbill below, which shows the adapted bill clearly.

In Phillip Miller's *Gardeners Kalendar* of 1771 we are instructed to sow seeds from the cones in February in a raised bed to keep them from soaking in rainwater in soggy soil. This bed should be where they receive the morning sun. Now we know to take a small handful of soil from beneath the mother tree when sowing seeds, to add the mycorrhizal fungi, which will help to support the tree as it grows.[2]

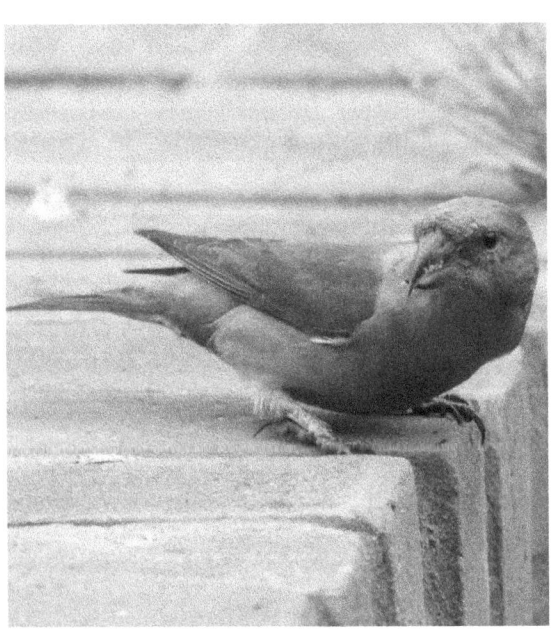

Crossbill. Photo David Papworth.

I was fortunate enough to be given a tiny seedling that had been planted as part of horticulture therapy for patients in a hospice a few months earlier. This has thrived for two years being re-potted annually and kept in shade out in the garden. At first it bore very little resemblance to the tall, upright trees that flourish in the surrounding countryside. Instead, it looked more like a bunch of windblown pine needles set into the pot. In the third year it has made considerable growth, becoming a recognisable sapling. As it grows I must remember that once unwanted branches are removed, this tree does not re-grow where it has been pruned. This may explain why the foliage of Scots pines is so often concentrated very high up the tree, with stumpy remains of branches lower down.

Many insects also flourish in contact with the pine. In the seventeenth century, that great garden writer John Evelyn recommended planting pines near to where bees were kept so that the bees would prosper.[3] Insects attracted by the tree are not all harmless. The gases from monoterpenes emitted by the trees attract a damaging pine shoot beetle (*Tomiscus pinperda*), which colonizes the new growth. As a result the tree releases verbenone. This is detected by other pine shoot beetles as they fly close to the tree giving them a message to look elsewhere.[4]

Pine burns particularly easily, hence the well known way of encouraging a recalcitrant fire into producing flames by adding pine cones. In Scotland a hundred years ago, the pine roots, which also contain sappy resin, were collected from boggy areas to use as torch lights. Since by experience it was found more resinous sap went down into the root when the moon was waning, trees were felled at full moon for boat building, in order to harvest stronger wood.[5] Pine is especially flammable from the content of resin that emerges from secretory ducts and canals in the wood, and there is oleoresin in the needles also. Terpenes in the oleoresin are the trees own defence against animals and insect attack.[6] Resin from pine is the base for rosin used for paper sizing, adhesives, and inks.

The wounding of the tree necessary to collect this resin stimulates greater production of ducts and more oleoresin. Distillation of the resin gives oil of turpentine, while the solid material left is called colophony. These resinous tears have been familiar to me for some years as they appear in historical recipes for fumigants. A tar distilled from the roots has been used in hair preparations but is not as well tolerated as tar from other trees and is no longer used.[7]

Pine needle extracts are commonly used in herbal bath supplements for treating a variety of nervous and rheumatic complaints, in addition to everyday aches and pains and fatigue. Extracts from the pine needles are made by distilling the essential oil and then extracting the water-soluble constituents, before thickening the remainder and adding the essential oil already distilled.[7] Essential oil of pine is used as an inhalant for sinus infections, to clear catarrh. Pine needles can also be infused for inhalations.

The delicious pine nuts sold in the shops are sadly not from this pine tree but the massive stone pines that grow in the Mediterranean area. When I visited Pompeii, I was astonished at their huge cones and the size of these trees, which dwarf even the Scots pine. A favourite healthy snack and garnish on many dishes today, the history of pine nuts in cookery in Britain goes back to medieval dishes. Later, in the eighteenth century they were being imported from Italy and the south of France. Thomas Hill recommended them at that period in the diet of consumptives as they were considered to be "balsamic and restorative" (p.497).[8]

Legends and Folklore. In Scotland, pine cones symbolized male fertility and the Scots pine was called the King of the forest and planted on warriors' graves. On the island of Orkney it was once traditional to purify mothers and newborn babies by whirling a pine-candle three times around the bed.[5]

Notes

1. Sterry P. *Collins Complete Guide to British Trees.* (Harper Collins. 2007). 118.
2. Adams M. *The Wisdom of Trees.* (Head of Zeus Ltd. 2014). 110.
3. Evelyn J. *Elysium Britannicum.* [1650–1700]. (University of Pennsylvania Press. 2001). 282.
4. Langenheim J.H. *Plant Resins, Chemistry Evolution Ecology Ethnobotany.* (Quote Byers et al. 1989). (Timber Press. 2003). 250.
5. Darwin T. *The Scots Herbal.* (Mercat Press. 1996). 63/4.
6. Sumner J. *The Natural History of Medicinal Plants.* (Timber Press. 2000). 89.
7. Weiss R.F. M.D. *Herbal Medicine.* (Thieme. 2nd edition revised and expanded 2000). 297, 321.
8. Hill J. M.D. 1751. *A History of the Materia Medica.* (London. 1751). 496.

SCOTS PINE – History of Medicinal Use

The tendency of this pine to grow in areas that became peat bogs has been particularly helpful for the preservation of prehistoric evidence. Submerged forest off the coast of South Wales at Ynyslas, and other sites from Shropshire to the Cleveland Hills, testify to the presence of early pine forests.[1] In southern England, archaeological excavations close to Stonehenge found evidence of pine support posts from pits dug in the Neolithic period. In a subsequent investigation, charcoal from pine in a pit dated to between 8,500 and 7,650 B.C. was found. This was earlier than the first outer ditch of Stonehenge.[2]

The Romans possibly tried to establish the Mediterranean Pine in Britain, which would have supplied them with larger edible pine-kernels during their occupation. The Mediterranean pine did not survive into the medieval period however, and the same Latin name was given to the similar native pine, known as the Scots pine in Scotland. Much of *Pinus sylvestris* in England was lost over the centuries of deforestation.

Pine resin for medicinal use has been extracted from a number of pines, including the Scots pine and *Picea abies. Pinus sylvestris* was also native across Europe. Use in applications such as plasters became widespread as recipes from the fifteenth century illustrate. These were applied to wounds, boils, and to aid new nail growth after the fingernail or toenail had died and come away.[3] Applying such plasters on areas with hairs clearly required caution as centuries later, Anne, Lady Blencowe used wax and rosin from the pine tree to remove unwanted hair.[4]

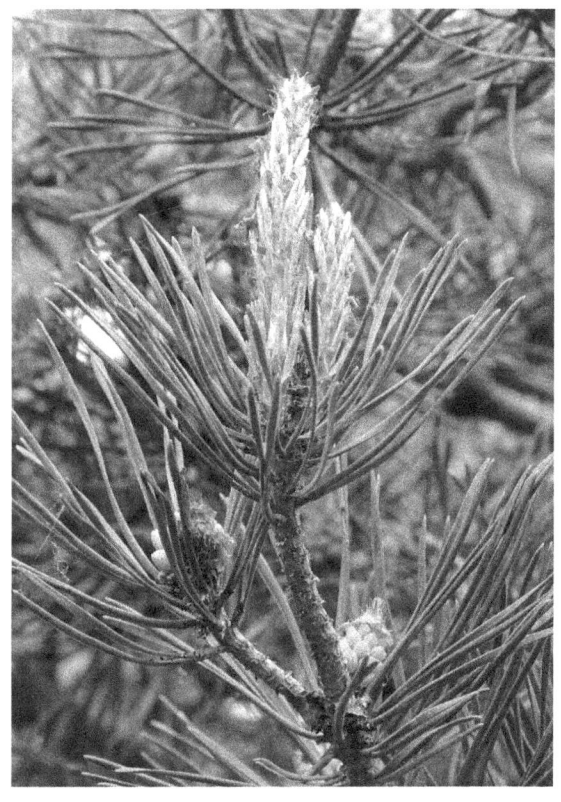

Scots pine flowers in April.

William Coles mentions no fewer than ten kinds of pine trees, his description of the medicinal pine is nevertheless an accurate one of the Scots pine. He follows this by saying, "The Bark of the Pine *Tree* is binding and drying: the *kernels* of the *Nuts* do concoct and moderately heat, being in a mean between cold and hot. The Leaves are cooling and asswage Inflammations"(p.10)[5]. As for the pine nuts, he thinks these are nourishing while they remain fresh, although eaten straight from the tree they prove hard to digest. To ease this he recommends steeping them for several hours in warm water to remove their "sharpnesse and oyliness". p.10)[5]

He further records that pine nuts were thought to stir up bodily lust and increase sperm when sweetened with honey or sugar. When made into an electuary, they were eaten to aid sore throats and wheezing chests, acting as an expectorant. They were considered "singularly good" for the thin person, helping them to put on weight. The distilled water of the needles was used as a wash to smooth wrinkles and to reduce the size of swollen breasts.[5]

In 1722, Joseph Miller quotes a Mr. Dale, writing in his *Pharmacologia* that the medicinal Burgundy Pitch was confirmed as being made from the turpentine after it has been boiled for a time, but before it became hard rosin and this was done in Saxony.[6]

Hills' History in 1751 tells us that pine kernels were brought "in sufficient Abundance from *Italy* and the South of *France*" (p.496). He then relates that they are rich in thin oil that is easily extracted, which resembles almond oil but lighter. These pine nuts were appreciated in food as well as medicine.[7] Such a reference might cast doubt on the origin of medicinal pine nuts in other herbals but certainly several definitely refer to the native tree.

Forty years later, William Meyrick makes it clear when he writes specifically about the *Pinus sylvestris* or Scots pine that the kernels or nuts have the same virtues as those of the other pines, being "excellent restoratives in consumptions, and after long illnesses". He gave them beaten up with barley water to make an emulsion, which also treated "heat of urine" (p.373) (urinary infections).[8]

In the 1740s the enthusiasm for taking tar water from the resin, a practice originating in North America, spread in Britain and was much debated. Applications ranged from treating wounds and ulcers, to rheumatism and the painful St. Anthony's fire.[9] Debate raged as Dr. Buchan in his advice on domestic medicine published in 1776, states "Though tar water falls greatly short of the character which has been given of it, yet it possesses some medicinal virtues. It sensibly raises the pulse, increases the secretions, and sometimes opens the belly, or occasions vomiting. A pint of it may be drank daily, or more, if the stomach can bear it" (pp.750/751).[10]

Tar ointment made of the tar melted with prepared mutton suet was used in particular against *Tinea capitis*, being applied to the shaven head as a plaster, with all the agony of removing hair roots as it was taken off.[11] This, and an oil prepared from the cones, was included in the Pharmacopoeias of the nineteenth century. Meanwhile, a more innocuous medicine was still recommended against scurvy. Several kinds of resins and turpentines went into plasters and ointments, also occasionally into pills.[12]

In 1879 a history of pharmacy details that the tar is obtained from two species, one of which is the *P. sylvestris*. Comment is then made that an ointment of tar is a common remedy for skin diseases and tar water is sometimes taken internally.[13] Mrs. Grieve adds that oil of turpentine and tar water were much used in veterinary practice, the first as an antiseptic and stimulant and the second internally and externally to kill parasites.[14] The essential oil is used today in blends for antiseptic and stimulating effects, and to treat osteoarthritis.[15]

Summary. As a native tree, the Scots pine has provided diverse medicinal products for many centuries. The most accessible are the young tops which have been infused to make a vitamin rich tea against scurvy. The pine kernels or nuts are smaller from trees growing in Britain than from other species, but have been eaten. These have been credited with being restorative after consumption (tuberculosis of the lungs), as well as good for coughs in removing phlegm and aiding the lungs and other organs. They might also be made into an emulsion, with almonds and barley water for the kidneys and urinary complaints. The astringency of the bark has been appreciated, as has the cooling anti-inflammatory effect of applying the needles.

In the twelfth century, we find pine resin used with other resins in a medicinal plaster. Resin, turpentine—which was distilled to produce oil of turpentine and vegetable tar obtained from distillation of the roots, as well as Burgundy pitch—were all ingredients in plasters applied to wounds, skin infections, and parasitic infestations. Drinking tar water and applying tar ointment became very popular in the eighteenth century, and oil of turpentine and tar water continued in veterinary practice. Use now concentrates more on the pine needle extract or distilled essential oil used in inhalants for catarrh. See Herbalists' Reference.

Recipe

Extracted from A Complete English Dispensatory. 1736. "*The Pectoral Electuary.* Take of the Juice of Liquorise, and of sweet Almonds, of each half an ounce; of Pine Leaves, 1 ounce; of Hyssop, Maiden-Hair, *Florentine* Orrice, Nettle Seeds, and round Birthwort, of each 1 dram and half: Seeds of Cresses, and Elecampane Root, of each half a dram; of Honey, 14 ounces; and make them into an Electuary. ... The Juice of Liquorise and sweet Almonds, are to be gradually softned with the Honey, in a Marble Mortar with a Wooden Pestle, and then the rest added in Powder. It is design'd for Distempers of the Breast, to soften, cool, and heal the Lungs" (p.437).[16]

Notes

1. Godwin Sir H. *History of the British Flora.* (Cambridge University Press. 2nd edition. 1975). 103, 105.
2. Pryor F. *Seahenge.* (Harper Collins. 2001). 91.
3. Dawson W. (ed), *A Leechbook of the XVth Century.* (Macmillan & Co. 1934). 113, (292), 199/200. (633).
4. Stapley C. (ed), *The Receipt Book of Lady Anne Blencowe.* (Heartsease Books. 2004). 114.
5. Coles W. *The Paradise of Plants.* (London. 1657). 10.
6. Miller J. *Botanicum officinale.* Bell. (London. 1722). 347.
7. Hill J. M.D. *A History of the Materia Medica.* (London. 1751). 496.
8. Meyrick W. *The New Family Herbal.* (Birmingham. 1790). 373.
9. Griggs B. *Green Pharmacy.* (Jill Norman and Hobhouse. 1981). 150/151.
10. Buchan W. M.D. *Domestic Medicine.* (London. 1776). 750/01.
11. Thornton R.J. *A New Family Herbal.* (London. 1810). 786/7.

12. Green T. *Universal Herbal or Botanical Dictionary.* 2 vols, (Caxton, London. 2nd edition. 1824). Vol 2. 322.
13. Flückiger & Hanbury. *A History of Drugs.* (Macmillan & Co. 2nd edition. 1879). 619, 623.
14. Grieve. M. *A Modern Herbal.* (1st published 1934 Jonathan Cape. Saavas. 1984). 634.
15. Worwood V.A. 1990. Th*e Fragrant Pharmacy.* (MacMillan. 1990). 127, 224, 377.
16. Quincy J. MD. *A Complete Dispensatory.* (10th edition. 1736). 437.

PINUS SYLVESTRIS – Herbalists' Reference

The Parts of Pine Used for Medicine – The leaves, or needles as they are also known, and young shoots with buds are collected in the spring. The essential oil is distilled from the pounded needles.

Dosage and Forms – Pine essential oil is used as an inhalation by adding several drops to hot water. Alternatively a handful of twigs may be soaked in 2.7 litre (4 pints) of water before simmering for five minutes. With either, sit so that bending over the steam, with the head covered by a towel you can inhale the steam for best effect.

For an infusion for internal use put ½ teaspoon of the twig to 1 cup of boiling water and infuse for ten to fifteen minutes. Tincture 1:20 in 90% alcohol, dose 5–10 drops in water three times daily.

Constituents – The volatile oil is rich in pinene. Other constituents include 1.8 cineole, caryophyllene, glucose, juniperic acid, quercetin, tannin, and resin.

Actions and Uses – Pine essential oil is generally regarded as strongly antiseptic. Properties of the herb in improving local blood flow and acting as a diuretic are useful in the treatment of urinary tract infections. It is also classified as antiarthritic and antirheumatic, as well as antieczemic, due to the same cleansing mechanism of the actions. When the volatile oil of pine is inhaled this produces a reflex vasoconstrictor reaction that opens the sinuses, acting as a decongestant, and is expectorant even with hard phlegm. The added antibacterial effects are particularly helpful in chronic bronchial and sinus infections and pneumonia. Pine is a herb of choice for asthma with adrenal hypofunctioning

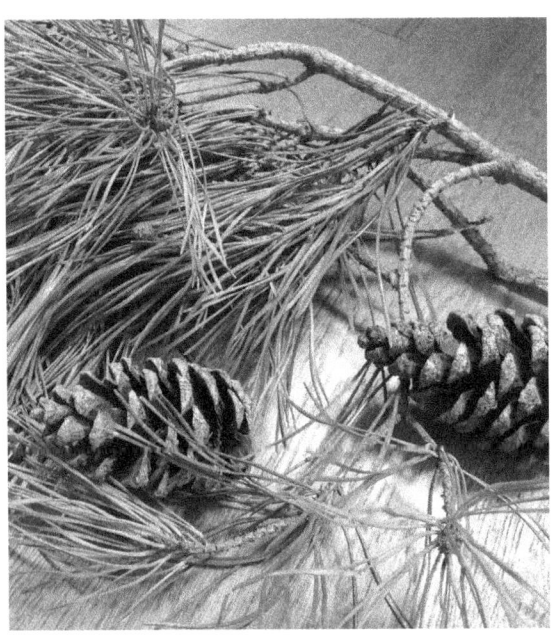

Scots pine flowers and cone.

and fatigue.[1] Commission E approved pine needle oil for catarrhal diseases of the respiratory tract, and externally only in analgesic ointments for rheumatic and neuralgic ailments.[2] These include lumbago, sciatica, neuralgia, and gout.

Topical Applications – Infusions may be applied as compresses by soaking a cloth in the liquid and applying, or added to hand or foot-baths. The essential oil may be an ingredient in creams and ointments. These might be rubbed on the chest for bronchial or sinus conditions. They are equally effective when applied to a painful joint or area as an analgesic. Other ingredients in the salve would vary according to intended use.

Contraindications and Precautions – No interactions are known. There are no restrictions in pregnancy or breast-feeding. Use is advised against when treating whooping cough and care noted with bronchial asthma patients.[3] Pine oil in massages and salves may be used for children over 3 years.[4] Cautions should include patch testing on anyone with sensitive skin if the herb is to be applied externally in any form.

Notes

1. Holmes P. *The Energetics of Western Herbs*. Vol. 1&2. (Snow Press. Boulder. Revised 3rd edition. 1989). Vol. 1.230.
2. Blumenthal et al. *Herbal Medicine. Expanded Commission E monographs*. (Integrative Medicine Commission. 2000). 305.
3. Duke J.A. *Handbook of Medicinal Herbs*. (CRC Press LLC. 2nd edition. 2002). 659.
4. McIntyre A. *The Herbal for Mother & Child*. (Element. 1992). 92–5.

Bibliography

Adams M. *The Wisdom of Trees.* (Head of Zeus Ltd. 2014).

Adams J. & Forbes S. (ed), *The Syon Abbey Herbal. A.D. 1517.* (AMCD Publishers Ltd. 2015).

Alcock J.P. *Food in Roman Britain.* (Tempus. 2001).

Anon. *A Collection of Receipts.* (Printed for the Executrix of Mary Kettilby. 1746).

Anon. *The Toilet of Flora.* (London. 1784).

Austin T. (ed), *Two Fifteenth Century Cookery Books.* (1888). (Oxford University Press. (Reprint) 1964).

A Virginia Farmer. (trans), *Roman Farm Management.* Treatises of Cato and Varro. (Macmillan. New York. 1916).

Aylett M. *Encyclopaedia of Home-Made Wines.* (Odhams Press Ltd. London. 1957).

Baker St. Barbe. *Trees A Book of the Seasons.* (Lindsay Drummond Ltd. 1948).

Barker J. *The Medicinal Flora of Britain and Northwestern Europe.* (Winter Press. 2001).

Barnes J. et al. *Herbal Medicines.* (Pharmaceutical Press. 2nd edition. 2002).

Bartram T. *Bartram's Encyclopedia of Herbal Medicine.* (Robinson. 1998).

Blochwich M. M.D. *Anatomy of the Elder Tree.* (London. 1677).

Blumenthal et al. *Herbal Medicine. Expanded Commission E monographs.* (Integrative Medicine Commission. 2000).

Bone K. *A Clinical Guide to Blending Liquid Herbs.* (Churchill Livingstone. 2003).

Bowman A.K. *Life and Letters on the Roman Frontier.* (The British Museum Press. 2003).

Bown D. *The RHS Encyclopedia of Herbs.* (Dorling Kindersley. 1996).

British Herbal Pharmacopoeia. (British Herbal Medicine Association. 1983).

Brodin G. *Agnus castus.* Upsala. (Harvard University Press. 1950).

Brook R. *Brook's Family Herbal.* (J.A. Brook, Richardson & Co. London. Revised edition. 1876).

Buchan W. M.D. *Domestic Medicine.* (London. 1776).

Buhner S.H. *Sacred and Herbal Healing Beers.* (Siris Books. 1998).

Buhner S.H. *Herbal Antibiotics.* (Storey Books. 1999).

Burlando B. et al. *Herbal principles in Cosmetics.* (CRC Press. 2010).

Campbell-Culver M. *The Origin of Plants.* (Headline Book Publishing. 2001).

Chapman G. & Tweddle M. (ed), *A New Herball.* William Turner (1551) (Carcanet Press. 1989).

Chiej R. *The Macdonald Encyclopedia of Medicinal Plants.* (Macdonald Publishing. London. 1984).

Coats. A.M. *Garden Shrubs and their Histories.* (Vista Books. London. 1963).

Coles W. *The Paradise of Plants.* (London. 1657).

Coles J. & Minitt S. *Industrious and Fairly Civilized.* (Somerset Levels Project. 1995).

Crockett L. *Healing Our Hormones Healing Our Lives.* (John Hunt Publishing O Books. 2009).

Culpeper N. *Culpeper's Complete Herbal and English Physician enlarged.* (1652). (London. 1815 edition).

Darwin T. *The Scots Herbal.* (Mercat Press. 1996).

Dawson W. (ed), *A Leechbook of the XVth Century.* (Macmillan & Co. 1934).

De Bairacli-Levy J. *The Complete Herbal Handbook for Farm and Stable.* (Faber and Faber, London. 1991).

De Bairacli-Levy J. *The Illustrated Herbal Handbook for Everyone.* (Faber and Faber. London. 1991).

DeCleene M. & Lejeune M.C. *Compendium of Symbolic and Ritual Plants in Europe.* (Man and Culture Publishers, Ghent. Belgium. 2003).

De Sloover J. & Goossens M. *Wild Herbs of Britain and Europe.* (David and Charles. 1994).

Doctor Dawa. *A Clear Mirror of Tibetan Medicinal Plants.* (Volume 1). (Tibet Domani. 1999).

Duke J.A. *Handbook of Phytochemical Constituents of GRAS herbs and other Economic Plants.* (CRC Press LLC. 2001).

Duke J.A. *Handbook of Medicinal Herbs.* (CRC Press LLC. 2nd edition. 2002).

Engel C. *Wild Health.* (Houghton Mifflin Co. 1979).

Erichson-Brown C. *Medicinal and other uses of North American Plants.* (Dover Publications. 1979).

Evelyn J. *Elysium Britannicum*. [1650–1700]. University of Pennsylvania Press. 2001.

Farrar L. *Ancient Roman Gardens*. (Budding Books. 1998).

Flückiger & Hanbury. *A History of Drugs*. 2nd edition. (Macmillan & Co. 1879).

Freethy R. *From Agar to Zenry*. (Crowood Press. 1985).

Frisk G. (ed), *A Middle English translation of Macer Floridus de Viribus Herbarum*. Harvard (University Press Cambridge, Mass. 1949).

Frőhne D. Pfander H. *A Colour Atlas of Poisonous Plants*. (Wolf Science. 1983).

Ghabru A. *Evaluation of Seabuckthorn byproducts for in vivo in vitro activities*. (Lambert Academic Publishing. 2019).

Gifford J. *The Celtic Wisdom of Trees*. (Godsfield Press. 2000).

Godwin Sir H. *History of the British Flora*. (2nd edition). (Cambridge University Press. 1975).

Green T. *Universal Herbal or Botanical Dictionary*. 2 vols, (2nd edition). (Caxton, London. 1824).

Grierson. S. *The Colour Cauldron*. (pub. Su Grierson. 1986).

Grieve. M. *A Modern Herbal*. (1st published 1934 Jonathan Cape. Saavas. 1984).

Griggs B. *Green Pharmacy*. (Jill Norman and Hobhouse. 1981).

Grigson G. *The Englishman's Flora*. (The Folio Society. 1987).

Gunther R.T. (ed), *Dioscorides Greek Herbal*. (Hafner. 1968).

Hagen A. *A Handbook of Anglo-Saxon Food*. (Anglo-Saxon books. 1992).

Hagen A. *Anglo-Saxon Food and Drink*. (Anglo-Saxon Books. 1995).

Hall A. & Barker A. *The National Botanic Pharmacopoeia*. (National Association of Medical Herbalists of Great Britain. 1932).

Hanmer Sir T. *The Garden Book of Sir Thomas Hanmer*. (mid 17th century). (Gerald Howe. 1944).

Harington Sir J. The School of Salernum. *Regimen Sanitatis Salerni*. (Ente Provinciale per Il Turismo. Salerno. Rome. 1957).

Harris M. *Botanica of North America*. (Harper Resource. 2003).

Hartley D. *Food in England*. (Futura. 1985).

Harvey J. *Early Gardening Catalogues*. (Phillimore & Co. 1972).

Harvey J. *Early Nurserymen*. (Phillimore & Co. 1974).

Harvey J. *Mediaeval Gardens*. (Batsford. 1981).

Healde T. M.D. F.R.S. *The Pharmacopoeia of the R.C.P. of London*. (1791).

Henslow G. Rev. Prof. M.A. *Medical Works of the Fourteenth Century*. (Burt Franklin. New York. 1972).

Hill J. M.D. *A History of the Materia Medica*. (London. 1751).

Hill Sir J. *The Family Herbal.* (Bungay edition. Brightly. 1812).
Hobby E. (ed), *The Birth of Mankind.* (1560). (Ashgate. 2009).
Hoffmann D. *The New Holistic Herbal.* (Element. 1990).
Holmes P. *The Energetics of Western Herbs.* Vol. 1&2. (Snow Press. Boulder. Revised 3rd edition. 1989).
Hort A. (trans), 1999. *Theophrastus Enquiry into Plants.* Loeb Classical Library.
Howkins C. *Rowan Tree of Protection.* (Howkins. 1996).
Johnson T. (ed), *The Herbal.* John Gerard. (1633 edition). (Dover Publications, New York. 1975).
Jones W.H.S. (trans), *Pliny Natural History* VI Books XX–XXIII. (Loeb Classical Library. 1989).
Keller Dr. F. (trans), Lee E. *The Lake Dwellings of Switzerland &c.* (Longmans Green & Co. 1878). Vols. 1 & 2.
Kelly W.J. (ed. director). *Nursing Herbal Medicine Handbook.* (Springhouse Corporation. 2001).
Langenheim J.H. *Plant Resins, Chemistry Evolution Ecology Ethnobotany.* (Timber Press. 2003).
Larkey S.V. (ed), *An Herbal* (1525), (Scholars Facsimiles and Reprints, New York. 1941).
Lewer H.W. (ed), *A Book of Simples.* (1700–1750). (Sampson Low, Marston & Co. Ltd. 1908).
Lewington A. *Plants for People.* (Eden Project Books. 2003).
Lyle T.J. A.M.M.D. 1897. *Physio-medical Therapeutics, Materia Medica and Pharmacy.* Ohio.
Mabey R. *The Gardener's Labyrinth* Thomas Hill. (1652 edition). (Oxford University Press. 1987).
Mabey R. *Flora Britannica* (concise edition). (Chatto & Windus. 1998).
Manniche L. *An Ancient Egyptian Herbal.* (British Museum Press. 1989).
McIntyre A. *The Herbal for Mother & Child.* (Element. 1992).
McLean T. *Medieval English Gardens.* (Barrie & Jenkins. 1989).
Meyrick W. *The New Family Herbal.* (Birmingham. 1790).
Miller J. *Botanicum officinale.* Bell. (London. 1722).
Miller J. F.R.S. *Gardener's Dictionary.* (London. 1771).
Miller A.B. *Shaker Herbs.* A History and a Compendium. (Potter. 1976).
Mills S. *Out of this Earth.* (Viking. Penguin. 1991).
Mills S. & Bone K. *Principles & Practice of Phytotherapy.* (Churchill Livingstone. 2000).

Mills S. & Bone K. *The Essential Guide to Herbal Safety*. (Elsevier Churchill Livingstone. 2005).

Moncrieff A.R. Hope. *Classical Mythology*. (Senate. 1994).

Nunn J.F. *Ancient Egyptian Medicine*. (British Museum Press. 2000).

Pasang Yonten Arya. Dr. *Dictionary of Tibetan Materia Medica*. (Motilal Banarsidass Publishing Delhi. 1998).

Pechey J. *The English Herbal of Physical Plants*. (London. 1694).

Phillips R. *Wild Food*. (Pan Books. 1983).

Philp R.B. *Herbal-Drug Interactions and Adverse Effects*. (McGraw Hill. 2004).

Piesse S.G. W. *The Art of Perfumery*. (1855). Echo Library. 2007.

Plat Sir H. *Delights for Ladies*. (1609). (Crosby Lockwood. 1948).

Pollington S. *Leechcraft*. (Anglo Saxon Books. 2000).

Power E. *The Goodman of Paris*. (orig. 1393). (Folio Society. 1992).

Pryor F. *Seahenge*. Harper (Collins. 2001).

Pughe J. (trans), *The Herbal Remedies of the Physicians of Myddfai*. (Llanerch. 1989).

Quincy J. M.D. *A Complete Dispensatory*. (10th edition. 1736).

Rackham O. *The History of the Countryside*. (Phoenix Paperback. 1986).

Reader's Digest. *Foods that Harm Foods that Heal*. (Reader's Digest General Books. 1999).

Riddle J.M. *Eve's Herbs*. (Harvard University Press. 1997).

Rosenman Leonard D. M.D. *A Medieval Surgical Pharmacopoeia and Formulary*. 1170–1325. (San Francisco. 1999).

Salmon W. *Comment on Bates Dispensatory*. (1794).

Samuelsson G. *Drugs of Natural Origin*. (Apotekarsocieteten.1999).

Schultz et al. *Rational Phytotherapy*. (Springer. 2004).

Scott. M. (ed), *An Irish Herbal*. K'Eogh. (1735). (Aquarian. 1986).

Scurrah J.W. F.N.A.M.H. *The National Botanic Pharmacopoeia*. Bradford. (1905).

Smith E. *The Compleat Housewife*. (London. 1739).

Spencer W.G. (trans), *Celsus De Medicina* 1 Books 1–1V. (Loeb Classical Library. 1971).

Spencer W.G. (trans), *Celsus De Medicina* 1 Books V–V1. (Loeb Classical Library. 1989).

Spindler K. *The Man in the Ice*. (Weidenfeld & Nicolson. 1994).

Stapley C. (ed), *The Receipt Book of Lady Anne Blencowe*. (Heartsease Books. 2004).

Stapley C. *Herbcraft Naturally*. (Heartsease Books. 1994).

Stapley C. *Herb Sufficient.* (Heartsease Books. 1998).

Stargrove et al. *Herb, Nutrient and Drug Interactions.* (Mosby Elsevier. 2008).

Sterry P. *Collins Complete Guide to British Trees.* (Harper Collins. 2007).

Stewart S. *Cosmetics & Perfumes in the Roman World.* (Tempus. 2007).

Stobart A. *The Medicinal Forest Garden Handbook.* (Permanent Publications. 2020).

Sumner J. *The Natural History of Medicinal Plants.* (Timber Press. 2000).

Teetgen A.B. *Profitable Herb-Growing and Collecting.* (London. 1916).

Thompson A. *Native British Trees.* (Wooden Books Ltd. 2005).

Thomson A.T. M.D. F.L.S. *The London Dispensatory.* (London. 4th edition. 1826).

Thornton R.J. *A New Family Herbal.* (London. 1810).

Throop P. (trans), *Hildegard von Bingen's Physica.* (Healing Arts Press. 1998).

Todd R.G. (ed), *Extra Pharmacopoeia Martindale.* (Pharmaceutical Press. 25th edition. 1967).

Togno J. Durand E. (trans) *A Manual of Materia Medica and Pharmacy.* (Philadelphia. 1829).

Trease & Evans W.C. *Pharmacognosy.* (W.B. Saunders. 14th edition. 1999).

Tudge C. *The Secret Life of Trees.* (Penguin Books. 2006).

Tusser T. *Five Hundred Points of Good Husbandry.* (Original 1573). (Oxford University Press. 1984).

Vickery R. *Oxford Dictionary of Plant-Lore.* (Oxford University Press. 1997).

Waller J. *Waller's New British Domestic Herbal.* Cox & Son. (London. 1822).

Warde W. & Anglosse R. (trans), *The Secretes of Maister Alexis of Piemont.* (Atenar. 2000).

Warren P. *British Native Trees, past and present uses.* (Wildeye. 2006).

Weeks N. & Bullen V. *The Bach Flower Remedies.* (C. W. Daniel & Co. Ltd. 1990).

Weiss R.F. M.D. *Herbal Medicine.* (Thieme. 2nd edition revised and expanded. 2000).

White G. Rev. M.A. The *Natural History and Antiquities of Selborne.* (1778). (Swan Sonnenschein & Co. 1911).

Woodville W. *Medical Botany.* 3 vols + Supplement. (London. 1790).

Worwood V.A. 1990. The *Fragrant Pharmacy.* (MacMillan. 1990).

Wren R.C. *Potter's Encyclopaedia of Botanical Drug and Preparations.* (Daniel, U.K. 1998).

Zeb A. *Sea Buckthorn: A Functional Food.* (Lambert Academic Publishing. 2014).

Biography for Christina Stapley

Christina Stapley has been researching the historical uses of herbs for over 40 years. Her first interest in herbs sprang from research for writing a novel set in the Elizabethan period. Her continued deep and practical research on medieval and Tudor medicine has provided original recipes for many historical herb workshops and presentations at a number of museums around the country. She has grown more than 300 herbs for over 30 years and her former third of an acre herb garden in Hampshire was featured on television on a number of occasions. In 2004, she qualified with a BSc in Phytotherapy and has practiced in Hampshire and Wiltshire, retiring recently. In 2010 Christina tutored a postgraduate course, Stillroom to Dispensary for NIMH in Reading. This involved making numerous historical recipes and discussing their suitability for use in modern Herbal Practice.

In celebration of the Millennium Year her historical workshops at the Weald and Downland Living Museum covered household and medicinal use of herbs over the past thousand years with a series of workshops, which also marked the introduction of important herbs from overseas. This included herbs taken abroad by the first settlers in America, in addition to those they found on their arrival. In 2011 she presented some of the latter in their native habitat during a week of herb workshops at Plimoth Plantation Museum near Boston, Massachusetts. Her workshops have included an A–Z of Medicinal Trees and Woodland Herbs.

A member of the Herbal History Research Network, Christina has given presentations at HHRN Seminars and helps to organise these events and support researchers. A speaker for the RHS and other registers, she gives many talks on varying aspects of herb use, historical and modern, and has written three books on growing and using herbs and edited a book of cookery and medicinal recipes from 1694 for the

Blencowe family. Her herbal practice has encouraged a growing enthusiasm for work in preventive medicine through herbs, diet, and lifestyle. This has led to writing both Interactive and Essentials courses on Ageing Successfully. She is a member of the College of Practitioners of Phytotherapy.

Christina now lives in Wiltshire and teaches History of Western Herbal Medicine, Pharmacognosy and Materia Medica for the School of Herbal Medicine in the south west. More details of her books, talks, and workshops can be found on www.christinastapley.co.uk. Over the past 27 years, she has developed over 120 different herb workshops and lists 35 available talks. In addition to having worked at 26 venues, she gives bespoke workshops by request for Craft Guilds and other groups.

Index

Acacia germanica 46, 47, 48.
Acorns 23, 179, 180, 183, 184, **186**.
Aelfric 162, 163, 193.
Aesculus hippocastanum
   see Horse Chestnut
Agnus castus 103, 104, 321.
Alder 118, 171.
Ales 29, 34, 72, 149, 151, 179, 196, 299, 317, 323.
Allergens 16, 29, 62, 77, 108, 157, 167, 173, 283, 305, 315, 317.
Almond 195, 196, 264, 285, 290, 338.
Alpinus 130, 131.
America 29, 32, 34, 38, 71, 81, 116, 126, 142, 159, 216, 217, 293, 297, 317, 321, 331, 336.
Amygdalin 41, 88, 203, 249.
Anglo-Saxon 12, 23, 33, 47, 55, 58, 67, 71, 103, 141, 143, 150, 183, 207, 208, 226, 228, 236, 237, 246, 247, 264, 288, 299, 321.
Animal feed 173, 288, 296, 309.
Anne Blencowe 88, 127, 263, **312**, 323, 335.
Antidotes 13, 151, 194, 226, 236.

Apollo 275.
Apple 204, 234, 236, 264.
Arabic medicine 92, 93, 104, 116.
Artemis 275.
Ash 7–17, 207.
Avicenna 129.

Bacchus 308.
Bach flower remedies 17, 78, 81, 111.
Banckes 104.
Barberry 19, 21, 29, 30, **125–135**.
Bark basketry 19, 21, 29, 30, 33, 169, 173, 261, 262, 331.
Basketry 8, 111, 112, 147, 273, 274, 283, 286, 305, 307.
Bates 13, **324**.
Bauhin 131.
Bay **273–281**, 286, 309.
Beech **19–27**. Beech tar 19, 24, 26, 27.
Bees 41, 87, 99, 111, 127, 170, 213, 295, 305, 333.
Berberine 125, 134.
Berberis vulgaris see Barberry
Betula alba, B. lenta see Birch

INDEX

Birch **29–39**, 149, 171, 281, 318, 332. Birch tar 29, 32, 33, 34, 38.
Birds 7, 10, 22, 29, 41, 54, 66, 189, 243, 295, 305, 307, 317, 318.
Bird-lime 297, 300.
Black Mulberry **137–145**.
Blackthorn **41–51**, 148, 204.
Blackberry 42, 44, 129, 148.
Blochwich M. 150, 151, **153**, 159.
Book of Bald 33, 46, 69, 116, 246, 310.
Boswellia 121, 221.
Brandy 67, 169, 224.
Brigantia 245.
Brigid 245.
Brook 44, 174, 228, 265, 300, 311,
Bronze Age 7, 33, 43, 173, 207, 216, 218.
Butser Ancient farm 112, 262, 285.
Butterflies 7, 10, 41, 42, 180, 295, 305, 306.

Canada 30, 217, 218, 252.
Castanea sativa see Sweet Chestnut
Cato 91, 308, 311.
Cattle 9, 21, 179, 305.
Celsus 141, 276, 309.
Celtic 32, 111, 149, 181, 182, 204, 243, 245, 246, 285, 286, 309, 319.
Charcoal 12, 20, 23, 31, 46, 58, 65, 69, 111, 114, 115, 171, 173, 236, 286, 298.
Charlemagne 162, 193.
Chaucer 224, 227, 236.
China 139, 253, 254, 255.
Chippewa 217.
Christmas 22, 44, 68, 101, 151, 191, 263, 273, 275, 295, 297, 307.

Cider 204, 210, 233, 234, 237.
Cinchona 81, 82, 117, 300.
Coffee substitute 21, 78, 179.
Coles 13, 24, 34, 46, 47, 59, 69, 71, 80, 82, 88, 92, 116, 129, 130, 149, 150, 163, 164, 184, 191, 194, 208, 209, 227, **228**, 234, 235, 237, 265, 266, 278, 289, 299, 309, 311, 322, 336.
Conserves 48, 55, 59, 100, 105, 125, 130, 131.
Cookery 41, 43, 53, 67, 87, 100, 141, 190, 215, 233, 234, 262, 263, 274, 273, 285, 317, 319, 334.
Cordial 53, 55, 94.
Corylus avellana See Hazel
Cosmetics 29, 41, 42, 54, 56, 60, 78, 99, 139, 148, 169, 170, 191, 283, 290, 311, 336.
Crab apple 44, 67, 148, **203–211**, 225.
Cramp bark **213–221**.
Crataegus oxycantha See hawthorn
Cree 217, 218.
Culpeper 13, 24, 34, 58, 68, 69, 92, 104, 116, 129, 142, 148, 150, 162, 164, 184, 225, 227, 228, 237, 247, 265, **266**, 273, 277, 278, 289, 297, 299, 308, 311, 322.
Cydonia vulgaris See Quince

Deer 8, 22, 296.
De Mondeville 91, 116, 183.
Diana 192.
Dioscorides 23, 91, 103, 115, 116, 143, 161, 171, 183, 194, 195, 207, 226, 236, 237, 264, 266, 288, 323.
Dionysius 308.

Distilled Waters 14, 41, 42, 48, 56, 59, 63, 69, 71, **72**, 96, 100, 101, 105, 108, 130, 174, 184, 194, 196, 208, 275, 280, 323, 336.
Doctrine of signatures 20, 34, 89, 129, 163, 194, 299, 300.
Dormouse
Dwale 58.
Dyes 7, 20, 29, 41, 44, 46, 55, 65, 66, 68, 77, 111, 114, 125, 137, 147, 148, 170, 179, 189, 190, 203, 233, 243, 251, 261, 283, 284, 305, 307, 331.

Ebers papyrus 115, 321.
Edible oils 7, 21, 26, 189, 194, 195, 198, 257, 283, **290**.
Egypt 46, 102, 115, 161, 308, 321, 323.
Elderflower **53–63**, 177, 213, 286.
Elderberry 145, **147–155**, 204, 240, 323.
Electuary 236, 249, 266, 336, **338**.
Essential Oil 32, 38, 100, 104, 108, 139, 280, 328, 331, 334, 337, 340.
Esus 181.
Etmuller 195.
Evelyn J. 80, 225, 333.

Fagus sylvatica See Beech
Ficus carica See Fig
Fig 139, **157–167**, 194, 196, 220, 264.
First nations 30, 38.
Flag Fen 181.
Folklore 8, 10, 14, 22, 32, 44, 56, 67, 68, 79, 89, 101, 102, 114, 139, 140, 149, 159, 171, 181, 191, 205, 224, 235, 245, 253, 263, 275, 286, 297, 308, 320, 334.
France 22, 81, 96, 174, 300, 323, 334, 336.
Fraoth 245.
Fraxinus excelsior See Ash
Freya 56, 171.
Fungi 7, 9, 20, 23, 33, 126, 179, 236, 237, 332.

Galen 92, 143, 162, 237.
Galls 179, 183, 184, **185**, 318.
Gall wasp 158, 159.
Gerard 13, 23, 24, 104, 116, 173, 174, 183, 194, 225, 237, 246, 247, 266, 289, 322.
Germany 71, 82, 245, 266, 320.
Gilbert White 10, 66, 174.
Gin 21, 43, 44, 88, 317, 318, 323.
Glastonbury Lake Village 46, 115, 207, 216.
Gluten-free flours 263, 283, 288.
Goats 8, 112, 251, 288, 301, 305, 309.   Goats milk 299.
Godwin 12, 264.
Goodyer J. 171.
Greek 181, 191, 275, 289, 310.
Green 43, 66, 70, 149, 190, 205, 208, 209, 235, 254, 311.
Grieve 81, 152, 174, 195, 209, 216, 300, 337.
Guaiacum 121.
Guelder rose 214, 216.
Gum 322.
Gunpowder 20, 171, 321.

Hair dye 19, 20, 114, 148, 163, 189, 191, 194, 195, 311.

INDEX

Hair treatments 9, 20, 24, 27, 38, 89, 93, 100, 114, **118**, 163, 194, 281, 283, 288, 289, **290**, 322, 337.
Hawthorn 42, 44, **65–75**, 148, 177, 221, 224, 285.
Hazel 10, 264, **283–293**.
Hedera helix See Ivy
Hedging 19, 42, 65, 66, 69, 126, 129, 147, 203, 213, 296, 306.
Herculaneum 157, 158.
Hildegard of Bingen 23, 33, 46, 141, 173, 194, 227, 236, 246, 247, 264, 265, 277, 289, 310, 322.
Hill Sir John 70, 174.
Hippophae rhamnoides see Sea buckthorn
Holly **295–303**.
Homoeopathic medicine 81, 131, 174.
Honey 20, 24, 31, 35, 61, 142, **143**, 149, 162, 166, 170, 191, 204, 219, 224, 234, 264, 285, 288, 336, 338.
Horses 54, 55, 77, 81, 171, 251, 252, 296, 305.
Horse chestnut **77–85**.
Hyldemoer 149.

Ice Age 33, 254, 298, 318.
Iceman 7, 33, 173, 285.
Ilex aquifolium See Holly
India 93, 94, 253, 254.
Ink 31, 41, 44, 147, 213, 215, 251, 333.
Insect repellents 54, 190, 275, 281.
Ireland 10, 14, 68, 136, 227, 238, 243, 245, 289, 311.
Iron Age 46, 115, 246.

Italy 99, 323, 334.
Ivy 163, 286, **305–315**.

Jay 19.
Juglans regia See Walnut
Juniperus Communis See Juniper
Juniper 151, **317–329**. Tar 337.
Jupiter 162, 181, 191, 264.

Lacnunga 46, 69, 116, 246, 277, **301**, 310.
Lake dwellings, Switzerland 207.
Lanfranche 183.
Langham W. 263, 265, 266.
Laurus nobilis See Bay
Leechbooks 23, 150, 183, 226, 288, 310, 321.
Leo 273, 277.
Limeflower **169–177**, 221.
Liqueurs 19, 41, 42, 43, 44, 89, 101, 147, 233, 274.

Macer 276, 278, 321.
Malus sylvestris See crab apple
Marmalade 50, 88, 92.
Mars 69, 159.
Marsh Elder see Guelder.
Matthiolus 13, 149.
Medlar 65, **223–231**, 264.
Membrillo 88.
Menominee 217.
Mercury 142, 286, 289.
Mesolithic 12, 33, 173.
Mespilus germanica See Medlar
Meyrick 14, 34, 47, 60, 93, 117, 130, 142, 208, 277, 290, 300, 336.

Mice 22, 66.
Miller Joseph 14, 47, 70, 92, 130, 151, 173, 195, 208, 238, 265, 336.
Miller Phillip 42, 66, 149, 205, 214, 216.
Milk (Nut) 88, 194, 196, 283, 285, 289, 290, 292.
Minerva 140.
Mithridate 163.
Moon 111.
Morus nigra See Mulberry
Moths 10, 66, 79, 101, 126.
Mulberry 8, **137–145**, 148, 163.
Myrrh 47.

National Association Medical Herbalists 35, 70, 81, 217, 218.
National Trust 137, 225.
Neckham A. 227.
Neolithic 69, 173, 183, 236, 246, 264, 288, 309, 335.
Nutmeg 13, 70, 106, 151, 204, 228, 278.

Oak 19, 23, 78, 163, **179–187**, 207, 242.
Oil 19, 21, 26, 32, 78, 189, 276, 278, 280, 317.
Olde English Herbarium 24, 310.
Oplontis 262.
Osiris 308.

Pear 65, **233–241**, 264.
Peach 236.
Pechey John 14, 34, 51, 92, 105, 130, 142, 151, 173, 194, 216, 218, 227, 247, 265, 277, 299, 322.

Perfumes 91, 111, 114, 275, 317, 321, 322.
Physicians of Myddfai 103, 247.
Physio-medicalists 217, 218.
Pickles 9, 13, 125, 127, 190.
Pinus sylvesttris See Scots Pine
Plague 13, 67, 92, 105, 131, 194, 195, 322.
Plat 34, 191, 234.
Pliny 23, 63, 91, 93, 143, 157, 173, 174, 182, 183, 194, 195, 207, 226, 236, 178, 266, 288, 309, 322.
Poisons 9, 143, 163, 194, 234, 236, 296, 302, 322.
Polish 21, 31, 189.
Pollen 23, 29, 33, 53, 62, 115, 127, 159, 173, 246, 254, 283, 284, 288, 322.
Pompeii 157, 334.
Port 44, 147, 148, 154.
Posset 72, **131, 164**, 299.
Preserves 44, 55, 65, 125, 127, 131, 152, 190, 203, 204, 213, 215, 223, 224, 230, 243, 249, 252.
Prunus spinosa See Blackthorn
Pyramus and Thisbe 140.
Pyrus communis See Pear

Quercus robur See Oak
Quince **87–97**, 140, 223, 229, 236, 264, 309.
Quincy 47, 70.

Ray 66, 130.
Rhasis 92.
Roman 55, 103, 112, 137, 140, 143, 150, 159, 162, 170, 191, 195, 204,

208, 224, 226, 234, 237, 246, 262, 264, 275, 276, 289, 10, 335.
Romulus and Remus 159.
Rope 31, 169, 173, 331.
Rosmarinus officinalis See Rosemary 67, **99–109**, 247, 278, 281, 290.
Rowan 148, 243, 249, 286.
Russia 32, 244, 253, 255.

Salerno 106, 116, 194, 224, 234, 236, 237.
Salicylates 32, 38, 107, 117, 118, 120.
Salix alba See Willow
Salmon W. 13, 324.
Sambucus nigra See Elder
Saturn 24, 92, 221, 227, 299.
Scandinavia 10, 149, 214, 243, 244, 254, 318, 331.
Scots Pine **331–341**. Tar 335, 336, 337.
Scotland 10, 26, 31, 32, 58, 67, 147, 150, 243, 244, 286, 318, 320, 331, 334.
Sea buckthorn **251–259**.
Seahenge 181.
Shakers 217, 218.
Shampoo 9, 31, 96, 99, 261, 275.
Sheep 251, 288, 296, 305, 308, 309.
Shrew 10.
Silkworms 137, 138, 139. Silk 139, 284, 307, 319.
Sloes see blackthorn.
Smith E. 234, 323.
Smoking Foods 31, 171, 274, 317.
Somerset levels 23, 112, 288, 299.
Soporific sponge 310, 312.
Sorbus aucuparia See Rowan

Spices 35, 88, 106, 151, 204, 207, 224, 228.
Squirrels 19, 22, 189, 224, 283, 284, 285.
Starr Carr 33.
Sweet Chestnut **261–269**.
Swiss Alps 7, 33, 150, 173, 207, 243, 285, 322.
Syon Abbey 139, 227.
Syrup 31, 42, 50, **60**, 92, 93, **94**, 96, 125, 127, 130, 131, 137, 142, 143, 145, 147, 148, 151, 154, 157, 166, 204, 234, 249.

Tanning 71, 111, 179, 286.
Tapping sap 31, 194.
Taranis 181.
Tea substitutes 8, 43, 44.
Teeth – treatments 26, 32, 104, 142, 195, 275, 310, 322.
Theodoric 12.
Theophrastus 158.
Theriac 195.
Thor 22, 181, 245.
Thomson 152, 154.
Thornton 60, 81, **82**, 93, 117, 131, 142, 323.
Tibet 253, 255.
Tilia europaea, T. cordata, T. platyphyllos See Limeflower
Tradescant J. 80.
Turnsole 137, 148.
Turner W. 139, 265.
Tusser T. 204, 285.

Venus 34, 58, 82, 89, 150, 237.
Verjuice 203, 204, 208.

Viburnum opulus See Cramp bark
Victorian 43, 77, 323.
Vinegar 13, 23, 54, 59, 79, 105, 142, 147, 184, 191, 203, 226, 276.
Vitamin C 14, 125, 157, 215, 240, 244, 247, 251, 252, 258, 337.

Wales 32, 104, 126, 182, 243, 244, 320, 335.
Waller 35, 117, 131, 152, 174, 195.
Walnut 163, **189–199**.
War- First 7, 14, 55, 70, 71, 77, 81, 112, 117, 131, 174, 218, 263, 266, 278.
War Second 77, 148.
Waxwings 66, 244.
Wayfaring tree 215, 216, 218.
Weald and Downland Living Museum 251, 297.
Withering W. 14, 47, 117.
Willow 12, **111–121.**

Wine 29, 34, 35, 44, 47, 51, 56, 65, 67, 69, 72, 88, 101, 105, **107**, 116, 125, 127, 137, 139, 148, 150, 151, **153**, 154, 170, 179, 181, 184, 194, 203, 205, 224, 230, 233, 243, 263, 301, 318, 322.
Wintergreen 32, 38.
Woman's book 91, 141, 183, 227, 323.
Woodville W. 81, 93, 117, 126, 131, 195, 323.
Writing tablets 20, 170, 171.

Xylitol 31.

Yeast 35, 68, 319.
York 264.

Zanthoxylum 221.
Zeus 181, 191.

www.ingramcontent.com/pod-product-compliance
Ingram Content Group UK Ltd.
Pitfield, Milton Keynes, MK11 3LW, UK
UKHW061918271025
464404UK00007B/211